Applications of Virtual and Augmented Reality for Health and Wellbeing

Kamal Kant Hiran
Sir Padampat Singhania University, India & Lincoln University College, Malaysia

Ruchi Doshi
Universidad Azteca, Mexico

Mayank Patel
Geetanjali Institute of Technical Studies, India

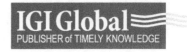

A volume in the Advances in Medical Technologies and Clinical Practice (AMTCP) Book Series

Published in the United States of America by
IGI Global
Medical Information Science Reference (an imprint of IGI Global)
701 E. Chocolate Avenue
Hershey PA, USA 17033
Tel: 717-533-8845
Fax: 717-533-8661
E-mail: cust@igi-global.com
Web site: http://www.igi-global.com

Library of Congress Cataloging-in-Publication Data

Names: Hiran, Kamal Kant, 1982- editor. | Doshi, Ruchi, editor. | Patel,
  Mayank, 1985- editor.
Title: Applications of virtual and augmented reality for health and
  wellbeing / edited by Kamal Hiran, Ruchi Doshi, Mayank Patel.
Description: Hershey, PA : Medical Information Science Reference, [2024] |
  Includes bibliographical references and index. | Summary: "Augmented
  Reality and Virtual Reality has tremendous opportunities in various
  domains and therefore exploring the ongoing research at both national
  and international level is necessary"-- Provided by publisher.
Identifiers: LCCN 2023054573 (print) | LCCN 2023054574 (ebook) | ISBN
  9798369311233 (hardcover) | ISBN 9798369311240 (ebook)
Subjects: MESH: Augmented Reality | Virtual Reality | Psychological
  Well-Being | User-Computer Interface | Health Promotion--methods
Classification: LCC R859.7.A78 (print) | LCC R859.7.A78 (ebook) | NLM W
  26.55.C6 | DDC 610.285--dc23/eng/20231220
LC record available at https://lccn.loc.gov/2023054573
LC ebook record available at https://lccn.loc.gov/2023054574

This book is published in the IGI Global book series Advances in Medical Technologies and Clinical Practice (AMTCP) (ISSN: 2327-9354; eISSN: 2327-9370)

British Cataloguing in Publication Data
A Cataloguing in Publication record for this book is available from the British Library.

All work contributed to this book is new, previously-unpublished material. The views expressed in this book are those of the authors, but not necessarily of the publisher.

For electronic access to this publication, please contact: eresources@igi-global.com.

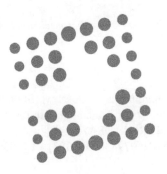

Advances in Medical Technologies and Clinical Practice (AMTCP) Book Series

Srikanta Patnaik
SOA University, India
Priti Das
S.C.B. Medical College, India

ISSN:2327-9354
EISSN:2327-9370

MISSION

Medical technological innovation continues to provide avenues of research for faster and safer diagnosis and treatments for patients. Practitioners must stay up to date with these latest advancements to provide the best care for nursing and clinical practices.

The **Advances in Medical Technologies and Clinical Practice (AMTCP) Book Series** brings together the most recent research on the latest technology used in areas of nursing informatics, clinical technology, biomedicine, diagnostic technologies, and more. Researchers, students, and practitioners in this field will benefit from this fundamental coverage on the use of technology in clinical practices.

COVERAGE

- Clinical Data Mining
- Clinical High-Performance Computing
- Biomedical Applications
- E-Health
- Clinical Studies
- Biometrics
- Biomechanics
- Medical Informatics
- Nursing Informatics
- Patient-Centered Care

IGI Global is currently accepting manuscripts for publication within this series. To submit a proposal for a volume in this series, please contact our Acquisition Editors at Acquisitions@igi-global.com or visit: http://www.igi-global.com/publish/.

Titles in this Series

For a list of additional titles in this series, please visit: http://www.igi-global.com/book-series/advances-medical-technologies-clinical-practice/73682

Approaches to Human-Centered AI in Healthcare
Veena Grover (Noida Institute of Engineering and Technology, India) Balamurugan Balusamy (Shiv Nadar University, India) Nallakaruppan M.K. (Vellore Institute of Technology, India) Vijay Anand (Vellore Institute of Technology, India) and Mariofanna Milanova (University of Arkansas at Little Rock, USA)
Medical Information Science Reference • copyright 2024 • 328pp • H/C (ISBN: 9798369322383) • US $380.00 (our price)

Future of AI in Medical Imaging
Avinash Kumar Sharma (Sharda University, India) Nitin Chanderwal (University of Cincinnati, USA) Shobhit Tyagi (Sharda University, India) and Prashant Upadhyay (Sharda University, India)
Medical Information Science Reference • copyright 2024 • 312pp • H/C (ISBN: 9798369323595) • US $390.00 (our price)

Multisector Insights in Healthcare, Social Sciences, Society, and Technology
Darrell Norman Burrell (Marymount University, USA)
Engineering Science Reference • copyright 2024 • 392pp • H/C (ISBN: 9798369332269) • US $545.00 (our price)

Change Dynamics in Healthcare, Technological Innovations, and Complex Scenarios
Darrell Norman Burrell (Marymount University, USA)
Medical Information Science Reference • copyright 2024 • 331pp • H/C (ISBN: 9798369335550) • US $495.00 (our price)

Intelligent Solutions for Cognitive Disorders
Dipti Jadhav (D. Y. Patil University (Deemed), Navi Mumbai, India & Ramrao Adik Institute of Technology, India) Pallavi Vijay Chavan (D. Y. Patil University (Deemed), Navi Mumbai, India & Ramrao Adik Institute of Technolgy, India) Sangita Chaudhari (D. Y. Patil University (Deemed), Navi Mumbai, India & Ramrao Adik Institute of Technology, India) and Idongesit Williams (CMI, Denmark & Aalborg University, Copenhagen, Denmark)
Medical Information Science Reference • copyright 2024 • 411pp • H/C (ISBN: 9798369310908) • US $355.00 (our price)

Intelligent Technologies and Parkinson's Disease Prediction and Diagnosis
Abhishek Kumar (Chitkara University Institute of Engineering and Technology, Chitkara University, Punjab, India) Sachin Ahuja (Chandigarh University, India) Anupam Baliyan (Geeta University, India) Sreenatha Annawati (University of New South Wales, Australia) and Abhineet Anand (Chandigarh University, India)

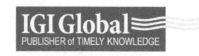

701 East Chocolate Avenue, Hershey, PA 17033, USA
Tel: 717-533-8845 x100 • Fax: 717-533-8661
E-Mail: cust@igi-global.com • www.igi-global.com

Table of Contents

Chapter 14
Blockchain Integration With the Digital Twin-Enabled Industrial Internet of Things Based on
*Rakshit Kothari, College of Technology and Engineering, Maharana Pratap University of
     Agriculture and Technology, India*
*Kalpana Jain, College of Technology and Engineering, Maharana Pratap University of
     Agriculture and Technology, India*
*Naveen Choudhary, College of Technology and Engineering, Maharana Pratap University of
     Agriculture and Technology, India*

Detailed Table of Contents

Chapter 1
C. Selvan, REVA University, India
K. Vidhya, Karunya Institute of Technology and Sciences, India
Senthil Kumar, Jain University, India
K. Veningston, National Institute of Technology, Srinagar, India

The virtual and augmented reality is a rapidly growing technology which focuses on visualization and recognition of 2D and 3D images using tools with bonded techniques (features). The virtual reality (VR) delivers only assumed digital world for viewers, but the expectations of viewers is real world with digital world. Thus, augmented reality (AR) has become popular to deliver enhanced view of VR. However, AR fulfilled the expectations of viewers but there is a gap between VR and AR. The intermediate gap is focused on enhanced visualization for controlling and manipulating VR and AR in parallel. In this chapter, the comparative study of VR, AR, and mixed reality (MR) are focused to expose different aspects of applications, performances, and tools requirements.

Chapter 2
Rajaprabakaran Rajendran, CMS Business School, Jain University (Deemed), Bengaluru, India
Yavana Rani Subramanian, CMS Business School, Jain University (Deemed), Bengaluru, India

Virtual reality (VR) technology has been gradually gaining traction in the healthcare industry and has the potential to significantly transform the way that patients receive medical care. VR technology delivers an immersive experience that may improve diagnosis, treatment, and overall patient outcomes by enabling patients and medical professionals to visualise and interact with medical data more effectively and intuitively. VR can help patients gain a better understanding of their medical diagnoses and treatments. Better health results may result from this and an improvement in the way care is delivered generally. In conclusion, VR technology creates an exceptional opportunity for medical practitioners to transform the way they treat patients. The field of digital health is an emerging discipline that integrates technology and healthcare to boost overall care, save costs, and improve patient outcomes.

This book chapter delves into the profound synergy between Biomedical Engineering and the burgeoning realm of augmented reality (AR) and virtual reality (VR) applications. Through a meticulous examination of state-of-the-art advancements and a forward-looking analysis of future prospects, this chapter endeavors to offer a comprehensive resource for a diverse audience, including dedicated researchers, seasoned healthcare practitioners, discerning educators, and aspiring students. The integration of these technologies has the potential to revolutionize medical training, patient education, surgical planning, and therapy delivery, ushering in an era of more personalized and effective healthcare solutions. This chapter serves as a guiding beacon in navigating this transformative landscape, ensuring that the adoption of AR/VR technologies is not only innovative but also ethically grounded and attuned to the highest standards of patient care.

Chapter 4

Virtual reality (VR) and augmented reality (AR) can revolutionize how individuals experience and perceive the world. Effective and engaging wellness practices are made possible by these technologies personalized, immersive experiences. The organization endeavors to foster empathy and understanding by attending to physical, mental, emotional, and social health. Nevertheless, ethical deliberations are of the utmost importance, including privacy, proper data handling, and secure data access. Education, support, and accessibility are critical determinants of user acceptance. Additional areas that warrant further investigation include treatment efficacy, diversity, long-term effects, and ongoing progress. A more inclusive, engaging, and productive approach to individual and communal health is anticipated due to the expanding use of AR and VR in well-being.

Image, audio, and video are rapidly evolving multimedia data, creating a platform for the creation, exchange, and storage of information in the modern era. Multiple techniques are available for content-based image, video, and audio retrieval using image processing methods to extract text features of the data. These methods produce similar text but not the same as per the user expectation. In this chapter, the authors offer an approach that uses edge map generation and Google tesseract-based text detection in image as well as in video. The accuracy of our method is 98% for speed video extraction, 100% for image/video/audio data.

Chapter 6

Ranjit Singha, Christ University, India
Surjit Singha, Kristu Jayanti College (Autonomous), India

By producing immersive, individualized, and captivating therapeutic experiences, augmented reality (AR) and virtual reality (VR) may significantly transform mental health treatment. These technologies provide efficacious resolutions for exposure therapy, augmenting conventional methodologies, mitigating social disapproval, and fortifying the therapeutic alliance. Virtual and augmented reality increase the accessibility and convenience of therapy by enabling highly individualized interventions. Training for mental health professionals, rigorous research, compliance with data privacy regulations, and adherence to ethical standards are essential for responsible use. Augmented reality (AR) and virtual reality (VR) can expand the accessibility of mental health services as costs decrease, thereby ultimately enhancing the welfare of those in search of assistance and recovery. Incorporating augmented reality and virtual reality into clinical practice may make mental health treatment more engaging, effective, and individualized.

Chapter 7

Bhupinder Singh, Sharda University, India
Christian Kaunert, Dublin City University, Ireland

Augmented reality (AR) and virtual reality (VR) modules are emerging as revolutionary tools for improving mindfulness, emotional intelligence, and mental health. These immersive technologies provide a one-of-a-kind and engaging platform for simulating real-life settings and guiding users through a variety of experiences aimed at regulating emotions and improving mental health. These modules can teach and reinforce mindfulness practices by immersing users in virtual worlds, allowing them to get a better awareness of their emotions, manage stress, and build emotional resilience. AR and VR modules are proving to be strong tools for personal growth and well-being, whether through guided meditation, stress reduction exercises, or interactive situations aimed at increasing empathy and self-awareness. This chapter comprehensively explores the transformational potential of AR and VR modules in building mindfulness, enhancing emotional intelligence, and contributing to overall mental well-being.

Chapter 8

Ranjit Singha, Christ University, India
Surjit Singha, Kristu Jayanti College (Autonomous), India

Investigating virtual reality (VR)-enhanced meditative movement reveals a promising strategy for improving mental and physical health. Virtual reality technology offers immersive, individualized experiences that effectively reduce tension, manage anxiety, and control pain, making it a valuable addition to conventional therapies. Research also demonstrates its efficacy in boosting motivation, maintaining an exercise regimen, and reducing stress. VR is an essential tool for treating mental health conditions such as anxiety and PTSD in clinical settings, with the potential to serve diverse populations. The significance of VR-enhanced mindful movement for overall well-being rests in its holistic approach, personalized experiences, and potential to revolutionize how individuals approach mental and physical health. With the ultimate goal of integrating VR into healthcare practices to enhance lives, a call to action includes additional research, ethical guidelines, accessibility efforts, and keeping abreast of emerging developments.

    Laura De Clara, MetaCare Srl, Italy

Recent advances in mental healthcare technology, especially in virtual reality (VR) and augmented reality (AR), have revolutionized psychiatry and psychology. This chapter critically examines these innovations' potential in treating various mental disorders, from anxiety and depression to PTSD and ADHD. It emphasizes the controlled and customizable nature of VR environments, which empower individuals to confront fears within personalized settings. Interdisciplinary collaboration is stressed, showcasing applications in psychology, from assessment to clinical treatment. The chapter explores neuropsychological impacts, detailing how VR modulates emotions, enhances neural plasticity in stroke rehabilitation, and alters neural networks. Despite promise, challenges like treatment standardization and ethical concerns persist, demanding careful consideration. The chapter advocates for ongoing research and global interdisciplinary cooperation to fully exploit these technologies' potential in mental healthcare.

    Gerardo Reyes Ruiz, Centro de Estudios Superiores Navales (CESNAV), Mexico

This chapter presents an augmented reality project applied to the study of cardiology, which is crystallized through a system known as service-oriented architecture (SOA). This system serves as an innovative and efficient learning platform for students interested in cardiology because it helps them to understand abstract concepts in cardiology, which require visual and manipulable objects that are difficult to obtain, due to the large space they occupy in magnetic media or because of the difficulty of obtaining their models in physical form. This system strengthened the process of anatomical identification of the human heart and allowed a better interaction with the student, i.e., the system enhanced the use of sight, hearing, and kinesthetic, which, together, allowed a better assimilation of knowledge. The effectiveness of this system was validated using a survey of 389 students from four public universities where the following aspects were verified: 1) Significant learning; 2) Motivation; 3) Ease of use, and; 4) Performance.

    Suyesha Singh, Department of Psychology, Manipal University Jaipur, India
    Vaishnavi Nambiar, Department of Psychology, Manipal University Jaipur, India

The application of AI in geriatric healthcare has become a revolutionary and essential solution to tackling the problems faced by older people. An important step toward providing patient-centered and cost-effective treatment, the integration of AI in geriatric healthcare will ultimately enhance the standard of life for older people. This chapter is a systematic review of the rapidly developing field of AI applications in geriatric healthcare. It provides a thorough analysis of the impact and potential of AI technologies in addressing the healthcare needs of the aging population. The review was conducted using PRISMA framework. Thirty-three articles were considered for final review from which five themes were deduced. The study will facilitate the development of relevant and inclusive solutions for healthcare of older individuals and hasten the possibility of greater wellbeing and inclusion of older adults in the technological innovativeness of the healthcare facilities.

Chapter 12

"Robotics Rx: A Prescription for the Future of Healthcare" provides a forward-thinking road plan for the implementation of robotics in the medical field. The purpose of this study is to investigate the revolutionary potential of robots in terms of boosting diagnostic accuracy, enhancing patient care, and revolutionising surgical procedures. This prescription illustrates a future in which artificial intelligence, machine learning, and precision robotics work together in a seamless manner with medical professionals, thereby enhancing their ability to perform and ultimately redefining the standards of medical practise. This is accomplished by delving into the advancements that have been made in these areas.

In recent years, the merging of augmented reality (AR) technology and gamification has received substantial attention, providing fresh pathways for engaging youngsters in encouraging healthy lifestyles and general well-being. This book chapter delves into the intersection of augmented reality and gamification as a novel method to addressing the growing concerns about childhood health issues. This chapter investigates how these technologies might effectively grab children's interest and empower them to make healthier choices by synergistically combining the immersive experiences of AR with the motivational features of gamification. This chapter elucidates the psychological underpinnings of gamification through a thorough assessment of relevant literature, emphasising its ability to inspire intrinsic motivation, foster skill development, and increase engagement. Furthermore, it delves into the pedagogical ideas that underpin great AR design, emphasising the significance of developing immersive and interactive experiences that smoothly integrate with real-world environments.

The industrial landscape is about to undergo a revolution thanks to the convergence of emerging technologies. Specifically, the integration of blockchain with the digital twin-enabled industrial internet of things (IIoT) within mixed reality environments has the potential to do just that. This chapter presents a thorough analysis of the applications, advantages, and difficulties of various technologies while examining their potential for synergy. The digital twin provides real-time data monitoring, analysis, and predictive maintenance capabilities. The industrial internet of things establishes connections between tangible objects and sensors, enabling smooth communication and interchange of data. This chapter investigates the use of mixed reality (MR) technology to integrate blockchain technology with the IIoT that is enabled by digital twins. The potential for improving data security, trust, and transparency in industrial applications through the integration of blockchain with IIoT and MR could aid in the development of the Industry 4.0 paradigm.

Foreword

In the ever-evolving landscape of technology, where innovation is a constant companion, few frontiers hold as much promise and potential as the convergence of Virtual and Augmented Reality with the delicate tapestry of healthcare and personal wellbeing. The pages you are about to explore are a testament to the transformative power of these immersive technologies, showcasing their applications as catalysts for positive change in the realms of health and wellness.

The advent of Virtual and Augmented Reality has ushered in a new era, redefining the possibilities within healthcare. As we grapple with the complexities of modern medicine and the ever-growing demand for innovative solutions, the intersection of these technologies offers a beacon of hope. This book, *Applications of Virtual and Augmented Reality for Health and Wellbeing*, serves as a comprehensive guide, shedding light on the myriad ways in which these technologies are reshaping the future of healthcare.

The journey begins with an exploration of virtual and augmented reality's foundational role in medical education and training. From immersive simulations that replicate surgical procedures to realistic scenarios that test the mettle of healthcare professionals, the applications are both diverse and profound. As you traverse these narratives, you will witness the democratization of knowledge and skill development, empowering the next generation of medical practitioners.

Moving beyond the confines of traditional medical practices, the book navigates through the uncharted territories of therapy and rehabilitation. Virtual and augmented reality have emerged as formidable allies in the pursuit of effective and personalized interventions. From aiding physical rehabilitation to providing therapeutic experiences for mental health, the potential for positive impact is awe-inspiring.

The chapters within these covers also delve into the integration of these technologies into preventive healthcare and wellness strategies. From gamified fitness experiences that inspire exercise to immersive mindfulness applications that promote mental wellbeing, the book explores the multifaceted ways in which virtual and augmented reality contribute to a holistic approach to health.

As we embark on this journey together, it is essential to acknowledge the diverse perspectives and expertise that our contributing authors bring to the table. Their insights, drawn from the fields of healthcare, technology, and academia, provide a rich tapestry of knowledge that enriches the reader's understanding of this dynamic landscape.

In conclusion, *Applications of Virtual and Augmented Reality for Health and Wellbeing* is more than a collection of chapters; it is a call to action. It invites readers to contemplate the implications, engage in dialogue, and actively participate in shaping a future where technology and humanity collaborate for the betterment of health and wellbeing. May this book be a source of inspiration and knowledge, guiding you through the immersive possibilities that lie ahead.

Patrick Acheampong
Ghana Communication Technology University, Ghana

Preface

In an era where technological advancements are reshaping the boundaries of what is possible, this book delves into the transformative impact of virtual and augmented reality on the landscape of healthcare and personal wellness.

The fusion of cutting-edge technologies, virtual and augmented reality, with the intricate intricacies of health and wellbeing opens up a fascinating frontier of possibilities. This book serves as a comprehensive exploration, offering insights into how these immersive technologies are revolutionizing healthcare practices, enhancing therapeutic interventions, and promoting overall wellness.

As we navigate through the pages of this volume, readers will embark on a journey that unravels the diverse applications of virtual and augmented reality in the healthcare ecosystem. From revolutionizing medical training and simulation to fostering breakthroughs in rehabilitation and therapy, the potential is vast and promising.

Through a careful examination of case studies, research findings, and expert perspectives, this book aims to bridge the gap between technology and its practical implementation in healthcare. It provides a nuanced understanding of the challenges and opportunities that arise when integrating virtual and augmented reality into the fabric of medical practices and personal wellbeing strategies.

Our contributors, comprising experts from the fields of healthcare, technology, and academia, have shared their valuable insights to illuminate the multifaceted dimensions of this evolving landscape. Whether you are a healthcare professional, a technology enthusiast, or someone intrigued by the intersection of innovation and wellness, this book offers a comprehensive exploration of the subject.

The ultimate goal of *Applications of Virtual and Augmented Reality for Health and Wellbeing* is to inspire a thoughtful dialogue and foster collaboration among diverse disciplines. As we stand on the cusp of a new era in healthcare, let this book be your guide to understanding the potential, navigating the challenges, and embracing the future where virtual and augmented reality converge to shape a healthier and more connected world.

ORGANIZATION OF THE BOOK

The book is organized in **14 chapters** written by researchers, scholars and professors from prestigious laboratories and educational institution across the globe. A brief description of each of the chapters in this section given below.

Chapter 1, "Comparative Overview of Augmented Reality, Virtual Reality and Mixed Reality," explores the differences and applications of three emerging technologies that manipulate reality: Augmented Reality (AR), Virtual Reality (VR), and Mixed Reality (MR). Chapter briefly describes the definitions and key concepts of Augmented Reality, Virtual Reality and Mixed Reality. They also done the comparative analysis of AR, VR and MR. Also elaborates the rise of Mixed Reality in the industry.

Chapter 2, "Revolutionizing Patient Care: The Impact of Virtual Reality in Healthcare," addresses the multifaceted applications of VR in healthcare, specifically delving into its transformative impact on various aspects of patient experience and treatment outcomes.

Chapter 3, "Integration of Biomedical Engineering in Augmented Reality and Virtual Reality Applications," explores the potential to revolutionize medical training, patient education, surgical planning, and therapy delivery.

Chapter 4, "Enhancing Well-being: Exploring the Impact of Augmented Reality and Virtual Reality," presents the engaging, and productive approach to individual and communal health is anticipated due to the expanding use of AR and VR in well-being. They explore the usage of AR/VR and investigate how they might impact various aspects of well-being in our lives.

Chapter 5, "Multimedia Text Extraction for Healthcare Applications," introduces an approach that uses Edge map generation and Google tesseract-based text detection in image as well as in video. They analyses the field of multimedia text extraction, focusing on techniques to effectively extract valuable textual content from diverse healthcare data sources.

Chapter 6, "Mental Health Treatment: Exploring the Potential of Augmented Reality and Virtual Reality," showcase that prevalence of mental health concerns continues to rise, there is a critical need for innovative and accessible treatment modalities. This paper explores the potential of Augmented Reality (AR) and Virtual Reality (VR) technologies to enhance mental health treatment, examining their unique capabilities and potential benefits in this evolving field.

Chapter 7, "Augmented Reality and Virtual Reality Modules for Mindfulness: Boosting Emotional Intelligence and Mental Wellness," analyses that how pressures of modern life can significantly impact mental well-being. This chapter explores the AR and VR technologies to address this growing concern.

Chapter 8, "Mindful Movement: VR-Enhanced Yoga and Exercise for Well-Being," throws light on the significance of VR-enhanced mindful movement for overall well-being rests in its holistic approach, personalized experiences, and potential to revolutionize how individuals approach mental and physical health.

Chapter 9, "The Neuropsychological Impact Of Immersive Experiences In The Metaverse And Virtual And Augmented Reality," explores neuropsychological impacts, detailing how VR modulates emotions, enhances neural plasticity in stroke rehabilitation, and alters neural networks.

Chapter 10, "The Study of Cardiology Through an Augmented Reality Based System," address the use of Augmented Reality in the study of cardiology. They also conducted the survey based on significant learning, Ease of use and Performance and conclude with the findings.

Chapter 11, "A Systematic Review of the Role of Gerontechnology and AI in Revolutionizing the Wellbeing Landscape for Aging Adults," presents a systematic review of the existing research on the role of gerontechnology and AI in revolutionizing the well-being landscape for aging adults. In this chapter they analyse the potential benefits and limitations, and identify future research directions in this critical domain.

Chapter 12, "Robotics Rx: A Prescription for the Future of Healthcare" investigate the revolutionary potential of robots in terms of boosting diagnostic accuracy, enhancing patient care, and revolutionising surgical procedures. They also explores the multifaceted potential of robots in revolutionizing various aspects of healthcare delivery, from diagnosis and treatment to rehabilitation and patient care.

Chapter 13, "Augmented Reality Gamification for Promoting Healthy Lifestyles and Wellbeing in Children," elves into the intersection of augmented reality and gamification as a novel method to addressing the growing concerns about childhood health issues. This chapter investigates how Augmented Reality effectively grab children's interest and empower them to make healthier choices by synergistically combining the immersive experiences with the motivational features of gamification.

Chapter 14, "Blockchain Integration with the Digital twin enabled Industrial Internet of Things Based on Mixed Reality," explores how blockchain technology can be integrated with digital twins (digital representations of physical assets) in an Industrial Internet of Things (IIoT) setting that utilizes mixed reality (MR). They investigate how this technological combination can revolutionize industrial operations by creating a secure, transparent, and data-driven ecosystem for managing physical assets.

Kamal Kant Hiran
Sir Padampat Singhania University, Udaipur, India & Lincoln University College, Petaling Jaya, Malaysia

Ruchi Doshi
Universidad Azteca, Chalco, Mexico

Mayank Patel
Geetanjali Institute of Technical Studies, Udaipur, India

Acknowledgment

The tireless support and endless contributions received from numerous individuals in the completion of this work must be duly acknowledged. This book would not have come to fruition without the invaluable support of IGI Global, USA. The team from IGI Global, namely Melissa Wagner, Elizabeth Barrantes, and Jocelynn Hessler, deserves our heartfelt gratitude for generously providing this exceptional opportunity and displaying unwavering cooperation since the inception of the notion for this book. Their distinct contributions, guidance, expertise, and unwavering endeavors have materialized this book.

With earnest gratitude and profound thanks, we would like to acknowledge the continuous guidance of Dr. N.S. Rathore, Campus Director, Geetanjali Institute of technical Studies, Udaipur, Rajasthan, India, Dr. Ricardo Saavedra, Universidad Azteca, Mexico, Prof.(Dr.) Prasun Chakrabarti, Director, Directorate of Research and Publications, Sir Padampat Singhania University, Udaipur, Rajasthan, India, Prof. Dr. Sandeep Poddar, Deputy Vice Chancellor (Research & Innovation), Lincoln University College, Malaysia for their time, dedication, expertise and continuous support in this publication journey. Special thanks to Col. Sanjay Sinha, Head of Education, JK Cement Education Vertical, India, Prof. Anders Henten, Prof. Kund Erik Skouby, Prof. Reza Tadayoni, Prof. Lene Tolstrup Sørensen, Anette Bysøe, Center for Communication, Media and Information Technologies (CMI), Aalborg University, Copenhagen, Denmark for providing in-depth scientific knowledge.

We express our profound gratitude to our esteemed institutions, namely Geetanjali Institute of Technical Studies in Udaipur, Rajasthan, India, Sir Padampat Singhania University (SPSU) in Udaipur, Rajasthan, India, Lincoln University College in Malaysia, and Universidad Azteca in Chalco, Mexico, for furnishing us with a nourishing scholarly and investigative milieu throughout this odyssey.

The Editorial Advisory Board has displayed an admirable gesture and unwavering support, which has deeply affected us. Since the inception of the concept of the edited book, we have been moved by their constant assistance. We would like to express our gratitude to all those who have contributed to this project, particularly the authors and reviewers who participated in the review process. Without their invaluable support, this publication would not have materialized.

The completion of this book could not have been possible without the contribution and support we got from our family, friends and colleagues. It is a pleasant aspect and we express our gratitude for all of them.

Acknowledgment

Kamal Kant Hiran
Sir Padampat Singhania University, Udaipur, India & Lincoln University College, Petaling Jaya, Malaysia

Mayank Patel
Geetanjali Institute of Technical Studies, Udaipur, India

Ruchi Doshi
Universidad Azteca, Chalco, Mexico

Chapter 1
Comparative Overview of Augmented Reality, Virtual Reality, and Mixed Reality

C. Selvan
https://orcid.org/0000-0003-4381-0284
REVA University, India

K. Vidhya
Karunya Institute of Technology and Sciences, India

R. Senthil Kumar
https://orcid.org/0000-0002-1393-756X
Jain University, India

K. Veningston
National Institute of Technology, Srinagar, India

ABSTRACT

The virtual and augmented reality is a rapidly growing technology which focuses on visualization and recognition of 2D and 3D images using tools with bonded techniques (features). The virtual reality (VR) delivers only assumed digital world for viewers, but the expectations of viewers is real world with digital world. Thus, augmented reality (AR) has become popular to deliver enhanced view of VR. However, AR fulfilled the expectations of viewers but there is a gap between VR and AR. The intermediate gap is focused on enhanced visualization for controlling and manipulating VR and AR in parallel. In this chapter, the comparative study of VR, AR, and mixed reality (MR) are focused to expose different aspects of applications, performances, and tools requirements.

DOI: 10.4018/979-8-3693-1123-3.ch001

Figure 1. XR Technologies (Vollmar, 2023)

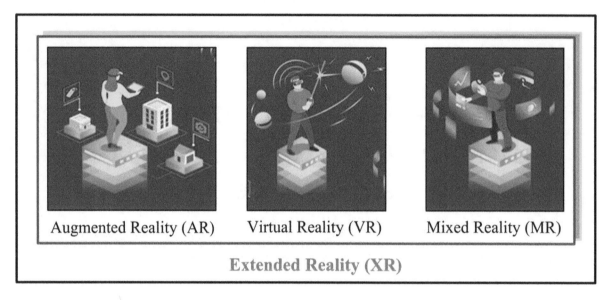

INTRODUCTION

Extended reality connects people, places, and experiences across distances. XR functions are being used for business leaders to address some of the most pressing issues. Whether it's for worker training, daily productivity, or immersive consumer experiences, extended reality allows businesses to rethink their operations without the constraints of distance. People, information, and experiences are becoming more accessible thanks to virtual and augmented reality technology, which are changing how people live and work.

Extended Reality (XR) is an emerging concept which encapsulates AR, VR and MR. Though, AR, VR and MR have their presence in today's world, XR is revolutionizing and gaining momentum in various corners such as consumer experiences, industrial manufacturing and healthcare, education and retail (Alnagrat et al., 2022). In a recent survey, XR would be the mainstream technology as more than 60% of respondents predicted it to happen in the next five years. The three key XR technologies: VR, AR, Mixed Reality (MR) is shown in Figure 1.

EXTENDED REALITY (XR)

Augmented Reality (AR)

In AR, both the real world and the content generated by the computer are combined to enhance the user experience. It comprises of real time interaction with combination of real and virtual world along with the 3 dimensional registrations of real and virtual objects (Al-Ansi et al., 2023). This can be envisioned using apps, software, some hardware devices such as AR glasses as depicted in Figure 2. A User adds digital attributes viz. photographs, animation, and text to the actual world. This makes the users to be connected to the outside world where he/she can still interact and experience in real time.

Figure 2. Augmented reality (UNCTAD, 2018)

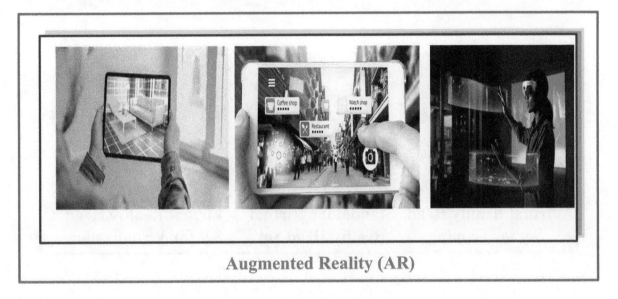

As an example of its realization, the Pokémon GO game, gives its users enhanced experience by using animals (digital) over the real environment, and Snapchat filters, uses the digital things like as spectacles or hats and places on user head.

Benefits of AR

- Interactive: The AR technology creates real time experience for the user by augmenting the digital content to real objects.
- It is used in marketing, product design for improved sales and return.
- It has huge contribution in healthcare.
- It is cost effective and a requirement of today's emerging technological development.

Virtual Reality (VR), Applications, and Benefits

Figure 3 depicts the examples of VR Headsets. In this the user put on a VR Headset with either a head mounted display or camera to experience the artificial world with 360-degree view. In this this individuals are fully engaged and immersed in the activity of their choice, like a VR Headset completed dedicated to enhance gaming experience in virtual world. The individuals are spellbound to feel that they are visualizing all as real like feeling of being onto the universe, walking on moon and so on (Hamad & Jia, 2022). Various sectors from entertainment to healthcare, gaming to education, manufacturing to sales, Military etc. are adopting the VR technology.

Benefits or advantages of VR

- VR provides an environment that is realistic.
- It allows consumers to discover new areas.
- VR makes the individuals the feeling of interacting with a virtual world.
- VR makes learning easier and more enjoyable

Figure 3. VR headset examples (Ivanova & Thorben, 2023)

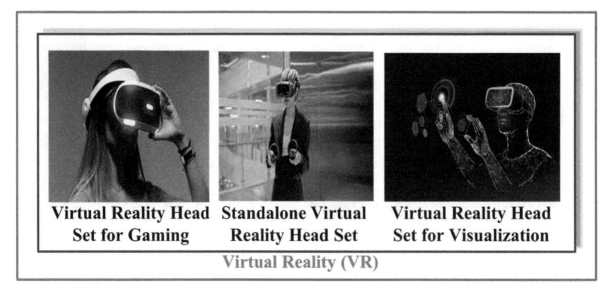

Mixed Reality (MR)

In mixed reality, digital and physical items exist side by side such that the interaction between them takes place in real time scenario. MR is one of the emerging and promising immersive technologies in today's time. To experience this technology an individual has to wear a MR headset which consists of advanced computing capability as against AR and VR Headset. Figure 4 shows some of the examples of MR Headsets. These headsets customize the user preferences in visualizing the virtual objects and hence give realistic feeling. Several companies are putting their effort to envision MR in product sales, military application, healthcare, education and so on (Farshid et al., 2018; Patel et al., 2022).

Advantages of Mixed Reality (MR)

- Reduce maintenance call-out times
- Improve quality control
- Improve staff training
- Reduce the skilled labor shortage

AMALGAMATION OF TECHNOLOGIES TO FORM XR

The components driving the XR technologies are VR, AR, and MR as shown in Figure 5.

The most basic of the three XR subcategories, augmented reality defines the amalgamation of a virtual experience with the real world and thus results in enhanced user visualization. The mobile game "Pokémon GO," which allows individuals to digitally put a character anywhere in their gaming environment, is a prominent example of augmented reality. The smartphone game accomplishes it by leveraging the camera of the mobile and screen, as shown in the Figure 5.

Figure 4. MR headset examples (Sridhar, 2023)

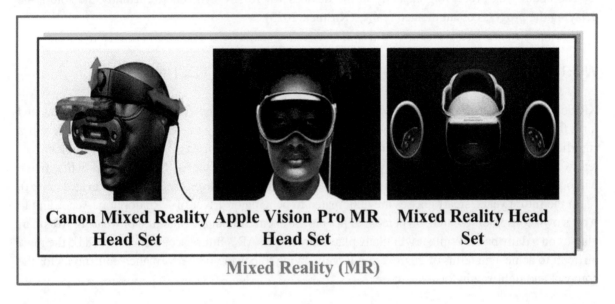

Figure 5. Components of XR technology (Bridges, 2022)

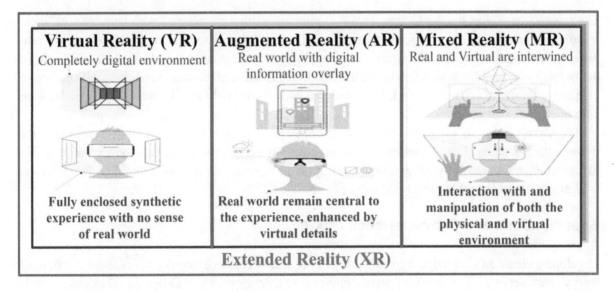

Beyond entertainment, AR is steadily finding it's place into retail, internet shopping, and manufacturing. Because it requires the least amount of computing, AR is likely the accepted among the available XR technologies because it can run on most mobiles and tablets. AR can occur in any setting which has two essential characteristics:

1. Camera: To take pictures of the surroundings
2. Processor: This is capable of comprehending the surroundings and dynamically simulating a virtual item put within it.

The underlying processing capacity in the devices where AR will run is currently the sole issue delaying the progress of augmented reality (Kastner, 2023).

WORKING AND FEATURES OF EXTENDED REALITY TECHNOLOGY

XR devices, whether developed for VR, MR, or AR, have similar needs. However, as use cases and form factors for wearable devices grow, these requirements are likely to differ dramatically. There is a significant distinction between AR and VR Headset. Microsoft HoloLens-2, is used to get a picture of real world or we may block it out in VR gaming Headset (Oculus Quest). These devices will emerge without dependency on the devices it is running like laptop, smartphone or a server (Çöltekin et al., 2020).

In the future years, smart glasses are anticipated to be a major driver of AR adoption. According to Arm's own consumer research, 58 percent of people are excited about the potential of wearing AR smart glasses on a daily basis. While it will likely play a key role in AR's future acceptance, it will be the most difficult to achieve in terms of engineering largely owing to power and performance constraints for the compact and lightweight form factor.

Features of XR

The capacity to explore the world or analyze the context-sensitive information with help of visual input techniques of object, gaze tracking, and the gesture is the key feature of the XR vision. Necessary requirement is the depth and location characteristics, mapping and perception. AR and VR distinguishes itself on the basis of types of experiences that each technology provides. 6DoF motion tracking, HD rendering pipeline, volumetric capture and facial expression capture is needed for VR immersive technology for entertainment experiences.

The smart glasses are used to provide always-on, easy, and secure navigation while users are on the move in the AR technology. AR technology requires in depth, semantics, occlusion (when one item in a 3D environment blocks the view of another), location, pose, orientation, position, and gesture with eye tracking, amongst the other aspects (Maran et al., 2022).

Specifications and Characteristics of XR

Developers create an immersive algorithm for a better user experience in order to accomplish extended reality characteristics. To construct a virtual environment, developers will also need 3D models and excellent computer vision. Extended Reality algorithms are created or designed in C, C++, Java, Python, and Swift. Developers employ smartphone cameras to record the surrounding scene with the aid of AR. We use augmented reality to scan the surroundings and overlay a digital item at a specified location.

Developers utilize trackers like GPS, infrared, and other sensors to locate the digital item in a precise area. Users may set the digital object wherever with the use of AR, but they cannot interact with it. As a result, we employ MR in situations when the user wishes to engage with a digital item. Virtual Reality allows users to see the virtual environment from all sides. It creates an immersive experience by using the user's touch, sight, and hearing senses (Teniou, 2019). The user's sensor must be able to be influenced by the VR headset. For the readers understanding, the Table 1 shows the key difference among AR, VR and MR.

Table 1. Key difference among AR, VR, MR (Li et al., 2018)

Features	Virtual Reality	Mixed Reality	Augmented Reality
Display device	Mostly using Special headset or smart glasses	Headsets optional	Headsets optional
Image source	Computer graphics or real images produced by a computer	Combination of computer-generated images and real-life objects	Combination of computer-generated images and real-life objects
Environment	Fully digital	Both virtual and real-life objects are seamlessly blended	Both virtual and real-life objects are seamlessly blended
Presence	Feeling of being transported somewhere else with no sense of the real world	Feeling of still being in the real world, but with new elements and objects superimposed	Feeling of still being in the real world, but with new elements and objects superimposed
Awareness	Perfectly rendered virtual objects that cannot be distinguished from real objects	Perfectly rendered virtual objects that cannot be distinguished from real objects	Virtual objects can be identified based on their nature and behavior, such as floating text that follows a user
Interaction	Joysticks and controller	Finger touch and tap interaction	Either controllers or gestures
Perspective	Virtual objects will change their position and size according to the user's perspective in the virtual world	Virtual objects behave based on user's perspective in the real world	Virtual objects behave based on user's perspective in the real world
Usage	Extensively used in games, education and training	Moderately used in games and training	Scarce usage
Consumer Adoption	Low due to high cost and complex hardware requirements	High due to low cost and ease of downloading application on mobile phones	Low due to high cost and complex hardware requirements

Extended Reality-Need and Importance

Although teleportation is not yet a reality, immersive experiences enabled by technology such as virtual and augmented reality are transporting us to far-flung locations and eradicating the concept of distance. We are here for XR, which is the first technology to "relocate" individuals in time and space. The fundamental changes to industry and society are obvious as immersive experiences extend across industries: the role of geography is vanishing.

XR is being used by business leaders to address some of the most pressing issues. Whether it's for worker training, daily productivity, or immersive consumer experiences, extended reality allows businesses to rethink their operations without the constraints of distance (Li et al., 2018).

Hundreds of talents from across the globe are available for businesses through immersive knowledge. Businesses may get knowledge in Immersive experiences are driving enterprises to not just think differently about what is possible, but also to design new solutions that circumvent the distance-based limitations they face today across sectors and applications.

APPLICATIONS OF EXTENDED REALITY

Health Care

XR is extremely important for the medical imaging, which has been proved by the recent use of the technology for MRIs and CT scans. Figure 6 shows an example of XR technology in dental study (Shaikh et al., 2022). XR make use of 3D portrayal rather than the standard 2D imaging of human bodies, which enhances the diagnostic efficiency as shown in Figure 6.

Figure 6. XR in dental study (Vyas, 2019)

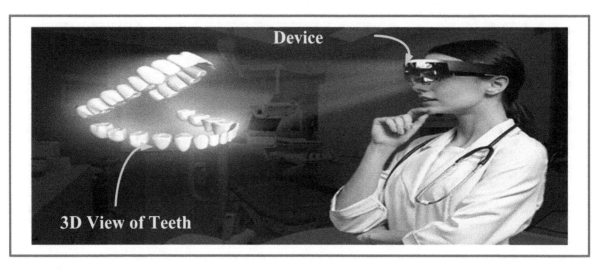

Entertainment Industry

Augmented reality technology is widely utilized in video games accounting for 34% of all sales in the gaming sector. There is no wonder, given that the ability to create a fully immersive experience is crucial for the success of such gaming businesses.

Moreover, the potential of XR technology in providing a holistic participation impact that it allow users to immerse into another world. People may visit the Louvre museum or watch the World Cup final while sitting at home and feeling thoroughly engaged in the event, rather than rushing through packed museums or stadiums. Concerts, exhibits, and sporting events may all benefit from AR, VR, and MR technology (Loeffler, 1993).

Taking different example consider the Denver Museum of Nature and Science, which already use augmented reality to properly communicate the message of its exhibit to visitors. Visitors can see dinosaurs rather than their fossils due to the technology. Figure 7 shows the application of XR in gaming.

Real Estate

XR may benefit the Real estate businesses greatly. Using XR technology, the consumers and the tenants inspect homes without physically being present at that venue. This is both time saving and cost effective solution for both the parties thereby decision making easy and comprehensive.

Architect and interior designers also use the immersive technology. Houzz, a design firm, uses augmented reality to let consumers see their future furniture. They've designed internet software that lets consumers acquire home remodeling suggestions (Lang & Sittler, 2012). The system will give professionals and their clients a complete picture of the project, reducing the risk of errors and unpleasant surprises. By the way, according to the agency, this software boosts the likelihood of a purchase by eleven fold.

Figure 7. XR in gaming (Carter, 2022)

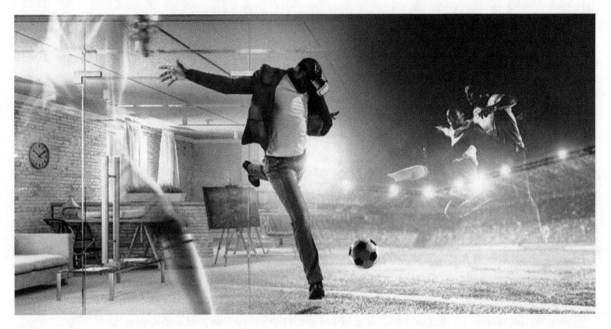

Manufacturing

A major producer (Komatsu) of construction, utility and mining, equipment, also used the XR for operator training. They give training for operators all around the world to minimize multi-million dollar losses caused by inappropriate usage of expensive technology. Also, the result of using AR-based assembly information, the General Electric has increased the efficiency of their workers by 34% who wire wind turbines (de Giorgio et al., 2023).

Education and Training

People who may work in high-risk situations might benefit from extended reality training. Teaching fresh students of aviation to fly real planes might be risky. Due to availability of digital simulations which provides immersive experiences, students can learn how to fly a plane effectively against any potential risk of an accident. Immersive technologies are also being used by medical students to acquire crucial skills. Getting hands-on experience with virtual patients is a fantastic example as shown in Figure 8.

Unique Uses of Extended Reality

1. Onboarding - Use augmented reality (AR) to operate new employees how to handle and maintain complex machines (Hiran et al., 2021).
2. Diversity and Inclusion (D&I) – It uses a 360° VR to simulate real-life scenarios and assess learner's reactions to micro aggressions
3. Customer Service Training - Place a simulated cash register in front of trainees and assess service abilities of their customer using AR plane detection

Figure 8. XR in education (Marr, 2021)

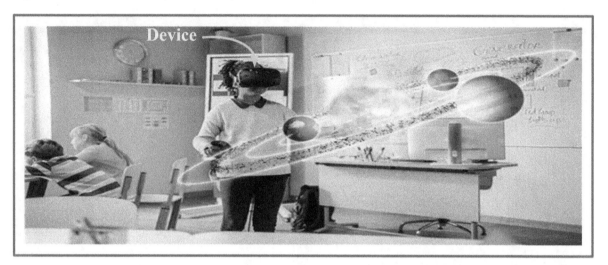

4.   Technical Training – It uses full VR to immerse learners in a realistic warehouse environment where the staffs can practice stacking boxes with the proper weight and orientation
5.   Leadership Training - Allow learners to experience having challenging talks with their teammates using 360° VR

In all industries, training and learning possibilities are one of the most common use cases for extended reality. The correct training is critical in fields like field service, where employees need assistance with everything from serving complicated customers to staying safe while on the go.

Professionals in field service may learn how to handle difficult requests quickly and conveniently with extended reality technologies, allowing them to feel more secure on the job. Staff can also benefit from training by avoiding possible pitfalls and discovering new upselling and cross-selling possibilities to boost income (Zwoliński et al., 2022).

For example, in the field service sector, warranties are seen as one of the most important aspects in producing additional income, with 93 percent of warranty specialists stating that warranty chain management is critical to corporate performance.

By detecting consumer mood in the present, a training system might teach personnel how to spot opportunities to upsell warranties and enhance profits.

Enhanced Customer Experiences

In today's digital world, customers are becoming more demanding. They expect to be able to get answers to their difficulties right away. Furthermore, many of the difficulties that clients confront now are significantly more complicated than they were previously. This puts a lot of pressure on field service employees to meet the most recent requirements. Extended reality tools can aid in a variety of ways to improve consumer interactions. For example, field service personnel might use augmented reality to remotely analyze and evaluate an issue from a machine without having to drive to the customer's location (Easwaran et al., 2022; Vaidyanathan & Henningsson, 2023). The same tools can assist that agent in guiding the customer through the process of performing their own repair in the shortest amount of time feasible.

When field service personnel are on the job, having access to augmented reality smart glasses may help them quickly locate a variety of critical bits of information. It's also feasible to get immediate assistance from team members and professionals. According to certain research, augmented reality and remote help solutions can enhance core customer satisfaction ratings by up to 30%.

Remote Work Opportunities

After the pandemic's constraints and problems, requirement of remote work has been in the option against work from office. Staff on site has always operated in a flexible setting, but augmented and virtual reality may make it much more so. For example, with AR smart glasses, a group of specialists might collaborate on the same problem with only one person on the floor.

Users can get vital feedback from professionals and distant triage teams using augmented reality glasses with streaming video. Technicians may use remote technology powered by augmented reality to view what clients are seeing from afar and address problems without having to visit the spot in person. When technicians are working with a difficult situation, this helps to reduce the amount of risk they face (Ratcliffe et al., 2021).

In-home visits might be drastically reduced thanks to augmented reality and remote troubleshooting options. These potential will only grow in the future as new technologies emerge, such as 5G and IoT.

Stronger Team Collaboration

Any team that wants to succeed has to collaborate. However, in the field services environment, dispersed and spread team members have made it difficult for experts to collaborate successfully. Extended reality settings, as briefly discussed above, enabling teams to get help from specialists and colleagues wherever they are. Teams may collaborate on inventive new goods and processes using virtual reality, or develop and explore digital twins of items. Staff employees may more readily obtain the guidance of their team members while on the road thanks to mixed and augmented reality. When dealing with a complicated gadget, for example, a member of the team might send video to an expert in another nation for assistance (Pereira et al., 2019).

Extended reality may also aid in the management of a scattered workforce, allowing company supervisors and managers to intervene and provide direction as needed, all while having full access to the situation's context. Using AR, the Lockheed Martin corporation cut onboarding and training time by 60% and enhanced new staff member proficiency by up to 70%.

Enhanced Employee Experiences

While boosting client experiences is a top priority for every business right now, it's equally critical not to overlook the value of staff experience. Employees that are happier are frequently more productive and capable of accomplishing a variety of tasks than their rivals. Team members that use extended reality have more access to the tools they need in the present to operate more efficiently. Staff can quickly obtain critical procedural and process information while still being able to do difficult activities with their hands free. Wearable devices in AR are smart glasses which are particularly useful for ensuring staff can easily access information without having to load up an app on a phone or tablet. With this the staff can address complex tasks with accuracy and be faster and with fewer issues.

Achievable Possibilities With Extended Reality

An Immersion Into Different Jobs

Companies are increasingly turning to XR to provide creative and safe training. This might include learning about a career, safety procedures professional practices and skill development. The importance of immersive technologies is ability to reproduce working environments and thus create a great number of scenarios, by offering a high degree of immersion and interactivity including ones that are risky or difficult to set up in reality (Papadopoulos et al., 2021).

The student progresses through an ultra-realistic site simulation or grasps a complex system while completing the assignments. The trainer will be able to evaluate the tactics used. Once in real-life situations, the individual who has been trained has a greater understanding of professional procedures and is able to apply them more readily.

Design and Production Assistance in the Factory of the Future

XR (AR, VR, MR) are used at all facets of the production chain, starting from the research and development while releasing items onto the market. This is assumed to be, and have been a strategic for industry 4.0.

They assist designers and engineers in the development and testing of industrial goods. Prototyping in virtual reality, for example, allows users to see 3D models of real products created with computer-aided design software, simulate their functioning in virtual reality, study the results, and improve their design. All the while, there's plenty of potential for collaborative work. The usage of virtual prototypes at an early stage of the development cycle minimises design costs and delays while simultaneously improving product quality by limiting prototypes and physical tests. In effect, they allow engineers to assess the performance of several models more quickly and to determine the optimum production techniques (Sow et al., 2017).

The Virtual Tour, a Major Asset for Estate Agents

Although 360-degree images allowed purchasers to receive a more accurate depiction of an interior, virtual reality takes it a step further by "teleporting" them into the property and allowing them to go from room to room. The owner may see a building in situ before it is erected thanks to augmented reality. They may travel onto the ground where construction is being done with their smartphone or tablet to imagine their future home or dwelling in 3D and actual dimensions (Hiran & Doshi, 2013).

Many experiences also allow you to customize the property from top to bottom. The estate agent may now show customers various plans (pulling down a wall to form an open-plan kitchen, creating a walk-in wardrobe, etc.) and customizing possibilities during a tour of an old property. With mixed reality, the buyer may even play interior designer by putting furniture in an empty space and experimenting with different floor and wall treatments (Miljkovic et al., 2023).

Training and education, maintenance and manufacturing processes, real estate, and so forth. These are only a handful of the possibilities. Medicine, e-commerce, advertising, leisure, and culture are just a few of the fields that are looking into the possibilities of virtual reality (Ramasamy et al., 2022).

CONCLUSION AND FUTURE SCOPE

The comparative study of VR, AR and MR which are the components of extended reality are focused to expose different aspect of applications, performances and tools requirements.

XR (extended reality) enthusiasts have envisioned long before about, played with, and accepted technology that immerse them in new worlds ones that are not constrained by physics or time. We feel the industry is at a crossroads, and now is the moment for businesses to act. This sector is fast evolving, and much has happened between the time of the interviews and the publishing of this article. However, we believe we have uncovered several key themes and forecasts about the Future of Extended Reality, as well as actionable insights for business executives all across the world.

Within five years, there will be hundreds of millions of VR systems sold throughout the world, and within ten years, it will be as popular as, if not more popular than, smartphones. In ten years, you'll be able to engage, take data, communicate, promote, and control 12 to 15 hours of XR screen time every day via a gadget on your head. It has the potential to be beneficial or harmful. In terms of the moral component of possessing such power, the system that underpins the global metaverse must be held accountable. When we have electroencephalogram (EEG) sensors in our gadgets, we may use them to send signals out to control things, but EEG signals can also be used the other way around. We might truly influence our thinking by sending impulses to your brain. People's perceptions can be altered even without EEG using immersive visual, auditory, and experiences. It has the potential to be the most powerful marketing tool ever. So, there's a lot of potential for good, but there's also a lot of potential for harm, and it's critical for industry and governments to be aware of it and prepare for it.

To provide great accessibility and prevent unscrupulous corporations from building exclusive walled gardens, some sort of interoperability legislation should be imposed. I believe we will require excellent privacy and identity protection, because consider how crucial your phone is in your everyday life right now, then double that by five or ten for the metaverse.

According to recent study, more than 60% of respondents anticipate that Extended Reality will become popular in the next five years. This demonstrates how quickly this technology is evolving and how eager the public is to accept it once it is ready and accessible on the market.

The consumer, enterprise, education, and healthcare markets all have different use cases. For example, DIY instruction is likely to be included in consumer training and guidance, whereas surgical training may be included in medical training. Some of these use cases, such as teaching and assistance in the corporate, education, and medical sectors, are already being seen in action on today's AR and VR head-mounted devices.

REFERENCES

Al-Ansi, A., Jaboob, M., Garad, A., & Al-Ansi, A. (2023). Analyzing augmented reality (AR) and virtual reality (VR) recent development in education. *Social Sciences & Humanities Open*, *8*(1), 100532. doi:10.1016/j.ssaho.2023.100532

Alnagrat, A., Che Ismail, R., Syed Idrus, S. Z., & Abdulhafith Alfaqi, R. M. (2022). A Review of Extended Reality (XR) Technologies in the Future of Human Education: Current Trend and Future Opportunity. *Journal of Human Reproductive Sciences*, *1*(2), 81–96. doi:10.11113/humentech.v1n2.27

Bridges. (2022). *From Virtual Reality to Extended Reality*. Bridges. https://www.bridges-horizon.eu/from-virtual-reality-to-extended-reality/

Carter, R. (2022). *Most Popular XR Gaming Reviews*. XR Today. https://www.xrtoday.com/mixed-reality/most-popular-xr-gaming-reviews-2022/

Çöltekin, A., Lochhead, I., Madden, M., Christophe, S., Devaux, A., Pettit, C., Lock, O., Shukla, S., Herman, L., Stachoň, Z., Kubíček, P., Snopková, D., Bernardes, S., & Hedley, N. (2020). Extended reality in spatial sciences: A review of research challenges and future directions. *ISPRS International Journal of Geo-Information*, *9*(7), 439. doi:10.3390/ijgi9070439

de Giorgio, A., Monetti, F. M., Maffei, A., Romero, M., & Wang, L. (2023). Adopting extended reality? A systematic review of manufacturing training and teaching applications. *Journal of Manufacturing Systems*, *71*, 645–663. doi:10.1016/j.jmsy.2023.10.016

Easwaran, B., Hiran, K. K., Krishnan, S., & Doshi, R. (Eds.). (2022). *Real-time applications of machine learning in cyber-physical systems*. IGI Global. doi:10.4018/978-1-7998-9308-0

Farshid, M., Paschen, J., Eriksson, T., & Kietzmann, J. (2018). Go boldly!: Explore augmented reality (AR), virtual reality (VR), and mixed reality (MR) for business. *Business Horizons*, *61*(5), 657–663. doi:10.1016/j.bushor.2018.05.009

Hamad, A., & Jia, B. (2022). How Virtual Reality Technology Has Changed Our Lives: An Overview of the Current and Potential Applications and Limitations. *International Journal of Environmental Research and Public Health*, *19*(18), 11278. doi:10.3390/ijerph191811278 PMID:36141551

Hiran, K. K., & Doshi, R. (2013). An artificial neural network approach for brain tumor detection using digital image segmentation. *Brain*, *2*(5), 227–231.

Hiran, K. K., Khazanchi, D., Vyas, A. K., & Padmanaban, S. (Eds.). (2021). *Machine learning for sustainable development* (Vol. 9). Walter de Gruyter GmbH & Co KG. doi:10.1515/9783110702514

Ivanova, D., & Thorben, P. H. S. (2023). Immersive imaginaries: Digital spaces as post place care. *Digital Geography and Society, 5*.

Kastner, K. (2023). Leveraging transdisciplinary engineering through the coalescence of digital twins and xr-technologies. In *Leveraging Transdisciplinary Engineering in a Changing and Connected World: Proceedings of the 30th ISTE International Conference on Transdisciplinary Engineering, Hua Hin Cha Am*. IOS Press,.

Lang, V., & Sittler, P. (2012). *Augmented reality for real estate*. In 18th Pacific-RIM Real Estate Society (PRRES) Conference, Adelaide, Australia.

Li, X., Yi, W., Chi, H. L., Wang, X., & Chan, A. P. (2018). A critical review of virtual and augmented reality (VR/AR) applications in construction safety. *Automation in Construction*, *86*, 150–162. doi:10.1016/j.autcon.2017.11.003

Loeffler, C. E. (1993). Distributed Virtual Reality: Applications for education, entertainment and industry. *Telektronikk*, *89*, 83–83.

Maran, P. L., Daniëls, R., & Slegers, K. (2022). The use of extended reality (XR) for people with moderate to severe intellectual disabilities (ID): A scoping review. *Technology and Disability*, *34*(2), 53–67. doi:10.3233/TAD-210363

Marr, J. (2021). Ten best examples of VR and AR in education. *Forbes*. https://www.forbes.com/sites/bernardmarr/2021/07/23/10-best-examples-of-vr-and-ar-in-education/?sh=13e5071e1f48

Miljkovic, I., Shlyakhetko, O., & Fedushko, S. (2023). Real Estate App Development Based on AI/VR Technologies. *Electronics (Basel)*, *12*(3), 707. doi:10.3390/electronics12030707

Papadopoulos, T., Evangelidis, K., Kaskalis, T. H., Evangelidis, G., & Sylaiou, S. (2021). Interactions in augmented and mixed reality: An overview. *Applied Sciences (Basel, Switzerland)*, *11*(18), 8752. doi:10.3390/app11188752

Patel, S., Vyas, A. K., & Hiran, K. K. (2022). Infrastructure health monitoring using signal processing based on an industry 4.0 System. *Cyber-Physical Systems and Industry*, *4*, 249–260.

Pereira, V., Matos, T., Rodrigues, R., Nóbrega, R., & Jacob, J. (2019). Extended reality framework for remote collaborative interactions in virtual environments. In *2019 International Conference on Graphics and Interaction (ICGI)*. IEEE. 10.1109/ICGI47575.2019.8955025

Ramasamy, J., Doshi, R., & Hiran, K. K. (2022, October). Detection of Brain Tumor in Medical Images Based on Feature Extraction by HOG and Machine Learning Algorithms. In *2022 International Conference on Trends in Quantum Computing and Emerging Business Technologies (TQCEBT)* (pp. 1-5). IEEE. 10.1109/TQCEBT54229.2022.10041564

Ratcliffe, J., Soave, F., Bryan-Kinns, N., Tokarchuk, L., & Farkhatdinov, I. (2021, May). Extended reality (XR) remote research: a survey of drawbacks and opportunities. In *Proceedings of the 2021 CHI Conference on Human Factors in Computing Systems* (pp. 1-13). IEEE. 10.1145/3411764.3445170

Shaikh, T. A., Dar, T. R., & Sofi, S. (2022). A data-centric artificial intelligent and extended reality technology in smart healthcare systems. *Social Network Analysis and Mining*, *12*(1), 122. doi:10.1007/s13278-022-00888-7 PMID:36065420

Sow, D., Imoussaten, A., Couturier, P., & Montmain, J. (2017). A Possibilistic Approach to Set Achievable and Feasible Goals while Designing Complex Systems. *IFAC-PapersOnLine*, *50*(1), 14218–14223. doi:10.1016/j.ifacol.2017.08.2094

Sridhar, S. (2023). *OPPO MR Glass Developer Edition*. Fone Arena. https://www.fonearena.com/blog/394919/oppo-mr-glass-developer-edition-features.html

Teniou, G. (2019). 3GPP achievements on VR & ongoing developments on XR over 5G. In *Proc. 3GPP/ VRIF/AIS 2nd Workshop VR Ecosyst. Standards, Immersive Media Meets*. IEEE.

UNCTAD. (2018). *Creative economy has new impetus in digital world*. UNCTAD. https://unctad.org/ news/creative-economy-has-new-impetus-digital-world

Vaidyanathan, N., & Henningsson, S. (2023). Designing augmented reality services for enhanced customer experiences in retail. *Journal of Service Management*, *34*(1), 78–99. doi:10.1108/JOSM-01-2022-0004

Vollmar, A. (2023). *Difference between VR and AR*. Hegias. https://hegias.com/en/knowledge/difference-vr-ar/

Vyas, B. (2019). *Top five use cases of extended reality in the healthcare sector*. Softweb Solutions. https:// www.softwebsolutions.com/resources/extended-reality-in-healthcare-sector.html

Zwoliński, G., Kamińska, D., Laska-Leśniewicz, A., Haamer, R. E., Vairinhos, M., Raposo, R., Urem, F., & Reisinho, P. (2022). Extended reality in education and training: Case studies in Management Education. *Electronics (Basel)*, *11*(3), 336. doi:10.3390/electronics11030336

Chapter 2
Revolutionizing Patient Care:
The Impact of Virtual Reality in Healthcare

Rajaprabakaran Rajendran

https://orcid.org/0009-0005-9272-5475

CMS Business School, Jain University (Deemed), Bengaluru, India

Yavana Rani Subramanian

CMS Business School, Jain University (Deemed), Bengaluru, India

ABSTRACT

Virtual reality (VR) technology has been gradually gaining traction in the healthcare industry and has the potential to significantly transform the way that patients receive medical care. VR technology delivers an immersive experience that may improve diagnosis, treatment, and overall patient outcomes by enabling patients and medical professionals to visualise and interact with medical data more effectively and intuitively. VR can help patients gain a better understanding of their medical diagnoses and treatments. Better health results may result from this and an improvement in the way care is delivered generally. In conclusion, VR technology creates an exceptional opportunity for medical practitioners to transform the way they treat patients. The field of digital health is an emerging discipline that integrates technology and healthcare to boost overall care, save costs, and improve patient outcomes.

INTRODUCTION

"Virtual" and "reality" are the foundational terms used to describe virtual reality. "Virtual" implies "near," while "reality" refers to having human experience. Thus, the ability to emulate a specific world is close to actuality. Computer technology is applied in VR to generate a simulated scenario. By simulating touch, hearing, and vision on a screen, it makes it possible for the user to interact with an artificial three-dimensional environment. This technology comprises a room-sized screen with a head-mounted display component. It utilises software to generate an artificial environment that is perceived as real. The primary application of this technology is to build a virtual world for training in a simulated environment and games with interactive stories. Using this technology, users can interact with virtual elements by

DOI: 10.4018/979-8-3693-1123-3.ch002

creating realistic visuals in a virtual world. Currently, it is utilised in driving guidance, aviation training, healthcare, architectural planning, and army training. It is employed to obtain significant knowledge and skills without the requirement for real-life experience. It is possible to promptly identify the number of undesired symptoms, such as pain, stress injuries, and other illnesses. It provides In-depth details about the anatomy and other bodily parts of the patient (Gold & Maher, 2018; Srinivasulu et al, 2022).

The Development of Virtual Reality (Hou et al., 2022)

The concept of virtual reality originally appeared in science fiction. Science fiction author Laurence Manning, a Canadian, released a collection of short stories in 1933, "The Man Who Awoke," which introduced the idea of virtual life. The "simulation simulator," originally developed by Morton Heiling in 1962, was the first attempt to allow users to transition from the physical world into the virtual world. Virtual reality begins to resemble the real world more and more as computer and virtual reality technology becomes more advanced. Based on theories developed and offered in the 1980s, and on proposals made in the 1960s, the initial phase of global virtual reality development commenced in the 1990s.

As illustrated in Figure 1, VR became the market's main emphasis when Facebook paid $2 billion to acquire Oculus in 2014. Manufacturers like Sony and HTC then introduced their own versions of virtual reality products. At the Game Developers Conference in 2014, Sony unveiled a virtual reality prototype of the gaming system. In 2015, HTC also showcased its VR device HTCVIVE, which helped to ignite the VR sector. The virtual reality market has expanded rapidly since 2016.

Virtual reality technology can be classified into two distinct categories: immersive and non-immersive. Non-immersive virtual reality, often known as desktop VR, is created using a computer, three-dimensional modelling applications, mouse, microphone, keyboard, and other peripheral tools. Either a virtual environment created in a window on the screen or another created from real photos that have been processed by computers and captured through photography. By utilising graphics processors and several control interface devices, immersive virtual reality can be created on computers. The creation of a virtual three-dimensional world by computer simulation, which allows users to experience visual, aural, tactile, and other sensations in a virtual setting, is known as the emulating real-life interaction.

Figure 1. Historical milestones in virtual reality
Adapted from (Molnár, 2017)

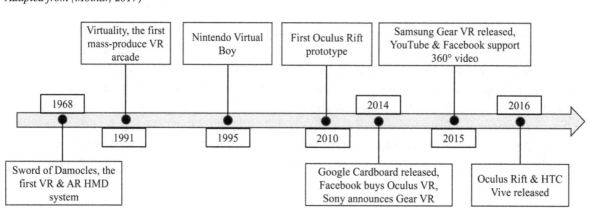

The Trajectory of Virtual Reality Development

VR is a technology that is developing gradually. Under continual modification and refinement during development, it has continuously advanced from far to near the top of the technical level. The main objective of virtual reality technology is to create a completely interactive artificial "world" that allows users to explore and interact with objects in the surroundings at any point in time. Immersive virtual reality is the most advanced form of virtual reality that can be achieved using a body motion tracker, data gloves, and specialist head-mounted display. In this way, users will be able to employ their senses of touch, hearing, and sight to fully engage with the virtual scenario. To enjoy the immersive nature of a virtual reality game world, it is anticipated that in the near future, gamers will be able to don gloves, helmets, and clothing designed specifically for the game. This development in technology will significantly advance technological advancement and profoundly change the landscape for existing players. The development concept of "low cost and high performance" will be pursued to explore virtual reality technology that is viewed through the lens of the VR development process (Hou et al., 2022).

VIRTUAL REALITY IN HEALTHCARE

The healthcare industry has been significantly impacted by the development of VR technology. VR provides significant potential for improving patient care, medical education, and overall digital health experiences by building immersive and engaging virtual worlds. VR is transforming how healthcare professionals provide care and how patients manage their well-being, from surgical simulations to mental health treatments (Portman et al., 2015).

The integration of virtual reality technology shows enormous potential for improving patient care, medical education, and overall well-being as the healthcare industry embraces digital transformation. Nevertheless, in order to ensure widespread adoption and optimise its advantages, challenges like cost, accessibility, and data security must be resolved. However, it is indisputable that the immersive and revolutionary potential of virtual reality technology will have a significant impact on healthcare in the future (Chen, 2015).

Designing Visual Communications for Virtual Reality (Yaqi, 2022)

The healthcare sector continually evolves due to advancements in technology and a greater emphasis on patient-centred care. VR is one of the cutting-edge techniques that has emerged in recent years and has the potential to completely transform several aspects of the healthcare sector. Creating visual messaging for the healthcare sector is one highly intriguing application for virtual reality. Virtual reality can enhance training, education, and communication in healthcare settings by providing a distinctive and immersive platform. To effectively convey complex facts to patients, healthcare professionals, and other stakeholders, effective visual communication is vital in the healthcare industry. Medical procedures and concepts have traditionally been made easier to understand through the utilisation of visual aids like charts, diagrams, and animations. However, these traditional two-dimensional representations frequently fall short of accurately depicting the complexities of the human body and medical procedures. Here is where virtual reality steps into play, providing an interactive, three-dimensional environment that makes it easier for users to explore and understand medical concepts in a realistic and intuitive way. The potential for enhancing patient education and engagement through the integration of VR-based visual communications is enormous (Yaqi, 2022).

Virtual reality provides a secure, controlled environment for trainees to hone their skills, refine techniques, and build confidence by simulating real-world medical scenarios. By bridging the gap between academic knowledge and actual application, this intensive training programme produces healthcare practitioners who are more competent and proficient. The development of visual communications is expected to be significantly enhanced by virtual reality as the healthcare industry continues to embrace cutting-edge technologies. Its ability to generate realistic, immersive, and interactive experiences could revolutionise training methods, enhance collaboration among healthcare professionals, and improve patient education. While the main purpose of packaging design is primarily to build a product or corporate image, public service advertising design aims to inform the public about a specific concept or set of information, etc (Beukelman & Mirenda, 2013; Hiran, 2013).

Furthermore, virtual reality enables improved communication and teamwork among medical practitioners. Surgeons, nurses, anaesthesiologists, and radiologists usually collaborate as a multidisciplinary team during complex medical procedures and surgeries. These specialists may work together to plan interventions, visualise the anatomy of the patient, model procedures, and interact effectively in a shared visual world that virtual reality offers. In addition to improving patient safety, this promotes efficient teamwork and minimises errors. Training programmes for medical professionals are also greatly impacted by virtual reality. Virtual reality offers students a secure and regulated environment to practise medical skills by simulating real-life situations. By bridging the gap between academic knowledge and practical application, this immersive training programme produces healthcare practitioners who are more knowledgeable and proficient.

Importance of VR in the Medical Industry

This technology was introduced in the medical field in the 1990s to ensure the appropriate grounding and successful surgeries. Improved coordination and communication are essential for fostering innovation in the medical sector among physicians, surgeons, scientists, researchers, and students. Virtual reality is a valuable tool that helps these groups work together to solve complex cases. It is essential to determine the ways in which a healthcare organisation could benefit from appropriate training and better preparedness. In the medical field, it appears to be an effective training aid (Javaid & Haleem, 2020).

DISTINCT ADVANTAGES OF VIRTUAL REALITY IN THE FIELD OF MEDICINE

The healthcare industry employs VR technology to enhance patient care since it facilitates the acquisition of new skills in a secure environment. It can train aspiring physicians and nurses in anatomy, surgical technique, and infection control (Gatica-Rojas & Méndez-Rebolledo, 2014). With the utilisation of virtual data, they can now effectively execute an operation and accurately comprehend a complex surgical procedure (Cano Porras et al., 2018; Javaid & Haleem, 2018). It aids in the development of skills and confidence refraining from inflicting any adverse effects. The numerous cutting-edge advantages associated with virtual reality in the field of medicine are shown in Figure 2.

Virtual reality offers an effective diagnostic platform that creates new opportunities for restorative procedures. The surgeon can use these virtual organs to prepare for the actual procedure by visually viewing a picture of the head of the patient with the aid of this technology. It assists in managing resources and lessens the cost of patient care. Connecting the real and virtual worlds is made possible by this effective instrument. New medical professionals may become more confident in their procedures and treatments. With the appropriate virtual knowledge, it manages complex processes with ease (Javaid & Haleem, 2020).

The application of this technology in research, training, clinical rehabilitation, and psychotherapy has made it feasible for students to virtually conduct secure and guided operations without any complications (Pan & Hamilton, 2018). Acquiring a life-saving skill is beneficial in emergency and accidental cases. VR also teaches patients how to lead a healthy lifestyle with a proper diet and exercise plan. Table 1 summarises several key implementations of virtual reality in the medical industry. Three-dimensional VR is a vital tool for practicing with medical instruments. The tool is close to the process, which aids in accurately measuring the body of the patient. It demonstrates insights-related attributes such as varying symptoms and changing vital signs. Virtual patient tissues are now accessible to engage with a medical expert. In the medical field, effective communication is essential to providing patients with improved care. It creates a cross-section in any plane, allowing for improved measurements and visualisation of the patient part. The clotting of a brain blood vessel is now visible to medical professionals. Virtual reality is currently being implemented by several surgeons to perform risky surgical procedures (Pizzoli et al., 2019; Hiran et al., 2013). It contributes to the development of a stable, secure, and effective environment that minimises inaccuracies produced in the surgical room. This technology also improves the professional setting for doctors and lowers training costs for medical trainees.

Figure 2. Advantages of virtual reality in medical sector
Adapted from (Javaid & Haleem, 2020)

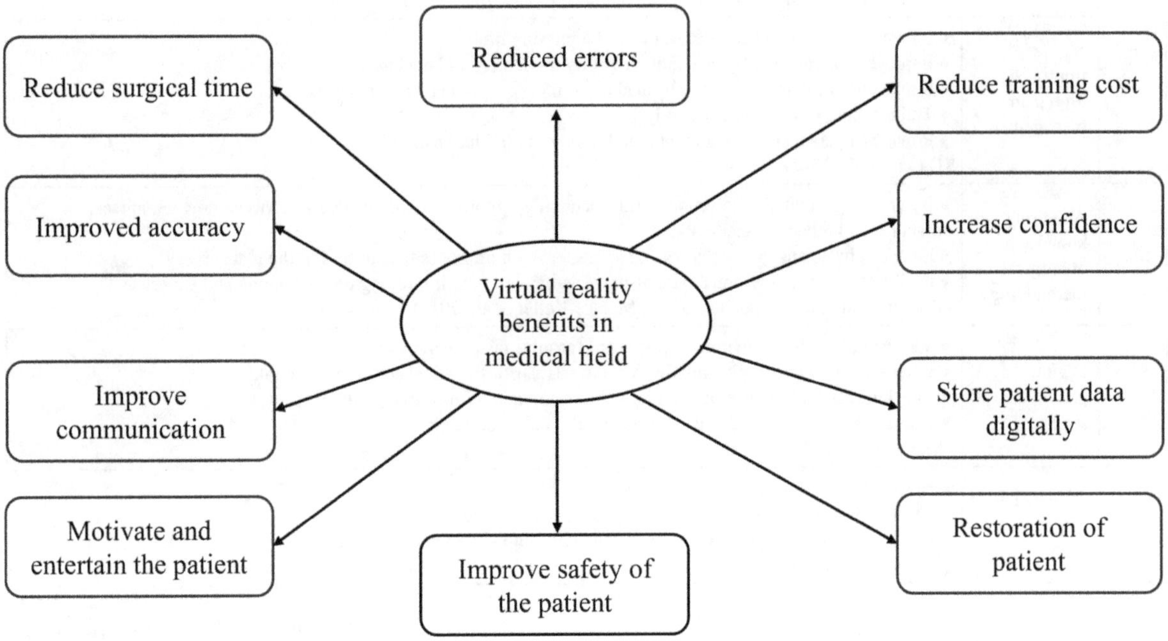

Table 1. Applications of virtual reality in the medical domain

S No	Medical area	Description
1	Virtual operation	• Virtual Reality is the ideal tool to simulate a surgical process • • Applied to deliver virtual surgery, which minimises risk and time • • Effective for assessing and analysing the amount of effort required to carry out the procedures. • Used for telesurgery, allowing the surgeon to execute the procedure from different locations. • Offers a clear image that facilitates improved practice and planning. (Diemer et al., 2015; Marco et al., 2013)
2	Preparation of medical procedures	• The surgeon can effectively plan and execute the procedure by using virtual 3D models. • It also improves communication within the medical community. • During the procedure, the technology creates an accurate scenario of the patient. • For performing the surgery, the surgeon utilises the latest virtual glasses in a three-dimensional environment. (Park et al., 2019 Li et al., 2017)
3	Medical diagnosis	• A valuable diagnostic tool that helps medical practitioners make accurate diagnoses. • Need for magnetic resonance imaging scans an computerised tomography is minimised. • Rapidly recognises the signs and symptoms of diseases • Compile patient data to ensure accurate diagnosis. (Cooper et al., 2018; HajesmaeelGohari et al., 2019)
4	Physiotherapy	• VR helps treatment accomplish enhanced outcomes during practical implementation. • Helpful to treat burn victims with mild pain. Helps quickly sort various cognitive issues safely and comfortably. • By utilising this technology, exercise is performed in a profoundly different way. • Has a major impact on physiotherapy when combined with appropriate, regular physical activity. (Parsons et al., 2017; Rothbaum et al., 2010)
5	Education and training	• Contributes to the development of the highest quality learning programme in medical training and education • Enhanced the understanding of learners on age-related issues and diseases • Presented an innovative approach for teaching and mentoring medical students. • Beneficial in practicing and planning complex surgical procedures with minimal risk (Drewett et al., 2019; Doshi et al., 2023; Bun et al., 2017)
6	Mental health treatment	• It facilitates social contact with virtual characters, which is beneficial for enhancing life skills • Beneficial for treating patients with psychological disorders • A device for changing the way exposure therapy is administered, which is advantageous for a range of psychological conditions • Offers an affordable treatment with a reduced probability of fatal complications (Chirico et al., 2016; Riva, 2011; Valmaggia et al., 2016)
7	Improved limb pain management	• Enhances the experience of movement of a missing limb • Improves patients' confidence in their ability to identify and manage pain • Simulates a limb to assess the physical discomfort experienced by the patient • Trains young physicians effectively • Provides a personalised treatment plan for every individual patient (Dascal et al., 2017)
8	Acquiring knowledge of surgical methodology	• By applying simulation techniques, this technology improves communication between doctors, nurses, surgeons, and other medical workers. • Enables physicians to practice virtual surgery, which improves the success of the real surgery • Facilitates three-dimensional patient-physician interaction, improving understanding and expertise (Du Sert et al., 2018; Gadelha, 2018); Maples-Keller et al., 2017)
9	Digital patient data storage	• VR technology has numerous applications for minimising paperwork • It helps in solving complex problems and treats various medical conditions digitally • This information can also be used for the development of new treatment protocols • Digital data storage is beneficial to potential medical services. (McIntosh et al., 2014; Flores et al., 2018)
10	Diagnosing respiratory problems	• Helps balance blood pressure and heart rate • Rapidly diagnoses breathing issues in patients and aids in treatment • Facilitates patients to view exercises virtually to improve medical conditions (De Luca et al., 2019)

continued on following page

Table 1. Continued

S No	Medical area	Description
11	Enhance the effectiveness of psychiatric counselling	• Considered to be a great technique for improving the effectiveness of psychotherapy • It has a great potential to cure various mental illnesses • Beneficial for regular interpersonal communication that can alter behaviours and solve relevant issues (Bergeron et al., 2015)
12	Alleviate mental depression	• Researchers and medical practitioners apply this technology to demonstrate that the rate of depression in young adults is lowering • The Well-being of adult and children is enhanced by the use of this technology (Biffi et al., 2017; Norouzi et al., 2019; Yildirim et al., 2018)
13	Monitor body motion	• VR has the potential to significantly impact a person suffering from depression • It may be a useful tool for monitoring the patient's body movements. • Offers patients an engaging rehabilitative training • Additionally, VR technology can provide outstanding opportunities to experience real-life scenarios. • It can instantly assess the way bones that move (Faric et al., 2019; Ventola, 2019)
14	Reduce trauma pain	• Patients can practise exercises virtually in a secured setting • They can effectively recuperate from trauma to carry out cognitive tasks. • This technology reduces pain when the patient engages virtually (Chan et al., 2018; Chen et al., 2018; Peeters, 2019)

Adapted from (Javaid & Haleem, 2020)

VR ADOPTION PROCESS IN THE MEDICAL INDUSTRY

VR programmes are utilised to accelerate the learning process without any exposure to danger or anxiousness. It is utilised in the medical field to treat many different types of illnesses. This application is helpful in enhancing the performance of the medical industry (Zhang et al., 2019). It is a practical and helpful technology to improve patient and trainee satisfaction. As seen in Figure 3, this technology leverages its approach to deliver an appropriate solution in the medical industry.

Figure 3. Method for implementing virtual reality in medical domain
Adapted from (Javaid & Haleem, 2020)

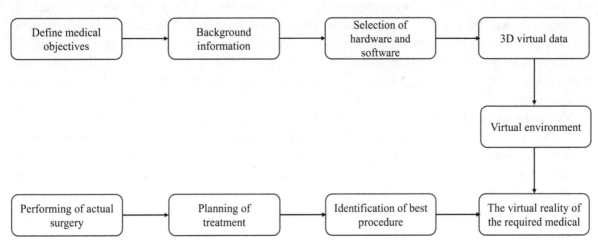

Virtual reality is an important innovation for the development phase which involves specially designed software and expensive hardware to operate. We can initially gather background data and specify the precise goal of the needed therapy. A 3D virtual environment is created by using various devices and programmes to generate three-dimensional digital information. The most effective approach is implemented to find and produce a simulated version of the relevant medical information. This method may assist with treatment planning and even in executing actual procedures (Javaid & Haleem, 2020).

APPLICATIONS OF VR TRAINING FOR MEDICAL PROFESSIONALS

Many VR platforms have been created and brought into practice in recent years to assist in training and teaching across many learning domains. It has been and still is a challenge for educators and developers to determine when learning in virtual environments (VEs) can truly add worth to conventional education and to comprehend the ways that promote the acquisition of various concepts and skills through the application and adaptation of virtual reality (Mantovani, 2003).

Traditionally, the majority of medical students learn anatomy through cadaveric dissection. Cadaveric orientation is not practical with the advent of modern imaging methods like ultrasound, CT scans, and MRI, despite the opportunity for hands-on learning (Gupta et al., 2022). As contrary to this, VR anatomy allows for the manipulation of the anatomical orientation. As a result, learning anatomy in virtual reality aids students in comprehending and acclimating to human anatomy more quickly. Nowadays, there are many different types of virtual training applications for healthcare. These include tele surgical applications (Satava & Jones, 1997), simulated environments for emergency training (to develop coping abilities in emergency scenarios), dynamic simulations of the human anatomy (to learn physioanatomical information), and many more (Small et al., 1999).

VR technology is being utilised by several international universities to train medical professionals. Medical procedures can then be performed in a virtual environment using VR equipment (Figure 4) (Hou et al., 2022).

Confidence among trainees is enhanced by virtual reality, which can be attributed to more individualised training, immediate feedback, and repeated practice (Buckley et al., 2012). Repeated use of VR could improve their knowledge and confidence to the point where an error made during training may be rectified without endangering any patients. Since virtual reality is a component of simulation-based education, trainee performance is improved and their learning curve is facilitated through feedback or debriefing (Van De Ridder et al., 2008). Another intriguing point is using VR training to manage stress. For instance, when a trainee is practicing driving an ambulance, the trainer can safely assess the trainee's emotional state and decision-making while they are in the comfort of the control room. By doing this, the risk that a real-world driving evaluation posed to the trainee and the trainers is eliminated (Ismail et al., 2022).

Medical and surgical training: Satava and Jones (1997) highlighted three areas in which virtual environments could be used for (medical) education and training: medical virtual prototyping, medical crisis training, and individual training. According to the authors, personalised training systems currently comprise a wide range of VR medical applications. These task-driven individualised healthcare trainers, sometimes referred to as "partial trainers," are designed to teach one or a limited set of skills with a remarkably accurate and anatomically precise simulation.

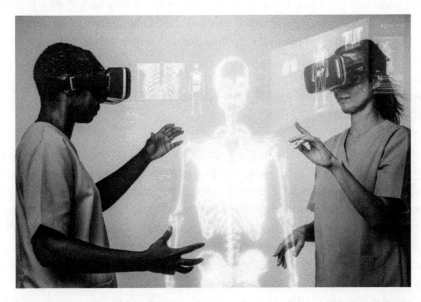

Kaufman (2001) addressed the possibility of VR-based partial instructors for educating and evaluating clinical skills that are specific to a specific task. Researchers from a wide range of clinical specialties are pursuing this potential field. These partial trainers are all focused on the specific skills and biological area: a virtual reality training programme for managing wounds caused by firearms (Delp et al., 1997), a virtual endoscopy simulator (Robb, 1997), a trainer for arthroscopic knee surgery (Mabrey et al., 2000), and a simulated training tool for palpating breast tumours under their outermost layer (Dinsmore et al., 2001). Virtual reality orthopaedic surgery (Tsai et al., 2001), VR based simulation of mastoidectomy (Agus et al., 2002), virtual reality open surgery simulation system (Bielser & Gross, 2002), VR guidance and Invasive neuroradiology preparatory planning, virtual reality esophageal intubation training (Kesawadas, 2002), and Training in VR and evaluation of laparoscopic techniques are some of the more recent examples.

Systems for emergency training: Programmes for training on medical crises emphasise challenging training assignments where the trainee must interact with the environment directly and physically and where the results of their actions can be quite subtle (like a change in skin tone).

Like a plane simulator, an emergency medical care instructor, was introduced by Small et al. (1999). Users operate on a mannequin that can be customised and has realistic anatomical features. A computerised monitoring system that determines the best possible medical condition and responses is interfaced with the mannequin. Other researchers (Stytz et al., 1997; Chi et al., 1996) developed a complete training scenario using software, in which a series of options allows the doctors and residents to engage with the device while dynamic virtual patients display changing physical conditions. U.S. Navy medical personnel can now learn emergency response techniques from a virtual reality patient simulation system designed by Freeman et al. (2001).

VR for the doctor-patient association: Letterie (2002) evaluated the effective use of VR to launch 3-dimensional instructors for surgical simulation and to reproduce interactions between individuals for training in social sciences and psychiatry under an array of circumstances. This shows that VR can aid in the development of technical abilities as well as a variety of other skills, such as the interpersonal aspects of patient care. For example, the author focuses on the potential use of VR as an educational modality in obstetrics and gynaecology, both for teaching the fundamentals of counselling and for learning surgical skills (from regular preoperative consent forms to intervention in more serious situations like domestic abuse or sexual assault).

Advantages and Rationale of Applying VR in Training and Education (Ismail et al., 2022)

Numerous advantages for healthcare teaching and training could result from the application of virtual environments, which offer features like 3D immersion, various viewpoints, and multisensory cues.

Experiential and active learning: Learning in virtual environments (VEs) necessitates interaction, which promotes active engagement rather than passivity. Users can experience new technology firsthand by using virtual reality. Learners and trainees consume information more effectively in a setting where they are free to wander around and engage in self-directed activities. They invest mental energy searching for and organising content on their own, building conceptual models that make them understand both the newly provided content and what they already know.

Visualization and reification: VEs offer an alternative approach to presenting content in novel ways. The utilisation of graphic symbols can be highly significant in fields that require information visualisation, like rearranging and manipulating data. It can also be beneficial in scenarios where it is essential to make perceptible the imperceptible, such as demonstrating biological and abstract physics concepts that are included in curricula for medical professionals.

Acquiring knowledge in environments too complex or unattainable in reality: VR makes it possible to observe and analyse objects and occurrences that are challenging to observe with traditional methods. (such as "travelling" inside the human body or moving between molecules). It also permits observation from a considerable distance as well as extremely close-up investigation of an object.

Evaluation and assessment: VR has a lot of potential as an assessment tool since it makes it easy for teachers and trainers to watch and record sessions in the virtual environment, which makes assessment tasks easier.

VR GAMES FOR PATIENT EDUCATION

In addition to training medical staff, serious games can be utilised for various aspects of patient care, including educating patients, their relatives, and the public about illnesses or clinical procedures. Serious games for health can take many forms. In an effort to treat chronic painful treatments such as anxiety (Michael & Chen, 2005), nausea during chemotherapy, pain during debridement of a burned wound, or other conditions that cause discomfort over time, the first category focuses on diverting the attention of the patients from their condition. Functional MRI (fMRI) has been used to scientifically validate the efficacy of VR and games in treating fears and diverting patients during burn treatment or chemotherapy. fMRI has revealed differences in brain activity between patients who use virtual reality and games to alleviate pain and those who do not. (Bergeron, 2006).

The second category, called "exergaming," incorporates a Wii, Kinect, joystick, or other special equipment (like GameWheels, which was created for patients in wheelchairs) to encourage physical exercise through gameplay (O'Connor et al., 2000). These games have been employed in traumatic brain injury (Caglio et al., 2009), stroke or limb shortage following trauma or stroke. They can be used to improve fitness or rehabilitation. Teaching the patient or their family about their condition and better ways to manage it comes under the third category.

According to Rossier Jr. et al. (2007), a game aimed at educating kids about asthma, for instance, requires them to stay away from triggers for Bronkie the Bronchiasaurus, or they can make an avatar of a covert agent monitoring asthma medication. Taking diabetic games as an additional example, consider how the user might influence patients' dietary choices by offering tips on managing insulin and overall nutrition (Harden, 1999). To help patients understand surgery, case studies and other games have been created. One interactive resource that could be used by patients is a description of students in a classroom undergoing intensive brain stimulation surgery or having an aneurysm repaired (Qin et al., 2010).

Impact of VR on Patient Safety

Furthermore, there is a correlation between the higher rate of errors and variables such as a heavy workload, time constraints, and the burnout that occurs. It has been challenging to address these underlying reasons since complex healthcare delivery systems tend to shift over time, resulting in new sources of failure. (Sentinel event alert 51, 2022). Most safety-enhancing measures already in place focus on the extremes of mistake. For example, the Accreditation Council for Graduate Medical Education necessitates multidisciplinary patient safety training and tasks, such as reporting patient safety events and root cause analyses, to be completed by residents, including surgical residents. This is evident that these requirements improve patient safety (Ferraro et al., 2017).

Furthermore, it seemed that attending surgeons' training through simulation minimised the number of malpractice lawsuits that followed. However, the majority of these initiatives concentrate on the technical skills and communication required to manage the error (e.g., communication and teamwork in the operation theatre). By contrast, there is a dearth of training on flawed error prevention systems (e.g., the Swiss cheese model [SCM]; Reason, 2000), patient safety culture, and the erratic thought processes and actions that cause people to commit errors or neglect to take preventative action (Bootman, 2000).

VR training is becoming a more practical and efficient teaching tool in the healthcare industry. Studies indicate that virtual reality training in the medical field can enhance both technical and nontechnical abilities (such as collaboration and teamwork), surgical planning and execution, and medical diagnosis (Pareek et al., 2018).

Researchers have frequently emphasised how virtual reality might improve patient safety (Kizil & Joy 2001). This can be provided either at pre- engagement or during patient engagement. Pre-engagement allows a surgeon to practise the procedure in advance of the procedure and refrain from doing surgical experiments on patients. A psychiatrist treating phobias in patients may avoid the trauma of real-life psychiatric intervention during patient interaction by utilising VR (Botella et al. 2017). It was thought that virtual reality training would ensure the safety of both trainers and trainees. By preventing novices from using real patients for practice, virtual reality has the potential to increase trainer-trainee safety both medically and legally. The findings of numerous research regarding the safety of trainers and trainees were consistent (Kizil & Joy 2001).

Consequences of Cybersickness in Immersive Virtual Reality (Li et al., 2023)

Exposure to immersive virtual worlds can induce a phenomenon known as "cybersickness," which can cause a variety of symptoms like nausea, oculomotor, and disorientation. This is a typical VR application challenge, and several factors can affect the severity of the impact. In order to design effective interventions to mitigate the impact of cybersickness on experiences of the users and encourage the safe usage of this technology, It is crucial to understand the fundamental causes and factors that cause cybersickness, especially in virtual rehab settings.

The demographic factor and the hardware and software of VR devices revealed that cybersickness conditions influenced the efficacy of the experiments. We should improve the rehabilitation approach considering the implications of the immersive background of the technological revolution. (Petrigna & Musumeci 2022). In view of the technology advancements, it is advantageous for us to improve the rehabilitation modality (Petrigna & Musumeci 2022). In addition, by comprehending VR technology more effectively, we will be able to develop equipment that is especially helpful for recovery (Yang & Lee, 2021; Garavand & Aslani, 2022).

Planning and execution are key to maximising the advantages of virtual reality therapy and minimising cybersickness. Larger or more informative studies should be the focus of future research since it is challenging to draw clear conclusions from small-scale studies that support the application of VR in rehabilitation. Immersive VR rehabilitation equipment continues to become more effective in FOV, latency, and realism. With the advancement of technology, further study needs to be done to assess the impact of cybersickness. A greater emphasis on rehabilitation symptoms is necessary for improved product engineering.

CHALLENGES WITH VIRTUAL REALITY TECHNOLOGY AND SOLUTIONS

Virtual reality technology has advanced over several decades, and as a result, more and more people can experience the realistic sensory experience that virtual reality technology offers due to the widespread use of headsets, controls, and other gadgets for commercial purposes. Virtual reality technology is still plagued by numerous issues, all of which require immediate remedial action (Wang et al., 2022).

The headgear is excessively heavy: Firstly, the virtual reality head-mounted display equipment is excessively huge because of its both weight and size, and it will make people feel fatigued when used for a long time, and the pressure on the face will become more obvious with the increase of use time. In addition, when the range of motion is too large, it may slide down due to too much weight, which affects the experience of use. In the hot weather season, wearing it for a long time will also make the user feel stuffy, especially in the closed environment of the eyes, which is easy to sweat, which affects the visual experience.

Inadequate interaction: Virtual reality gadgets mostly rely on the sensors and the head-mounted device, and gesture recognition is used in a few applications. The lack of interaction is a big problem for game developers and hardware manufacturers right now.

Limitation on utilising the venue: If a player is engrossed in the action and moves swiftly, it is possible to hit the wall in reality, and there are more actions, such as dodging, jumping, jumping, diving, climbing, etc. There will be limitations of physical venues, and it is impossible to truly achieve an immersive experience. Some external devices can mimic specific aspects of the experience, like driving seats that can simulate turning, driving, and so on.

Compatibility of VR Devices: While there is already a plethora of VR devices out there, consumers have more choices. Although VR devices are currently widely available, consumers have more alternatives. Nevertheless, VR equipment from different manufacturers is incompatible with one another. The need to create several versions of games for various VR devices compels game developers to incur additional costs during the production process.

Easily become fatigued: In the virtual reality scene, frequent visual changes tend to fatigue viewers. Viewers of virtual reality head-mounted displays are more likely to experience visual fatigue when they move with the virtual world since they are fully engaged in it. The movement of the screen and the body of the user can even induce dizziness. Furthermore, extended usage will exacerbate eye fatigue due to the limitation of the refresh rate.

LIMITATIONS

Virtual reality in the medical field has several drawbacks and limitations. Avatars are not exceptionally convincing in their present form, which could impede the ability of medical professionals to fully immerse in the scenario. Compared to a real person, doctors could feel more comfortable refusing an avatar. An increase in funding might lead to more advanced technology, including speech recognition and more natural facial expressions. More funding is needed to create avatars with greater quality, which presents another implementation challenge. Thus far, the scenarios have merely facilitated behaviour observation; they have not demonstrated behaviour modification. The results could have been less meaningful if clinicians acted differently knowing they were participating in research as opposed to receiving training in communication skills. More research is required to further investigate challenges with implementation and assess the relative efficacy of virtual reality over role performers in training.

The main limitation of this technique is its high cost, which prevents its commercial implementation in medical settings. VR intervention requires a long time and involves a lot of hardware and software support. For high-resolution patient data, additional costs apply. In order to store data, VR imagery demands an enormous amount of storage capacity. Currently, this technology is ineffective in detecting the signs of emerging ailments. Its scope is restricted to understanding specific cases, and appropriate treatment that necessitates appropriate motion of the body part. It is confined to the demonstration, and only the body motion of the patient and specific areas is covered by the VR headgear. But with more research and integration with other technology, this will be very beneficial to the general public (Javaid & Haleem, 2020).

FUTURE OPPORTUNITIES

VR applications in healthcare will ultimately proliferate in the future. Any complex procedure can be carried out accurately and safely by doctors and surgeons. The surgical team should be able to examine both the hard and soft tissues inside the body of a patient to ensure that the surgery is successful. It has the potential to develop into an advanced gadget and an effective instrument that produces a superior visual tool. In addition to other necessary disciplines, the medical field may enhance knowledge, skills, and habits. Buildings, industries, and hospitals with optimised designs will be constructed using this technology. The next couple of years will witness it rise in intelligence, which will aid in bringing all medical procedures into the digital age. VR presents potentially advantageous techniques for protecting and enhancing the patient's life. This immersive tool creates the training of the operating room environment at any moment and any place. Doctors can quickly determine the accurate and inaccurate status of the sickness with the use of this technology. It guides medical professionals on the biological processes of the body. With the application of this technology, realistic and precise virtual world simulations can be generated (Javaid & Haleem, 2020).

Virtual reality is set to become the predominant method of teaching and preparing aspiring surgeons, as well as assisting seasoned professionals in learning novel techniques. The next development is expected to be the integration of virtual reality with holographic projection, which will enhance the three-dimensional image (Custură-Crăciun et al., 2013). The integration of autonomous cybernetic systems and VR will lead to the development of advanced virtual research software, autonomous surgical robots, autonomous education systems, and autonomous rehabilitation systems for the disabled, which may even have the potential to manage themselves and self-supporting their existence (Graur, 2014).

According to the law of supply and demand, virtual reality technology will become affordable over the years (Gale, 1955). A change in mindset is another obstacle that calls for attention. Those who are potential users, administrators, supervisors, and trainers frequently have a pessimistic attitude and are resistant to change. Although it was generally believed that senior trainers were reluctant to use virtual reality, recent research indicates that this unfavourable mindset appears to be prevalent across rank and age in the academic area (Shao & Lee, 2020). A further concern that needs to be addressed is the potential side effects of VR use. Despite the limited number of people affected, the issue nevertheless exists.

Cybersickness can include nausea, vertigo, dry eyes, dizziness, headaches, loss of vision, disorientation, eye pain, and seizures, among other symptoms (Huygelier et al., 2019; Lewis, 2018). To increase VR adoption, these problems must be resolved. There are several methods to navigate around this problem, such as setting time limits for VR exposure and only utilising VR when absolutely necessary. The ecosystem needs significant collaboration between the subject matter expert and VR technology expert for VR to become more widespread (Morvan, 2019).

The lack of awareness or understanding of VR resources must be addressed promptly because neither institutional administrators nor potential users can see VR in practice. The lack of knowledge exhibited by trainers and institutional administration is impeding the expansion of the virtual reality industry. VR, however, has enormous potential, particularly in surgical specialties and related fields. The implementation of VR technology in healthcare requires stronger cooperation between VR technologists and healthcare subject matter experts, as well as more funding, a positive outlook, increased exposure, and an understanding of available resources (Ismail et al., 2022).

It is anticipated that this field will develop as a result of the developing Web facilities the growing accessibility of top-notch devices, and their enormous processing capability. It is advisable to consider future research guidelines due to the rapid development in this field. As VR eyeglasses become more affordable and widely available, greater possibilities emerge for comprehensive virtual reality immersion (Mazurek et al., 2019).

VR With Artificial Intelligence

The majority of VR research and clinical applications in the last few decades have focused on areas of inexpensive technology, particularly the development of a realistic 3-D area with stringent restrictions on experiential components above basic motions and modifications in the surroundings. When it comes to virtual reality, there is less of a need for interaction because the user can be progressively exposed to the fearful setting, which can help with issues like agoraphobia, claustrophobia, and more (Trahan et al., 2019).

Examples of scenarios in which this might be helpful include practicing counselling a virtual person experiencing the same problems, learning how to deal with bullies, practicing for a job interview, or expressing trauma in a cathartic way to an avatar that represents an aggressive character (Talbot et al., 2012, Rizzo et al., 2014).

When AI is employed with animated characters, it may independently diagnose serious depression on its own after a 15–20-minute interview with a high degree of sensitivity (~ 90%). It truly depends on how user-friendly, how well they engage with users, and how useful people think these AI technologies are before they are adopted by them (Sarangi & Sharma, 2018). Studying the human aspects of these interactions and learning the appropriate ways to communicate with humans through AI framework swill be important as these frameworks develop. Ethical AI usage standards are essential to protect client confidentiality, autonomy, and safety (Stratou & Morency 2017).

CONCLUSION

Virtual reality generates a virtual 3D environment that brings up new possibilities and makes treatment a pleasant experience for the patient. It provides an improved understanding of the surrounding environment. This technique can be used to treat illnesses associated with stress-associated disorders and provides numerous applications across the fields of neuroscience, psychiatry, physical and occupational therapy, and other intervention modalities. This technology development promises to be an appropriate solution for the medical industry, since it may enable situations to be fully immersed. It could reduce the length of therapy consultations. Dealing with challenging and unique patient cases is now feasible with the aid of this technology. In recent years, there has been rapid exploration of the application of this technology, leading to significant advancements. Thus, the medical industry successfully employs VR technology to achieve these goals through the delivery of effective treatment outcomes. Virtual reality appears to be an effective instrument to minimise overall treatment costs. By employing this technology, the patient reduces overall stress and focuses on the real world. Virtual motion and expertise provide experiences to the human brain (Ramasamy et al., 2022). This technology offers a more efficient and effective approach to stress management that improves patient outcomes and may even save the life of the patient.

The utilisation of VR technology in the healthcare sector is opening the door to a new phase of advancement and innovation. VR has the potential to transform patient care, medical education, and digital health experiences with its dynamic and immersive virtual environments. It provides healthcare professionals with realistic simulations and bridges the gap between theory and practice, enabling them to deliver effective and individualised care. By providing trainee healthcare professionals with practical, practical experiences in an appropriate setting, virtual reality technology has already demonstrated its value in the field of medical training and education. Ultimately, this enhances patient safety by improving their skills and decision-making processes. VR also has a significant effect on therapy and patient care, especially in the areas of pain management and mental health services. VR can help with pain relief, anxiety reduction, and mental health promotion through distraction, relaxation, and exposure therapies. The delivery of healthcare is also transforming as a result of the incorporation of VR technology in telemedicine and remote patient monitoring. Through remote examinations, virtual consultations, and real-time vital sign monitoring, patients can receive timely medical advice and diagnoses from the comfort of their own homes. This optimises patient outcomes and efficiency in addition to improving accessibility. However, to maximise VR advancements in the healthcare sector, challenges like cost, accessibility, and data security must be successfully managed. VR solutions should be accessible and affordable to healthcare organisations of all sizes. In addition, to protect patient data and ensure privacy, robust data security protocols need to be implemented. The transformational impact of VR technology is undeniably pertinent to the future of healthcare, regardless of the challenges that it poses. VR has the potential to completely transform patient care, medical education, and overall wellness as the sector continues its digital transformation. We can anticipate even more cutting-edge VR healthcare applications in the future, raising the standard for patient care globally and improving patient outcomes with continuous research and innovations. VR therapy showed promise for improvement in both patient-clinical outcomes and patient-reported experiences of individuals undergoing the surgical procedure. Future virtual reality solutions have to consider patient acceptability and implementation viability into account in acute care settings.

REFERENCES

Agus, M., Giachetti, A., Gobbetti, E., Zanetti, G., Zorcolo, A., John, N. W., & Stone, R. J. (2002). Mastoidectomy simulation with combined visual and haptic feedback. In *Medicine Meets* [IOS Press.]. *Virtual Reality (Waltham Cross)*, *02/10*, 17–23.

Bergeron, B. (2006). Developing Serious Games. Charles River Media. Inc, Hingham, MA.

Bergeron, M., Lortie, C. L., & Guitton, M. J. (2015). Use of virtual reality tools for vestibular disorders rehabilitation: A comprehensive analysis. *Advances in Medicine*, *2015*, 2015. doi:10.1155/2015/916735 PMID:26556560

Beukelman, D. R., & Mirenda, P. (2013). *Augmentative and alternative communication: Supporting children and adults with complex communication needs*. Paul H. Brookes Pub.

Bielser, D., & Gross, M. H. (2002). Open surgery simulation. In *Medicine Meets* [IOS Press.]. *Virtual Reality (Waltham Cross)*, *02/10*, 57–63.

Bielser, D., & Gross, M. H. (2002). Open surgery simulation. In *Medicine Meets* [IOS Press.]. *Virtual Reality (Waltham Cross)*, *02/10*, 57–63.

Biffi, E., Beretta, E., Cesareo, A., Maghini, C., Turconi, A. C., Reni, G., & Strazzer, S. (2017). An immersive virtual reality platform to enhance walking ability of children with acquired brain injuries. *Methods of Information in Medicine*, *56*(02), 119–126. doi:10.3414/ME16-02-0020 PMID:28116417

Bootman, J. L. (2000). To err is human. *Archives of Internal Medicine, 160*(21), 3189–3189. doi:10.1001/archinte.160.21.3189 PMID:11088077

Botella, C., Fernández-Álvarez, J., Guillén, V., García-Palacios, A., & Baños, R. (2017). Recent progress in virtual reality exposure therapy for phobias: A systematic review. *Current Psychiatry Reports, 19*(7), 1–13. doi:10.1007/s11920-017-0788-4 PMID:28540594

Buckley, C., Nugent, E., Ryan, D., & Neary, P. (2012). Virtual reality–a new era in surgical training. *Virtual reality in psychological, medical and pedagogical applications, 7*, 139-166.

Buń, P. K., Wichniarek, R., Górski, F., Grajewski, D., Zawadzki, P., & Hamrol, A. (2016). Possibilities and determinants of using low-cost devices in virtual education applications. *Eurasia Journal of Mathematics, Science and Technology Education, 13*(2), 381–394. doi:10.12973/eurasia.2017.00622a

Caglio, M., Latini-Corazzini, L., D'agata, F., Cauda, F., Sacco, K., Monteverdi, S., Zettin, M., Duca, S., & Geminiani, G. (2009). Video game play changes spatial and verbal memory: Rehabilitation of a single case with traumatic brain injury. *Cognitive Processing, 10*(S2), 195–197. doi:10.1007/s10339-009-0295-6 PMID:19693564

Caglio, M. A. R. C. E. L. L. A., Latini-Corazzini, L., D'Agata, F., Cauda, F., Sacco, K., Monteverdi, S., Zettin, M., Duca, S., & Geminiani, G. (2012). Virtual navigation for memory rehabilitation in a traumatic brain injured patient. *Neurocase, 18*(2), 123–131. doi:10.1080/13554794.2011.568499 PMID:22352998

Cano Porras, D., Siemonsma, P., Inzelberg, R., Zeilig, G., & Plotnik, M. (2018). Advantages of virtual reality in the rehabilitation of balance and gait: Systematic review. *Neurology, 90*(22), 1017–1025. doi:10.1212/WNL.0000000000005603 PMID:29720544

Chan, E., Foster, S., Sambell, R., & Leong, P. (2018). Clinical efficacy of virtual reality for acute procedural pain management: A systematic review and meta-analysis. *PLoS One, 13*(7), e0200987. doi:10.1371/journal.pone.0200987 PMID:30052655

Chen, H. (2015). Research of virtools virtual reality technology to landscape designing. *The Open Construction & Building Technology Journal, 9*(1), 164–169. doi:10.2174/1874836801509010164

Chen, Y., Fanchiang, H. D., & Howard, A. (2018). Effectiveness of virtual reality in children with cerebral palsy: A systematic review and meta-analysis of randomized controlled trials. *Physical Therapy, 98*(1), 63–77. doi:10.1093/ptj/pzx107 PMID:29088476

Chi, D. M., Clarke, J. R., Webber, B. L., & Badler, N. I. (1996). Casualty modeling for real-time medical training. *Presence (Cambridge, Mass.), 5*(4), 359–366. doi:10.1162/pres.1996.5.4.359 PMID:11539375

Chirico, A., Lucidi, F., De Laurentiis, M., Milanese, C., Napoli, A., & Giordano, A. (2016). Virtual reality in health system: Beyond entertainment. a mini-review on the efficacy of VR during cancer treatment. *Journal of Cellular Physiology, 231*(2), 275–287. doi:10.1002/jcp.25117 PMID:26238976

Cima, R. R., Kollengode, A., Garnatz, J., Storsveen, A., Weisbrod, C., & Deschamps, C. (2008). Incidence and characteristics of potential and actual retained foreign object events in surgical patients. *Journal of the American College of Surgeons, 207*(1), 80–87. doi:10.1016/j.jamcollsurg.2007.12.047 PMID:18589366

Cooper, N., Milella, F., Pinto, C., Cant, I., White, M., & Meyer, G. (2018). The effects of substitute multisensory feedback on task performance and the sense of presence in a virtual reality environment. *PLoS One*, *13*(2), e0191846. doi:10.1371/journal.pone.0191846 PMID:29390023

Custură-Crăciun, D., Cochior, D., Constantinoiu, S., & Neagu, C. (2013). Surgical virtual reality-highlights in developing a high performance surgical haptic device. *Chirurgia (Bucharest, Romania: 1990), 108*(6), 757-763.

Dascal, J., Reid, M., IsHak, W. W., Spiegel, B., Recacho, J., Rosen, B., & Danovitch, I. (2017). Virtual reality and medical inpatients: A systematic review of randomized, controlled trials. *Innovations in Clinical Neuroscience*, *14*(1-2), 14. PMID:28386517

De Luca, R., Manuli, A., De Domenico, C., Voi, E. L., Buda, A., Maresca, G., & Calabrò, R. S. (2019). Improving neuropsychiatric symptoms following stroke using virtual reality. *Case Reports in Medicine*, *98*(19). PMID:31083155

Delp, S. L., Loan, P., Basdogan, C., & Rosen, J. M. (1997). Surgical simulation: An emerging technology for training in emergency medicine. *Presence (Cambridge, Mass.)*, *6*(2), 147–159. doi:10.1162/pres.1997.6.2.147

Diemer, J., Alpers, G. W., Peperkorn, H. M., Shiban, Y., & Mühlberger, A. (2015). The impact of perception and presence on emotional reactions: A review of research in virtual reality. *Frontiers in Psychology*, *6*, 26. doi:10.3389/fpsyg.2015.00026 PMID:25688218

Doshi, R., Hiran, K. K., Gök, M., El-kenawy, E. S. M., Badr, A., & Abotaleb, M. (2023). Artificial Intelligence's Significance in Diseases with Malignant Tumours. *Mesopotamian Journal of Artificial Intelligence in Healthcare*, *2023*, 35–39.

Drewett, O., Hann, G., Gillies, M., Sher, C., Delacroix, S., Pan, X., Collingwoode-Williams, T., & Fertleman, C. (2019). A discussion of the use of virtual reality for training healthcare practitioners to recognize child protection issues. *Frontiers in Public Health*, *7*, 255. doi:10.3389/fpubh.2019.00255 PMID:31608266

Du Sert, O. P., Potvin, S., Lipp, O., Dellazizzo, L., Laurelli, M., Breton, R., Lalonde, P., Phraxayavong, K., O'Connor, K., Pelletier, J.-F., Boukhalfi, T., Renaud, P., & Dumais, A. (2018). Virtual reality therapy for refractory auditory verbal hallucinations in schizophrenia: A pilot clinical trial. *Schizophrenia Research*, *197*, 176–181. doi:10.1016/j.schres.2018.02.031 PMID:29486956

Fari, N., Yorke, E., Varnes, L., Newby, K., Potts, H. W., Smith, L., & Fisher, A. (2019). Younger Adolescents' Perceptions of Physical Activity, Exergaming, and Virtual Reality: Qualitative Intervention Study. *JMIR Serious Games*, *7*(2).

Ferraro, K., Zernzach, R., Maturo, S., Nagy, C., & Barrett, R. (2017). Chief of residents for quality improvement and patient safety: A recipe for a new role in graduate medical education. *Military Medicine*, *182*(3-4), e1747–e1751. doi:10.7205/MILMED-D-16-00179 PMID:28290953

Flores, A., Linehan, M. M., Todd, S. R., & Hoffman, H. G. (2018). The use of virtual reality to facilitate mindfulness skills training in dialectical behavioral therapy for spinal cord injury: A case study. *Frontiers in Psychology*, *9*, 531. doi:10.3389/fpsyg.2018.00531 PMID:29740365

Freeman, K. M., Thompson, S. F., Allely, E. B., Sobel, A. L., Stansfield, S. A., & Pugh, W. M. (2001). A virtual reality patient simulation system for teaching emergency response skills to US Navy medical providers. *Prehospital and Disaster Medicine, 16*(1), 3–8. doi:10.1017/S1049023X00025462 PMID:11367936

Gadelha, R. (2018). Revolutionizing Education: The promise of virtual reality. *Childhood Education, 94*(1), 40–43. doi:10.1080/00094056.2018.1420362

Gale, D. (1955). The law of supply and demand. *Mathematica Scandinavica, 3*, 155–169. doi:10.7146/math.scand.a-10436

Garavand, A., & Aslani, N. (2022). Metaverse phenomenon and its impact on health: A scoping review. *Informatics in Medicine Unlocked, 32*, 101029. doi:10.1016/j.imu.2022.101029

Gatica-Rojas, V., & Méndez-Rebolledo, G. (2014). Virtual reality interface devices in the reorganization of neural networks in the brain of patients with neurological diseases. *Neural Regeneration Research, 9*(8), 888. doi:10.4103/1673-5374.131612 PMID:25206907

Gohari, S. H., Gozali, E., & Kalhori, S. R. N. (2019). Virtual reality applications for chronic conditions management: A review. *Medical Journal of the Islamic Republic of Iran, 33*, 67. PMID:31456991

Gold, J. I., & Mahrer, N. E. (2018). Is virtual reality ready for prime time in the medical space? A randomized control trial of pediatric virtual reality for acute procedural pain management. *Journal of Pediatric Psychology, 43*(3), 266–275. doi:10.1093/jpepsy/jsx129 PMID:29053848

Graur, F. (2014). *Virtual reality in medicine–going beyond the limits. Thousand Faces Virtual Real*. InTech.

Gupta, A. K., Srinivasulu, A., Hiran, K. K., Sreenivasulu, G., Rajeyyagari, S., & Subramanyam, M. (2022). Prediction of omicron virus using combined extended convolutional and recurrent neural networks technique on CT-scan images. *Interdisciplinary Perspectives on Infectious Diseases, 2022*, 2022. doi:10.1155/2022/1525615 PMID:36562006

Haleem, A., Javaid, M., & Khan, I. H. (2020). Virtual reality (VR) applications in dentistry: An innovative technology to embrace. *Indian Journal of Dental Research, 31*(4), 666–667. doi:10.4103/ijdr.IJDR_501_19 PMID:33107476

Harden, R. M. (1999). What is a spiral curriculum? *Medical Teacher, 21*(2), 141–143. doi:10.1080/01421599979752 PMID:21275727

Hiran, K. K., & Doshi, R. (2013). An artificial neural network approach for brain tumor detection using digital image segmentation. *Brain, 2*(5), 227–231.

Hiran, K. K., & Doshi, R. (2013). Robust & secure digital image watermarking technique using concatenation process. *International Journal of ICT and Management*.

Hou, Y., Song, J., & Wang, L. (2022, October). P-2.6: Based on the status quo of virtual reality and prospects for future development. In *SID Symposium. Digest of Technical Papers, 53*(S1, No. S1), 640–642. doi:10.1002/sdtp.16049

Huygelier, H., Schraepen, B., Van Ee, R., Vanden Abeele, V., & Gillebert, C. R. (2019). Acceptance of immersive head-mounted virtual reality in older adults. *Scientific Reports, 9*(1), 4519. doi:10.1038/s41598-019-41200-6 PMID:30872760

Ismail, M. S., Hisham, I. M., Alias, M., Mahdy, Z. A., Nazimi, A. J., Ixora, K. A., Nazir, A. M., & Ismawira, M. I. M. (2022). Challenges in Embracing Virtual Reality from Healthcare Professional's Perspective: A Qualitative Study. [Universiti Kebangsaan Malaysia]. *Medicine & Health (Kuala Lumpur, Malaysia), 17*(2), 256–268. doi:10.17576/MH.2022.1702.19

Javaid, M., & Haleem, A. (2018). Additive manufacturing applications in orthopaedics: A review. *Journal of Clinical Orthopaedics and Trauma, 9*(3), 202–206. doi:10.1016/j.jcot.2018.04.008 PMID:30202149

Javaid, M., & Haleem, A. (2020). Virtual reality applications toward medical field. *Clinical Epidemiology and Global Health, 8*(2), 600–605.

Javaid, M., & Haleem, A. (2020). Virtual reality applications toward medical field. *Clinical Epidemiology and Global Health, 8*(2), 600–605. doi:10.1016/j.cegh.2019.12.010

Kaufmann, C. R. (2001, January). Computers in surgical education and the operating room. *Annales Chirurgiae et Gynaecologiae, 90*(2), 141–146. PMID:11459260

Kesawadas, T., Joshi, D., Mayrose, J., & Chugh, K. (2002). A virtual environment for esophageal intubation training. In *Medicine Meets* [IOS Press.]. *Virtual Reality (Waltham Cross), 02/10*, 221–227.

Kizil, M. S., & Joy, J. (2001). *What can virtual reality do for safety*. University of Queensland.

Krizek, T. J. (2000). Surgical error: Ethical issues of adverse events. *Archives of Surgery, 135*(11), 1359–1366. doi:10.1001/archsurg.135.11.1359 PMID:11074896

Letterie, G. S. (2002). How virtual reality may enhance training in obstetrics and gynecology. *American Journal of Obstetrics and Gynecology, 187*(3), S37–S40. doi:10.1067/mob.2002.127361 PMID:12235439

Letterie, G. S. (2002). How virtual reality may enhance training in obstetrics and gynecology. *American Journal of Obstetrics and Gynecology, 187*(3), S37–S40. doi:10.1067/mob.2002.127361 PMID:12235439

Lewis, C. (2018). The negative side effects of Virtual Reality. *Resource Magazine.*

Li, L., Yu, F., Shi, D., Shi, J., Tian, Z., Yang, J., & Jiang, Q. (2017). Application of virtual reality technology in clinical medicine. *American Journal of Translational Research, 9*(9), 3867. PMID:28979666

Li, X., Luh, D. B., Xu, R. H., & An, Y. (2023). Considering the Consequences of Cybersickness in Immersive Virtual Reality Rehabilitation: A Systematic Review and Meta-Analysis. *Applied Sciences (Basel, Switzerland), 13*(8), 5159. doi:10.3390/app13085159

Mabrey, J. D., Cannon, W. D., Gillogly, S. D., Kasser, J. R., Sweeney, H. J., Zarins, B., & Poss, R. (2000). Development of a virtual reality arthroscopic knee simulator. In *Medicine Meets* [IOS Press.]. *Virtual Reality (Waltham Cross), 2000*, 192–194.

Mantovani, F., Castelnuovo, G., Gaggioli, A., & Riva, G. (2003). Virtual reality training for healthcare professionals. *Cyberpsychology & Behavior, 6*(4), 389–395. doi:10.1089/109493103322278772 PMID:14511451

Maples-Keller, J. L., Bunnell, B. E., Kim, S. J., & Rothbaum, B. O. (2017). The use of virtual reality technology in the treatment of anxiety and other psychiatric disorders. *Harvard Review of Psychiatry*, *25*(3), 103–113. doi:10.1097/HRP.0000000000000138 PMID:28475502

Marco, J. H., Perpiñá, C., & Botella, C. (2013). Effectiveness of cognitive behavioral therapy supported by virtual reality in the treatment of body image in eating disorders: One year follow-up. *Psychiatry Research*, *209*(3), 619–625. doi:10.1016/j.psychres.2013.02.023 PMID:23499231

Mazurek, J., Kiper, P., Cieślik, B., Rutkowski, S., Mehlich, K., Turolla, A., & Szczepańska-Gieracha, J. (2019). Virtual reality in medicine: A brief overview and future research directions. *Human Movement*, *20*(3), 16–22. doi:10.5114/hm.2019.83529

McIntosh, K. S., Gregor, J. C., & Khanna, N. V. (2014). Computer-based virtual reality colonoscopy simulation improves patient-based colonoscopy performance. *Canadian Journal of Gastroenterology & Hepatology*, *28*(4), 203–206. doi:10.1155/2014/804367 PMID:24729994

Michael, D. R., & Chen, S. L. (2005). *Serious games: Games that educate, train, and inform*. Muska & Lipman/Premier-Trade.

Morvan, L. (2019). Waking up to a new reality. *Accenture*.

Norouzi, N., Bölling, L., Bruder, G., & Welch, G. (2019). Augmented rotations in virtual reality for users with a reduced range of head movement. *Journal of Rehabilitation and Assistive Technologies Engineering*, *6*, 2055668319841309. doi:10.1177/2055668319841309 PMID:31245034

O'Connor, T. J., Cooper, R. A., Fitzgerald, S. G., Dvorznak, M. J., Boninger, M. L., VanSickle, D. P., & Glass, L. (2000). Evaluation of a manual wheelchair interface to computer games. *Neurorehabilitation and Neural Repair*, *14*(1), 21–31. doi:10.1177/154596830001400103 PMID:11228946

Pan, X., & Hamilton, A. F. D. C. (2018). Why and how to use virtual reality to study human social interaction: The challenges of exploring a new research landscape. *British Journal of Psychology*, *109*(3), 395–417. doi:10.1111/bjop.12290 PMID:29504117

Pareek, T. G., Mehta, U., & Gupta, A. (2018). A survey: Virtual reality model for medical diagnosis. *Biomedical & Pharmacology Journal*, *11*(4), 2091–2100. doi:10.13005/bpj/1588

Park, M. J., Kim, D. J., Lee, U., Na, E. J., & Jeon, H. J. (2019). A literature overview of virtual reality (VR) in treatment of psychiatric disorders: Recent advances and limitations. *Frontiers in Psychiatry*, *10*, 505. doi:10.3389/fpsyt.2019.00505 PMID:31379623

Parsons, T. D., Gaggioli, A., & Riva, G. (2017). Virtual reality for research in social neuroscience. *Brain Sciences*, *7*(4), 42. doi:10.3390/brainsci7040042 PMID:28420150

Peeters, D. (2019). Virtual reality: A game-changing method for the language sciences. *Psychonomic Bulletin & Review*, *26*(3), 894–900. doi:10.3758/s13423-019-01571-3 PMID:30734158

Petrigna, L., & Musumeci, G. (2022). The metaverse: A new challenge for the healthcare system: A scoping review. *Journal of Functional Morphology and Kinesiology*, *7*(3), 63. doi:10.3390/jfmk7030063 PMID:36135421

Pizzoli, S. F. M., Mazzocco, K., Triberti, S., Monzani, D., Alcañiz Raya, M. L., & Pravettoni, G. (2019). User-centered virtual reality for promoting relaxation: An innovative approach. *Frontiers in Psychology*, *10*, 479. doi:10.3389/fpsyg.2019.00479 PMID:30914996

Portman, M. E., Natapov, A., & Fisher-Gewirtzman, D. (2015). To go where no man has gone before: Virtual reality in architecture, landscape architecture and environmental planning. *Computers, Environment and Urban Systems*, *54*, 376–384.

Qin, J., Chui, Y. P., Pang, W. M., Choi, K. S., & Heng, P. A. (2009). Learning blood management in orthopedic surgery through gameplay. *IEEE Computer Graphics and Applications*, *30*(2), 45–57. PMID:20650710

Ramasamy, J., Doshi, R., & Hiran, K. K. (2022, October). Detection of Brain Tumor in Medical Images Based on Feature Extraction by HOG and Machine Learning Algorithms. In *2022 International Conference on Trends in Quantum Computing and Emerging Business Technologies* (TQCEBT) (pp. 1-5). IEEE. 10.1109/TQCEBT54229.2022.10041564

Reason, J. (2000). Human error: Models and management. *BMJ (Clinical Research Ed.)*, *320*(7237), 768–770. doi:10.1136/bmj.320.7237.768 PMID:10720363

Riva, G. (2011). The key to unlocking the virtual body: Virtual reality in the treatment of obesity and eating disorders. *Journal of Diabetes Science and Technology*, *5*(2), 283–292. doi:10.1177/193229681100500213 PMID:21527095

Rizzo, A. A., Hartholt, A., Rothbaum, B. O., Difede, J., Reist, C., Kwok, D., . . . Buckwalter, J. G. (2014, January). Expansion of a VR Exposure Therapy System for Combat-Related PTSD to Medics/Corpsman and Persons Following Military Sexual Trauma. In MMVR (pp. 332-338).

Robb, R. A. (1997). Virtual endoscopy: evaluation using the visible human datasets and comparison with real endoscopy in patients. In *Medicine Meets Virtual Reality* (pp. 195–206). IOS Press.

Rodziewicz, T. L., Houseman, B., & Hipskind, J. E. (2018). *Medical error reduction and prevention*.

Rothbaum, B. O., Rizzo, A. S., & Difede, J. (2010). Virtual reality exposure therapy for combat-related posttraumatic stress disorder. *Annals of the New York Academy of Sciences*, *1208*(1), 126–132. doi:10.1111/j.1749-6632.2010.05691.x PMID:20955334

Sarangi, S., & Sharma, P. (2018). *Artificial intelligence: evolution, ethics and public policy*. Taylor & Francis. doi:10.4324/9780429461002

Satava, R. M., & Jones, S. B. (1997). Virtual environments for medical training and education. *Presence (Cambridge, Mass.)*, *6*(2), 139–146. doi:10.1162/pres.1997.6.2.139

Shao, D., & Lee, I. J. (2020). Acceptance and influencing factors of social virtual reality in the urban elderly. *Sustainability (Basel)*, *12*(22), 9345. doi:10.3390/su12229345

Small, S. D., Wuerz, R. C., Simon, R., Shapiro, N., Conn, A., & Setnik, G. (1999). Demonstration of high-fidelity simulation team training for emergency medicine. *Academic Emergency Medicine*, *6*(4), 312–323. doi:10.1111/j.1553-2712.1999.tb00395.x PMID:10230983

Srinivasulu, A., Gupta, A. K., Hiran, K. K., Barua, T., & Sreenivasulu, G. (2022). Omi-cron Virus Data Analytics Using Extended RNN Technique. *Int J Cancer Res Ther*, *7*(3), 1-3.

Stratou, G., & Morency, L. P. (2017). MultiSense—Context-aware nonverbal behavior analysis framework: A psychological distress use case. *IEEE Transactions on Affective Computing*, *8*(2), 190–203.

Stytz, M. R., Garcia, B. W., Godsell-Stytz, G. M., & Banks, S. B. (1997). A distributed virtual environment prototype for emergency medical procedures training. In *Medicine Meets Virtual Reality* (pp. 473–485). IOS Press.

Talbot, T. B., Sagae, K., John, B., & Rizzo, A. A. (2012). Sorting out the virtual patient: How to exploit artificial intelligence, game technology and sound educational practices to create engaging role-playing simulations. [IJGCMS]. *International Journal of Gaming and Computer-Mediated Simulations*, *4*(3), 1–19.

Trahan, M. H., Smith, K. S., & Talbot, T. B. (2019). Past, present, and future: Editorial on virtual reality applications to human services. *Journal of Technology in Human Services*, *37*(1), 1–12. doi:10.1080/1 5228835.2019.1587334

Tsai, M. D., Hsieh, M. S., & Jou, S. B. (2001). Virtual reality orthopedic surgery simulator. *Computers in Biology and Medicine*, *31*(5), 333–351. doi:10.1016/S0010-4825(01)00014-2 PMID:11535200

Valmaggia, L. R., Latif, L., Kempton, M. J., & Rus-Calafell, M. (2016). Virtual reality in the psychological treatment for mental health problems: An systematic review of recent evidence. *Psychiatry Research*, *236*, 189–195. doi:10.1016/j.psychres.2016.01.015 PMID:26795129

Van De Ridder, J. M., Stokking, K. M., McGaghie, W. C., & Ten Cate, O. T. J. (2008). What is feedback in clinical education? *Medical Education*, *42*(2), 189–197. doi:10.1111/j.1365-2923.2007.02973.x PMID:18230092

Ventola, C. L. (2019). Virtual reality in pharmacy: Opportunities for clinical, research, and educational applications. *P&T*, *44*(5), 267. PMID:31080335

Wang, S., Lim, S. H., & Aloweni, F. B. A. B. (2022). Virtual reality interventions and the outcome measures of adult patients in acute care settings undergoing surgical procedures: An integrative review. *Journal of Advanced Nursing*, *78*(3), 645–665.

Wang, S., Lim, S. H., & Aloweni, F. B. A. B. (2022). Virtual reality interventions and the outcome measures of adult patients in acute care settings undergoing surgical procedures: An integrative review. *Journal of Advanced Nursing*, *78*(3), 645–665. doi:10.1111/jan.15065 PMID:34633112

Yang, J. O., & Lee, J. S. (2021). Utilization exercise rehabilitation using metaverse (vr· ar· mr· xr). *Korean Journal of Sport Biomechanics*, *31*(4), 249–258.

Yaqi, M. (2022). Designing Visual Communications Virtual Reality matters in healthcare industry. *Journal of Commercial Biotechnology*, *27*(4).

Yildirim, G., Elban, M., & Yildirim, S. (2018). Analysis of use of virtual reality technologies in history education: A case study. *Asian Journal of Education and Training*, *4*(2), 62–69. doi:10.20448/ journal.522.2018.42.62.69

Zhang, J. F., Paciorkowski, A. R., Craig, P. A., & Cui, F. (2019). BioVR: A platform for virtual reality assisted biological data integration and visualization. *BMC Bioinformatics*, *20*(1), 1–10. doi:10.1186/s12859-019-2666-z PMID:30767777

Chapter 3
Integration of Biomedical Engineering in Augmented Reality and Virtual Reality Applications

Jaya Rubi
 https://orcid.org/0000-0001-6988-149X
Vels Institute of Science Technology and Advanced Studies, India

A. Vijayalakshmi
 https://orcid.org/0000-0003-3594-6691
Vels institute of Science Technology and advanced Studies, India

Shivani Venkatesan
 https://orcid.org/0009-0008-3140-3415
Vels Institute of Science Technology and Advanced Studies, India

ABSTRACT

This book chapter delves into the profound synergy between Biomedical Engineering and the burgeoning realm of augmented reality (AR) and virtual reality (VR) applications. Through a meticulous examination of state-of-the-art advancements and a forward-looking analysis of future prospects, this chapter endeavors to offer a comprehensive resource for a diverse audience, including dedicated researchers, seasoned healthcare practitioners, discerning educators, and aspiring students. The integration of these technologies has the potential to revolutionize medical training, patient education, surgical planning, and therapy delivery, ushering in an era of more personalized and effective healthcare solutions. This chapter serves as a guiding beacon in navigating this transformative landscape, ensuring that the adoption of AR/VR technologies is not only innovative but also ethically grounded and attuned to the highest standards of patient care.

DOI: 10.4018/979-8-3693-1123-3.ch003

INTRODUCTION

Recent technological developments have led to new changes in health care, changing treatments, and improving patient care. Augmented reality (AR) and virtual reality (VR) are revolutionary technologies that are getting a lot of attention. Today's technologies hold great promise in many industries, and their combination with biomedical engineering is leading to a paradigm shift in healthcare. Combining biomedical engineering skills with the great potential of AR and VR, doctors can now explore new areas in medical education, patient care, diagnosis, and rehabilitation (Pourmand et al., 2017).

Biomedical Engineering is located at the intersection of engineering and medicine and includes disciplines such as diagnostics, biosensors, medical devices, biomechanics, and more. Its main goal is to produce innovative solutions to complex problems in the healthcare industry. With the advent of AR and VR, the potential applications of biomedical engineering have greatly expanded and ushered in a new era of health awareness.

Medical education and training have traditionally been based on textbooks, lectures, and practical experience (Mishra et al., 2022). However, these methods often have limitations in replicating real-world situations and complex medical procedures. AR and VR streamline the transformation process by providing immersive and interactive experiences.AR and VR technology change the rules of the game in medical vision and diagnosis. By combining skills in biomedical engineering with AR/VR interfaces, medical imaging technology has reached a new level of accuracy and interactivity. Advanced visualization tools enable physicians to interpret complex medical data to provide more accurate diagnoses and personalized treatment plans.

In addition, real-time biosensors integrated into AR/VR applications can provide continuous health monitoring and enable patients to take an active role in managing their own health. Physical therapy and physical therapy have also made significant advances thanks to the integration of AR and VR technology. Biomedical engineering principles play a role in designing interactive and engaging exercises for patients undergoing rehabilitation. AR/VR services facilitate engagement, engagement, and advancement, ultimately leading to better and more effective treatments (Letterie, 2002).

The AR/VR revolution did not neglect mental health and wellness. Biomedical engineering expertise helps create an immersive environment for the treatment of mental disorders, anxiety, and phobias. Patients can achieve better results by confronting their fears in a controlled virtual environment. In addition, AR/VR apps provide relaxation exercises, mindfulness, and stress relief techniques to support mental health in a digitally connected world.

The integration of AR and VR into healthcare is problematic as technology evolves rapidly. Ensuring the security of personal data, addressing user security concerns and promoting customer acceptance are key areas of focus. Accountability and ethics are crucial to harnessing the potential of this technology while prioritizing patient safety and health (McCradden et al., 2020).

Against this background, this section of the book aims to explore the integration of AR and VR applications into biomedical engineering and healthcare. By analyzing recent developments, contracts, challenges, and future prospects, we hope to see the impact of changes in this hand on the stock. Through this analysis, we aim to help understand the potential of AR and VR to transform healthcare, improve patient outcomes and pave the way for better health, drinking cleaner, and connecting with the future.

Role of Biomedical Engineering in Healthcare Industry

Biomedical engineering has influenced healthcare culture, leading to new innovations that transform nursing, medical research, and medicine. This interactive course uses architectural models and techniques to solve problems in medicine and biology and their implications for clinical practice. In this narrative, we explore the many ways biomedical engineering creates and improves health (Nanthakumar and Sivakumaran, 2018).

1. Medical Research and Treatment

Biomedical engineering has played an important role in the development of medical imaging such as magnetic resonance imaging (MRI), computed tomography (CT), positron emission tomography (PET), and ultrasound.

These tests provide a detailed and non-invasive view of body structure, facilitating early detection, diagnosis and monitoring of diseases. With continuous research and development, medical imaging has become clearer, faster and safer, allowing doctors to make accurate diagnoses and develop treatment plans.

2. Prosthetic and Assistive Devices

Biomedical Engineering has made significant advances in the design and manufacture of prosthetic and assistive devices. Thanks to the integration of new materials, sensors and robots, prostheses have become more functional, wearable and functional.

Lost patients can now regain strength and independence, and some advanced artificial intelligence can exercise physical control through brain-computer interfaces (BCI). In addition, assistive devices such as hearing aids and vision aids are very effective and improve the quality of life of people with intellectual disabilities.

3. Medical devices and equipment

Biomedical Engineering drives innovation in a variety of medical devices and equipment used in diagnosis, treatment and patient care. Examples include infusion pumps, defibrillators, pacemakers, and cardiac stents, among others.

This device is designed to be safe, effective and precise, helping to improve patient outcomes and reduce the risk of complications during the treatment process.

4. Regenerative medicine and tissue engineering

Regenerative medicine is a branch of biomedical engineering that focuses on the repair and regeneration of damaged tissues and organs. In the process of tissue engineering, scientists create organs, blood vessels, and tissues that can replace the need for transplants and reduce the number of organs. This area of research holds great promise for personalized medicine, as tissues and organs created with the patient's brain can reduce the risk of rejection and increase transplant success.

5. Drug Delivery and Nanomedicine

Biomedical Engineering contributes to the development of new drug delivery systems, especially in the nanomedicine industry. Nanoparticles and nanocarriers can be designed to deliver drugs directly to cells or tissues, increasing drug efficacy while reducing side effects. These drug delivery plans have the potential for better treatment and improved patient compliance.

6. Telemedicine and Health Technology

Advances in biomedical engineering and health technology have led to recent advances in telemedicine. Telemedicine platforms allow patients to talk to doctors remotely, facilitating access to medical advice and reducing the burden on hospitals. In addition, wearable devices and remote monitoring systems can enable individuals to take control of their health by enabling continuous health monitoring (Rubi et al., 2023).

7. Data analytics and artificial intelligence

Biomedical engineering uses data analytics and artificial intelligence (AI) to process large volumes of medical data to enable better disease prediction, patient risk stratification, and treatment optimization.

Artificial intelligence algorithms analyze patient data, medical images, and genetic data to identify patterns and patterns that help doctors make informed decisions and improve patient outcomes.

8. Surgical Innovation and Robotics

Biomedical Engineering contributes to surgical innovation and the development of robot-assisted surgery. Advanced diagnostics and minimally invasive techniques led by robotics reduce surgical complications, shorten recovery time, and increase patient satisfaction. Surgical robots are more efficient, stable and flexible, making complex surgeries easier and more successful.

9. Health Information Systems

Biomedical Engineering has played an important role in the development and implementation of medical records, electronic health records (EHR), and medical information management systems (Li et al., 2020). This system simplifies clinical work, improves communication between physicians, and increases accessibility to patient information, leading to better collaboration and increasing patient safety.

In conclusion, biomedical engineering has had a profound impact on culture, providing new and technological advances in many areas of medicine. From screening and diagnostics to regenerative medicine, drug delivery, and telemedicine, this partnership continues to shape the future of healthcare by delivering better treatments, better patient outcomes, and improving the quality of life for people around the world. As technology and science continue to advance, the potential for biomedical engineering to benefit healthcare remains unlimited. The field of biomedical engineering continues to witness significant advances and cutting-edge research. Here are some insights into some professional research areas in biomedical engineering:

Neural Engineering and Brain-Computer Interfaces (BCI)

Researchers are actively investigating the development of advanced BBAs that can communicate directly between the human brain and external devices. These brain-computer interfaces hold great promise in helping people with mobility impairments by allowing them to use their senses to control joints, limbs, and other assistive devices.

Tissue Engineering and Regenerative Medicine

Advances in tissue engineering and regenerative medicine have paved the way for the development of stem cells, tissues, and biomaterials. Scientists are working to create functional organs in the lab using 3D bioprinting and stem cell research that can be transplanted and make up for a shortage of donor organs.

Artificial Intelligence and Machine Learning in Healthcare

The integration of AI and machine learning algorithms is changing all aspects of healthcare, including diagnostics, drug discovery, and personalized medicine. AI-powered systems can analyze large volumes of medical data and assist with early disease detection, optimal treatment, and treatment decisions (Vaishya et al., 2020).

Wearable Medical Devices and Sensors

Advances in technology and biosensors have led to the development of new medical devices for continuous health monitoring. The wearable monitors vital signs, blood sugar levels, water and other body metrics, providing users and doctors with health information.

Nanomedicine and Drug Delivery

Nanotechnology has been widely studied for its potential in drug delivery and precision medicine. Nanoparticles and nanocarriers can deliver therapeutic drugs directly to cells or tissues, reducing side effects and improving treatment.

Biomedical Imaging and Visualization

Innovations in medical imaging modalities such as MRI, CT, PET, and ultrasound are improving diagnosis. Researchers are working to develop new differential agents, imaging techniques, and AI-driven image analysis tools to improve early disease detection and treatment planning.

Gene Editing and Gene Therapy: Gene editing technologies such asCRISPR-Cas9 are opening up new possibilities for the treatment of hereditary diseases and inherited diseases. Scientists are exploring the potential of gene therapy to repair faulty genes and correct genetic diseases at the molecular level (Barrangou and May, 2015).

Biomechanics and Rehabilitation Engineering

Research in biomechanics focuses on understanding the mechanics of the human body to design aesthetic devices, orthoses, and medical devices. These advances are designed to improve mobility, improve performance, and provide a better quality of life for people with physical disabilities.

Bedside Diagnosis and Telemedicine: Advances in bedside diagnostic devices provide fast, accurate diagnosis at the patient's bedside or remote locations. In addition, technology has facilitated communication in remote areas and improved access to healthcare, especially in underserved areas.

Augmented Reality

Augmented reality (AR) is a technology that brings digital information or virtual content to the real-world environment, thereby improving the user's perception of reality. Unlike virtual reality (VR), which creates a purely virtual environment, AR places digital content above the physical world, allowing users to interact with real and virtual content simultaneously. AR is often experienced on a variety of devices such as smartphones, tablets, smart glasses, and headphones, making it useful for a variety of applications (Liono et al., 2021). Here are some applications of augmented reality in healthcare:

1. Medical education and training: AR enables medical students and doctors to participate in realistic experiments and interactive learning. Medical training provides physical models, surgical simulations, and teaching techniques, allowing users to practice complex medical procedures and hone their skills in a risk-free environment.
2. Surgical Navigation: The AR-assisted surgical navigation system places real-time images and patient information in the surgeon's field of view during surgery. This helps surgeons see important anatomical structures, surgical targets, and tumors, making surgery more efficient and effective.
3. Diagnostic and medical visualization: AR enhances medical visualization by presenting diagnostic images (such as CT or MRI scans) of the patient's body during surgery or interventions. The machine makes it easy to understand the location and helps doctors make decisions.
4. Patient Education and Engagement: AR apps can educate patients about their condition, treatment options, and post-operative care. By viewing medical information in an interactive and accessible way, patients can better understand their health and participate in care (Higgins, Larson, and Schnall, 2017).
5. Treatment of Phobias and Anxiety: AR-based therapy can help people confront and manage phobias and anxiety. In a controlled virtual environment, patients can face their fears, become increasingly desensitized and contribute to the improvement of treatment.
6. Rehabilitation and Physical Therapy: AR apps provide interactive and rehabilitation programs to support patients during their recovery. These interventions promote adherence to treatment and improve overall recovery outcomes.
7. Medical equipment and care training: AR helps train doctors in the use and care of medical equipment and supplies. By placing instructions and visual aids in the system, users can learn and solve problems effectively.
8. Teleconferencing: AR helps improve healthcare by enabling remote communication between doctors and patients. Doctors can effectively diagnose patients, view medical records, and provide real-time medical advice, reducing the need for face-to-face visits.

9. Preoperative Planning: AR allows surgeons to make preoperative planning by viewing the patient's anatomy and the outcome of the surgery in 3D. This will help to better understand complex problems and develop appropriate surgical strategies.

10. Health and wellness monitoring: AR-supported wearables can display health-related information such as vital signs and consumption metrics directly based on user time. This makes it easy for people to keep track of their health and well-being (Mishra et al., 2020).

The use of AR in healthcare continues to expand as technology evolves and researchers explore new possibilities. Augmented reality holds great promise for improving healthcare, patient outcomes, and medical education, ultimately helping to improve healthcare delivery and personalized care everywhere.

Virtual Reality

Virtual reality (VR) is a technology that creates a computer-generated three-dimensional (3D) environment in which users can interact and explore as if they were physically in that virtual world. VR often uses head-mounted displays and tracking devices to engage people in a simulated environment to provide a realistic interactive experience. Unlike augmented reality (AR), which places virtual elements above the real world, VR replaces the user's physical environment with a completely computer-generated one (Jain and Hiran, 2024).

Virtual reality in healthcare has emerged as a powerful tool with many applications to improve clinical education, patient care, treatment, and research. Here are some important uses of virtual reality in healthcare:

1. Clinical training and simulations: Virtual reality provides realistic simulations for medical students and doctors. It allows surgeons to hone their skills without putting real patients at risk by performing complex procedures in a safe and controlled virtual environment. VR simulations are also used to train emergency medical personnel and improve their planning and decision-making.

2. Medical Management: VR is used as a medical intervention to patients who are sick during treatment or treatment. By engaging patients with positive and meaningful experiences such as virtual environments or games, VR can reduce pain and stress and provide better treatment outcomes.

3. Physical Therapy: Using virtual reality in physical therapy and rehabilitation to make exercises more effective and motivating for patients. VR-based rehabilitation encourages patients to repeat exercises with pleasure, resulting in better performance and recovery.

4. Treatment: VR is used in therapy for people with phobias, post-traumatic stress disorder (PTSD), and anxiety. By allowing patients to experience and manage stress in a safe environment, clinicians can create controlled virtual situations that gently expose patients to fear.

5. Patient Education: VR facilitates patient education by providing interactive information about medical imaging, treatment options, and surgical procedures. Patients can better understand medical information, improve their knowledge of their own health, and intervene.

6. Surgical planning and visualization: Virtual reality helps surgeons pre-plan by seeing the patient's unique anatomy in 3D. This detailed view helps develop effective surgical strategies and improve patient outcomes (Ujiie et al., 2021; Doshi and Hiran, 2023).

7. Post-Traumatic Stress Disorder (PTSD) Therapy: VR treats PTSD sufferers by recreating traumatic events in a virtual environment.Under the guidance of a doctor, patients can revisit symptoms to help them process and resolve their emotions.

8. Cognitive rehabilitation: VR-based cognitive rehabilitation programs are used to assist people with brain damage or intellectual disability. These services support cognitive recovery and independence by focusing on memory, maintenance, and function.

9. Medical research: Virtual reality is used in medical research to explore human behavior, knowledge, and understanding. VR provides a controlled experimental environment that allows scientists to more accurately examine various situations and events.

10. Pain assessment and biofeedback: VR with biofeedback technology can measure the patient's pain and stress. By monitoring physical activity in real time, doctors can tailor pain management to the patient.

The adoption of virtual reality in healthcare is growing, with research and innovation expanding its applications. As technology and virtual reality become more accessible, the potential to transform leadership, patient care, and healthcare becomes more and more apparent (Goel et al., 2023).

Role of Biomedical in AR and VR

The role of biomedical engineering in augmented reality (AR) and virtual reality (VR) can help improve treatment and patient outcomes. Experience in biomedical engineering helps integrate AR and VR technology into medical education, patient care, diagnosis and therapy. AR and VR simulations in medical education provide immersive and interactive learning experiences that allow medical students and physicians to practice complex procedures and cook their skills in a safe and controlled environment. Use the principles of biomedical engineering to create realistic anatomical models and surgical simulations and provide valuable training to dedicated surgeons. AR and VR applications in patient care improve visualization and diagnosis by projecting medical images onto the patient's body during procedures and interventions.

This real-time image increases spatial awareness, guiding the surgeon to make precise decisions during the operation. In addition, AR and VR technologies facilitate patient education, visualize clinical and treatment interactions, and facilitate greater patient understanding and engagement. In addition, in rehabilitation and treatment, biomedical engineering plays an important role in the creation of interactive and gamification interventions to encourage patients to participate in the healing process. The combination of biomedical engineering and AR/VR technology is paving the way for new medical treatments that change practice and ultimately improve patient quality (Riener and Harders, 2012).

Biomedical engineering plays an important role in enabling the successful integration of AR and VR technology into all aspects of healthcare, helping to improve medical education, patient care, diagnosis, and treatment.

Medical Education:AR and VR simulations provide immersive and interactive learning experiences that provide medical students and clinicians with a safe environment to perform complex procedures and hone their skills. Biomedical engineering skills are essential to creating realistic anatomical models, surgical simulations and diagnostics, providing accurate and efficient training. These simulations allow students to gain hands-on experience and confidence before working on real patients, ultimately improving the quality of medical education.

Nursing: Biomedical Engineering advances nursing with AR and VR applications that improve visualization and diagnosis. Augmented reality places medical information on the patient's body during procedures and interventions, allowing surgeons to better visualize anatomical structures and surgical plans in real time (Srinivasulu et al., 2022). Biomedical engineering professionals work to create clear labels and visual strategies to ensure the relationship between virtual data and the real world. This better understanding of the environment can guide surgeons to make better decisions, reduce risk, and improve the outcome of surgery (Kim et al., 2011).

Patient Education: AR and VR technologies provide valuable tools for patient education. Biomedical engineering professionals create interactive visualizations of diseases, treatments, and surgical procedures that make medical information more complex and understandable for patients. Patients can interact with 3D models to explore their bodies and understand their health and potential effects. This allows patients to make informed decisions about their treatment and to be partners in their treatment.

Rehabilitation and Therapy: Biomedical engineering expertise contributes to the development of AR and VR interactive exercises and gamification interventions for rehabilitation and therapy. These practices encourage patients to participate in the healing process, improve recovery, and work effectively. Biomedical engineers collaborate with doctors to create personalized treatments that fit a patient's needs and goals.

Medical Research and Innovation: In medical research, biomedical engineering plays an important role in exploring the potential of AR and VR technology to advance medical knowledge and innovation. Researchers are using this technology to study human behavior, cognition and perception in controlled laboratories. Biomedical engineering professionals facilitate the development of experimental protocols and data analysis methods that influence discoveries and advances in medicine.

Collaboration between biomedical engineering and AR/VR technology is changing healthcare and enabling new solutions for medical education, patient care and treatment. As these technologies continue to evolve, biomedical engineering professionals will continue to be at the forefront of driving innovation in the healthcare industry, ultimately benefiting both patients and doctors (Mylrea and Siverston, 1975).

Challenges of Using AR and VR in Healthcare

While augmented reality (AR) and virtual reality (VR) have many advantages and changes in healthcare, they also have some disadvantages and challenges. Some of the disadvantages of using AR and VR in healthcare are:

1. Cost and availability: Using AR and VR technology in healthcare can be expensive, especially for small clinics or facilities with limited resources. The cost of high-quality VR equipment, AR equipment, and required infrastructure will affect their widespread adoption. In addition, ensuring accessibility for all patients, including the disabled or elderly, can be problematic.
2. Application limitations: AR and VR technologies are developing rapidly, but still have some limitations. VR can cause pain, dizziness or eye strain for some users, especially when used for long periods of time. Latency or latency issues can disrupt the experience in AR apps and affect real-time interactions.
3. Education and Learning Curve: Integrating AR and VR into clinical training and clinical operations will require specific training for clinicians and staff. Learning how to manipulate and interpret data from AR and VR systems can take a long time, and some users may find it difficult to adapt to this new technology.

4. Data privacy and security: AR and VR applications in healthcare often involve the handling and storage of sensitive patient information, including medical images and documents, and personal medical records. Securing personal information and security measures to protect patient privacy and comply with regulations is important but can be difficult.

5. Lack of design: AR and VR medical facilities are still young and lack good modelling of hardware, software and development content. Collaboration issues between different devices and platforms can hinder integration with existing healthcare systems.

6. Ethical considerations: The use of AR and VR in healthcare raises ethical concerns, particularly in areas such as virtual therapy and patient consent. It is important to ensure that patients are fully aware of the consequences and potential risks of using technology in their care

7. Over-reliance on technology: While AR and VR can improve clinical education and training, there is a risk of over-reliance on technology that ignores the importance of hands-on work and traditional teaching methods (Fahim et al., 2022).

8. Bias and Representation: AR and VR content may contain biases or inaccuracies that affect the representation of certain demographic or medical conditions.

Making sure the content created is inclusive and relevant is important to avoid encouraging false ideas or information. Despite these disadvantages, continued research and advancement in AR and VR technologies, with a better understanding of their applications and limitations, can help solve these problems and unlock the full potential of these technologies in healthcare. It is important to carefully consider the balance of pros and cons for the role and effective integration of AR and VR in healthcare.

Future Applications of AR and VR in Healthcare

As immersive technologies continue to evolve and become more integrated into medical practice, future applications of augmented reality (AR) and virtual reality (VR) in healthcare are promising. Here are some promising futures for AR and VR in healthcare:

1. Surgical planning and guidance: AR and VR could revolutionize surgical planning by providing real-time, patient-specific 3D images of the body during surgery. Surgeons can use AR layers to improve the perception of space and accuracy during surgery, improve the outcome of surgery, and reduce risk (Volonté et al., 2011; Nankani et al., 2022).

2. Telesurgery and Telemedicine: Advances in AR and VR could lead to telesurgery, where surgeons operate remotely using robotic systems guided by real-time AR vision. This development could expand access to surgical specialists in underserved and emergency areas this will improve the telehealth experience and provide a more collaborative and personalized approach to telehealth services.

3. Personalized medicine and treatment planning: AR and VR can support personalized medicine by combining patient-specific information such as genetic information and medical history. Doctors can see how different treatments will affect the patient's anatomy and physiology, allowing for better treatment planning.

4. Virtual Rehabilitation and Therapy: AR and VR-based treatments are more effective and customizable, allowing patients to tailor treatment to their needs and development. These interventions can facilitate recovery and engage patients

5. Medical Education and Teaching: AR and VR promise to revolutionize medical education and training by providing practical and realistic experiences for medical students and physicians. Future applications may include collaborative virtual learning, which allows students to interact with and learn from international experts.

6. VR-Based Mental Health Interventions: VR can play an important role in mental health interventions by providing a comfortable environment for clinical and cognitive behavioural interventions. Virtual reality can be customized to each patient's needs and supports the treatment of anxiety, PTSD, phobias and more.

7. Telemedicine support and care: AR and VR can be used to provide telemedicine services and home care for sick or recovering patients. Virtual assistants and remote monitoring tools can provide real-time feedback and assistance, improving patient compliance and clinical outcomes (Pereira et al., 2020; Gupta et al., 2022).

8. AR-enabled diagnostics and diagnostics: AR overlays can improve the interpretation of medical images by presenting diagnostic information directly to the patient during the examination. Radiologists and clinicians can benefit from increased knowledge and improved decision-making.

9. Augmented reality health apps: As smartphones and wearables become more accessible to AR technology, health-focused AR apps may become popular (Rubi and Dhivya, 2022).

These apps can provide personal health information, exercise guidance, nutritional recommendations, and real-time health services through an AR interface. Although many future applications are still in the early stages of development, continued research and technological advances in AR and VR are paving the way for richer, patient-centered experiences in healthcare. As these technologies continue to evolve and shape the future of healthcare, ethical considerations, patient safety, data privacy, and regulatory compliance will be critical issues to address.

CONCLUSION

In conclusion, the integration of biomedical engineering with augmented reality (AR) and virtual reality (VR) applications has great potential to transform clinical practice and improve patient outcomes. Today's interactive applications reflect the development of this technology in every aspect of healthcare. Biomedical engineering has played an important role in advancing the use of AR and VR in medical education and training. The creation of realistic anatomical models, surgical simulations, and interactive learning enable medical students and physicians to hone their skills in a safe and controlled environment. In addition, AR and VR provide new solutions for patient care, superimposing medical data in real-time, and helping surgeons make clear decisions during surgeries and interventions, thereby improving the outcome of surgery. The potential for patient education is also clear, as AR and VR technology provide interactive visuals that make complex medical information accessible and understandable. Patients can participate in their health and treatment choices, resulting in more informed decisions and greater patient involvement in care. The impact of AR and VR extends to rehabilitation and therapy, where personal intervention and exercise can increase patient motivation and improve recovery outcomes. This technology will play an important role in the treatment of mental disorders with a positive environment that supports clinical and cognitive behavior. Looking ahead, AR and VR have the potential to support collaboration in telemedicine, personalized medicine, and virtual education, facilitating access to specialist doctors and medical care for patients around the world (Rubi, Hemalatha, and Janney, 2023). As with any change, challenges must be faced. Issues such as cost, regulatory constraints, data privacy, and ethical considerations need to be carefully considered to ensure the responsible and ethical use of AR and VR in therapy. As a result, the integration of biomedical engineering with AR and VR applications is at the forefront of medical advancement, nursing, and medical education. With continuous research and technological development, these technologies are poised to become the future of healthcare, delivering new personal, interactive, and patient-centered information that has the potential to transform the healthcare environment for the better. By striking the balance between innovation and responsible use, the integration of biomedical engineering with AR and VR will lead to positive change in healthcare, ultimately benefiting patients, physicians, and the medical community as a whole.

REFERENCES

Barrangou, R., & May, A. (2015). Unraveling the potential of CRISPR-Cas9 for gene therapy. *Expert Opinion on Biological Therapy*, *15*(3), 311–314. doi:10.1517/14712598.2015.994501 PMID:25535790

Doshi, R., & Hiran, K. K. (2023). Decision Making and IoT: Bibliometric Analysis for Scopus Database. *Babylonian Journal of Internet of Things*, *2023*, 13–22. doi:10.58496/BJIoT/2023/003

Fahim, S., Maqsood, A., Das, G., Ahmed, N., Saquib, S., Lal, A., Khan, A., & Alam, M. (2022). Augmented Reality and Virtual Reality in Dentistry: Highlights from the Current Research. *Applied Sciences (Basel, Switzerland)*, *12*(8), 3719. doi:10.3390/app12083719

Goel, P., Jhanwar, N., Jain, P., Khatri, S., & Hiran, K. K. (2023, August). Efficient Blood Availability for Targeted Individuals Through Cloud Computing Web Application. In *2023 International Conference on Emerging Trends in Networks and Computer Communications (ETNCC)* (pp. 1-7). IEEE. 10.1109/ETNCC59188.2023.10284940

Gupta, A. K., Srinivasulu, A., Hiran, K. K., Sreenivasulu, G., Rajeyyagari, S., & Subramanyam, M. (2022). Prediction of omicron virus using combined extended convolutional and recurrent neural networks technique on CT-scan images. *Interdisciplinary Perspectives on Infectious Diseases*, *2022*, 2022. doi:10.1155/2022/1525615 PMID:36562006

Higgins, T., Larson, E., & Schnall, R. (2017). Unraveling the meaning of patient engagement: A concept analysis. *Patient Education and Counseling*, *100*(1), 30–36. doi:10.1016/j.pec.2016.09.002 PMID:27665500

Jain, R. K., & Hiran, K. K. (2024). BIONET: A Bio-Inspired Neural Network for Consensus Mechanisms in Blockchain Systems. In Bio-Inspired Optimization Techniques in Blockchain Systems (pp. 78-100). IGI Global. doi:10.4018/979-8-3693-1131-8.ch004

Kim, S., Hong, J., Joung, S., Yamada, A., Matsumoto, N., Kim, S., Kim, Y., & Hashizume, M. (2011). Dual Surgical Navigation Using Augmented and Virtual Environment Techniques. *International Journal of Optomechatronics*, *5*(2), 155–169. doi:10.1080/15599612.2011.581743

Letterie, G. (2002). How virtual reality may enhance training in obstetrics and gynecology.. *American journal of obstetrics and gynecology*, *187*(3), S37-40 . doi:10.1067/mob.2002.127361

Li, R., Chen, Y., Ritchie, M., & Moore, J. (2020). Electronic health records and polygenic risk scores for predicting disease risk. *Nature Reviews. Genetics, 21*(8), 493–502. doi:10.1038/s41576-020-0224-1 PMID:32235907

Liono, R., Amanda, N., Pratiwi, A., & Gunawan, A. (2021). A Systematic Literature Review: Learning with Visual by The Help of Augmented Reality Helps Students Learn Better. *Procedia Computer Science, 179*, 144–152. doi:10.1016/j.procs.2020.12.019

McCradden, M., Joshi, S., Anderson, J., Mazwi, M., Goldenberg, A., & Shaul, R. (2020). Patient safety and quality improvement: Ethical principles for a regulatory approach to bias in healthcare machine learning. *Journal of the American Medical Informatics Association : JAMIA, 27*(12), 2024–2027. doi:10.1093/jamia/ocaa085 PMID:32585698

Mishra, R., Narayanan, M., Umana, G., Montemurro, N., Chaurasia, B., & Deora, H. (2022). Virtual Reality in Neurosurgery: Beyond Neurosurgical Planning. *International Journal of Environmental Research and Public Health, 19*(3), 1719. doi:10.3390/ijerph19031719 PMID:35162742

Mishra, T., Wang, M., Metwally, A., Bogu, G., Brooks, A., Bahmani, A., Alavi, A., Celli, A., Higgs, E., Dagan-Rosenfeld, O., Fay, B., Kirkpatrick, S., Kellogg, R., Gibson, M., Wang, T., Hunting, E., Mamić, P., Ganz, A., Rolnik, B., & Snyder, M. (2020). Pre-symptomatic detection of COVID-19 from smartwatch data. *Nature Biomedical Engineering, 4*(12), 1208–1220. doi:10.1038/s41551-020-00640-6 PMID:33208926

Mylrea, K., & Sivertson, S. (1975). Biomedical Engineering in Health Care - Potential Versus Reality. *IEEE Transactions on Biomedical Engineering, BME-22*(2), 114–119. doi:10.1109/TBME.1975.324429 PMID:1123239

Nankani, H., Mahrishi, M., Morwal, S., & Hiran, K. K. (2022). A Formal study of shot boundary detection approaches—Comparative analysis. In *Soft Computing: Theories and Applications: Proceedings of SoCTA 2020,* Volume 1 (pp. 311-320). Springer Singapore.

Nanthakumar, R., & Sivakumaran, N. (2018). Role of Biomedical Engineering for Diagnose and Treatment. *Role of Biomedical Engineering for Diagnose and Treatment., 4*(11), 94–112. doi:10.31695/IJASRE.2018.32944

Pereira, M., Prahm, C., Kolbenschlag, J., Oliveira, E., & Rodrigues, N. (2020). Application of AR and VR in hand rehabilitation: A systematic review. *Journal of Biomedical Informatics, 103584*, 103584. doi:10.1016/j.jbi.2020.103584 PMID:33011296

Pourmand, A., Davis, S., Lee, D., Barber, S., & Sikka, N. (2017). Emerging Utility of Virtual Reality as a Multidisciplinary Tool in Clinical Medicine. *Games for Health Journal, 6*(5), 263–270. doi:10.1089/g4h.2017.0046 PMID:28759254

Riener, R., &Harders, M. (2012). *VR for Medical Training,* 181-210. Springer. . doi:10.1007/978-1-4471-4011-5_8

Rubi, J., A., V., Kanna, K. R., & G., U. (2023). Bringing Intelligence to Medical Devices Through Artificial Intelligence. Recent Advancements in Smart Remote Patient Monitoring. *Wearable Devices, and Diagnostics Systems,* 154–168. doi:10.4018/978-1-6684-6434-2.ch007

Rubi, J., & Dhivya, A. J. A. (2022). Wearable Health Monitoring Systems Using IoMT. The *Internet of Medical Things (IoMT),* 225–246. doi:10.1002/9781119769200.ch12

Srinivasulu, A., Gupta, A. K., Hiran, K. K., Barua, T., & Sreenivasulu, G. (2022). Omi-cron Virus Data Analytics Using Extended RNN Technique. *Int J Cancer Res Ther, 7*(3), 122, 129, 1-3.

Ujiie, H., Yamaguchi, A., Gregor, A., Chan, H., Kato, T., Hida, Y., Kaga, K., Wakasa, S., Eitel, C., Clapp, T., & Yasufuku, K. (2021). Developing a virtual reality simulation system for preoperative planning of thoracoscopic thoracic surgery. *Journal of Thoracic Disease, 13*(2), 778–783. doi:10.21037/jtd-20-2197 PMID:33717550

Vaishya, R., Javaid, M., Khan, I., & Haleem, A. (2020). Artificial Intelligence (AI) applications for COVID-19 pandemic. *Diabetes & Metabolic Syndrome, 14*(4), 337–339. doi:10.1016/j.dsx.2020.04.012 PMID:32305024

Volonté, F., Pugin, F., Bucher, P., Sugimoto, M., Ratib, O., & Morel, P. (2011). Augmented reality and image overlay navigation with OsiriX in laparoscopic and robotic surgery: Not only a matter of fashion. *Journal of Hepato-Biliary-Pancreatic Sciences, 18*(4), 506–509. doi:10.1007/s00534-011-0385-6 PMID:21487758

Chapter 4
Enhancing Well–Being:
Exploring the Impact of Augmented Reality and Virtual Reality

Ranjit Singha
ⓘ https://orcid.org/0000-0002-3541-8752
Christ University, India

Surjit Singha
ⓘ https://orcid.org/0000-0002-5730-8677
Kristu Jayanti College (Autonomous), India

ABSTRACT

Virtual reality (VR) and augmented reality (AR) can revolutionize how individuals experience and perceive the world. Effective and engaging wellness practices are made possible by these technologies personalized, immersive experiences. The organization endeavors to foster empathy and understanding by attending to physical, mental, emotional, and social health. Nevertheless, ethical deliberations are of the utmost importance, including privacy, proper data handling, and secure data access. Education, support, and accessibility are critical determinants of user acceptance. Additional areas that warrant further investigation include treatment efficacy, diversity, long-term effects, and ongoing progress. A more inclusive, engaging, and productive approach to individual and communal health is anticipated due to the expanding use of AR and VR in well-being.

INTRODUCTION

This chapter probed into the domain of virtual and augmented reality (VR and AR) and their significant influence on improving overall health. To establish clarity, we shall begin by defining well-being and underscoring its profound importance in our existence. It explores the critical significance of virtual reality (VR) and augmented reality (AR) technologies in fostering an enhanced state of self-being. Well-being, alternatively referred to as state of being, is a multifaceted notion that incorporates a range of facets from an individual's existence and indicates their overall quality of life. Wellness encompasses

DOI: 10.4018/979-8-3693-1123-3.ch004

an individual's mental, emotional, physical, and social well-being and is frequently linked to satisfaction, equilibrium, and contentment. Well-being is an all-encompassing notion that considers multiple facets of an individual's being; its importance is substantial, influencing individuals and society at large (Simons & Baldwin, 2021; Ruggeri et al., 2020; Proctor, 2014). This dimension pertains to the physical well-being of an individual, encompassing aspects such as physical fitness, proper nutrition, absence of illness or infirmity, and general physical vitality. Mental health encompasses both the affective and cognitive dimensions of existence. This concept includes mental health, cognitive functioning, emotional stability, and psychological resilience. Emotional well-being pertains to an individual's emotional health and capacity to regulate and control their emotions efficiently (Ruggeri et al., 2020; Pinar, 2018; Oades & Mossman, 2017). This dimension pertains to an individual's interpersonal relationships, social connections, and sense of community affiliation. It comprises both the depth and character of social interactions. Environmental well-being examines the influence that an individual's immediate environment has on their holistic state of being. Access to pure air, water, green spaces, and a secure and encouraging environment are all components of this concept. Economic well-being comprises income, financial security, and economic prospects that facilitate a life of ease and comfort (Pinar, 2018; Linton et al., 2016).

Well-being and mental and physical health are intricately intertwined. Individuals with elevated levels of well-being generally exhibit reduced levels of stress, improved physical health, and an enhanced sense of contentment and life satisfaction. Intense well-being is frequently associated with greater resilience in life's difficulties. They possess enhanced capabilities to manage tension, obstacles, and setbacks. Elevated levels of well-being can enhance productivity and performance across various domains, such as professional and personal spheres (Oades & Mossman, 2017). Well-being is correlated with enhanced interpersonal connections and the capacity to establish and sustain significant rapport with others. A society's collective well-being can impact its social cohesion, economic stability, and overall health. Enhancements in life quality and a more profound sense of purpose and meaning can be attributed to a heightened state of well-being (Au et al., 2023). Environmental well-being is of paramount importance for the planet's sustainability, as it entails the adoption of environmentally mindful behaviours and the safeguarding of the natural environment. In essence, well-being is an indispensable notion incorporating various physical, mental, emotional, social, environmental, and economic aspects. Its importance transcends individual well-being, health, and resiliency, as well as social interactions and the collective prosperity of society. The comprehension and advancement of well-being are fundamental objectives in numerous disciplines, including public policy, healthcare, psychology, and education (Oades & Mossman, 2017). The potential for Augmented Reality (AR) and Virtual Reality (VR) to positively influence an individual's physical, mental, and emotional health is extensive and encompasses a wide range of dimensions (Au et al., 2023). These immersive technologies provide novel and inventive approaches to augmenting well-being across multiple dimensions:

Application development in AR and VR can generate interactive and captivating fitness experiences. Engaging in virtual routines, sports simulations, and physical challenges enables users to augment the enjoyment and motivation derived from exercising. Physical therapy and rehabilitation programs may incorporate VR. By engaging in activities and exercises in a virtual environment, patients can accelerate and improve their recovery. Virtual reality (VR) distractions have been implemented in medical procedures to mitigate pain and discomfort, reducing the need for analgesics and tension (Longo et al., 2023; Benjamin et al., 2022). Augmented reality (AR) can furnish individuals with health metrics and real-time health information via wearable devices. It is especially beneficial for individuals managing chronic health conditions (Canali et al., 2022; Zhao et al., 2021; Channa et al., 2021). VR provides calming environments, nature simulations, and immersive relaxation experiences that can aid in the reduction of tension and anxiety.

Post-traumatic stress disorder (PTSD), phobias, and anxiety disorders are some of the mental health conditions that are treated with virtual reality (VR) therapy, which provides a controlled and immersive environment for desensitization and therapeutic exposure. Cognitive training and rehabilitation for people with cognitive impairments, such as Alzheimer's disease and attention disorders, can be aided by augmented reality and virtual reality applications. By incorporating positive emotions and mood enhancements into virtual reality environments and experiences, a form of emotional support can be provided. Virtual reality (VR) enables users to establish connections in digital social environments, facilitating social interaction and surmounting the challenges posed by geographical separation. It is especially beneficial in remote work or isolation (Gambella et al., 2022).

By superimposing digital information onto the physical world, augmented reality can improve communication by rendering it more expressive and interactive. By increasing awareness of environmental issues and encouraging sustainable behaviour, virtual reality can cultivate a sense of environmental responsibility. Virtual reality can allow individuals to engage with wildlife conservation efforts and natural environments, even in cases where physical travel is not feasible. Applying AR and VR technologies to skill development and job training can improve an individual's economic opportunities and employment prospects. By facilitating more flexible and productive work hours, AR-enabled remote collaboration and work management applications may help individuals achieve a healthier work-life balance (Scurati et al., 2021). Augmented reality (AR) and virtual reality (VR) technologies can substantially augment well-being in multiple facets, including but not limited to physical health, mental health, social connections, and economic prospects. These technologies are in a constant state of development and hold the potential to enhance the quality of life for communities and individuals as a whole. Additional investigation and advancement in this domain are probable to reveal groundbreaking approaches through which augmented and virtual reality can enhance overall welfare.

ENHANCING PHYSICAL WELL-BEING

The integration of Augmented Reality (AR) and Virtual Reality (VR) applications is on the rise in healthcare and rehabilitation environments, providing novel approaches to patient care, medical education, and therapy. VR can divert the attention of patients enduring arduous medical procedures. Utilizing tranquil and engaging virtual environments can diminish patients' perception of pain, thereby reducing their reliance on pain medication. For surgical training, surgeons and medical professionals utilize VR simulations. Employing these simulations, one can hone surgical skills and practice complex procedures in a secure and authentic setting. By superimposing 3D anatomical models onto physical objects or the human body, augmented reality applications facilitate medical students' comprehension of intricate anatomical structures. AR can be utilized to educate patients about medical conditions and treatment alternatives. Healthcare providers can enhance patient comprehension by superimposing digital information, including animations or 3D models, onto printed materials or the patient's body using augmented reality. Virtual reality can generate stimulating and motivational exercises for physical therapy patients. Tailored to the specific requirements of each patient, these exercises may facilitate recovery from surgical procedures, neurological disorders, or traumas. VR applications enhance coordination and assist patients in regaining motor skills. Patients can engage in virtual activities that present physical challenges in supervised and encouraging settings (Meena, 2021; Doshi, 2023). Individuals afflicted with neurode-generative diseases, brain injuries, or cognitive impairments may benefit from the cognitive rehabilitation capabilities of VR. Engaging and adaptive cognitive training exercises are provided (Clarke, 2021; Wiederhold & Wiederhold, 2007).

Especially in patients with veins that are difficult to locate, augmented reality technology can assist medical personnel in locating veins with greater ease, thereby reducing the discomfort associated with needle insertion. Individuals with chronic pain conditions, such as fibromyalgia or chronic back pain, may benefit from VR experiences that offer immersive relaxation and pain diversion. VR can facilitate remote consultations by enabling patients to interact with healthcare providers in a virtual environment. Providing care to patients in remote areas or during a health crisis is incredibly beneficial. VR is utilized to treat phobias, anxiety disorders, and post-traumatic stress disorder (PTSD) as part of exposure therapy. By permitting patients to confront their anxieties in a controlled virtual environment, the therapeutic process is rendered more tolerable. AR applications can deliver educational content and medication reminders, enhancing patient adherence to treatment plans. Virtual reality gaming and fitness applications promote physical activity by enhancing the enjoyment of exercise and fostering greater adherence to fitness regimens. By providing real-time data on blood sugar levels, diet management, and insulin administration, augmented reality (AR) applications have the potential to assist people with diabetes in effectively managing their condition. AR can engage and interact with patients while educating them about asthma triggers, inhaler techniques, and asthma management (Rajkumar et al., 2023; Brea-Gómez et al., 2021). Potential benefits of integrating AR and VR technologies in healthcare and rehabilitation include enhanced medical training, improved patient outcomes, and more engaging and accessible healthcare. These applications are anticipated to grow in scope as technology progresses, providing the healthcare industry with even more inventive resolutions. Virtual fitness and exercise programs, frequently utilizing Virtual Reality (VR) technology, provide individuals with a novel and captivating method to engage in physical activity and uphold their physical health (Siani & Marley, 2021). By offering personalized exercise experiences, interactive challenges, and immersive routines, these programs enhance the enjoyment and motivation of physical activity. Key characteristics and advantages of virtual fitness and exercise programs include the following:

Virtual fitness programs employ VR headsets to engross users in various exercise environments, including virtual gyms and picturesque landscapes. This level of immersion enriches the workout experience and increases the enjoyment derived from it. By incorporating physical movements into the gameplay, virtual reality fitness games transform exercise from a burden to an enjoyable and engaging experience. Gamification elements, including challenges, rewards, and scoring, encourage users to remain active. Numerous VR fitness programs provide individualized exercise regimens tailored to the user's fitness level, objectives, and preferences. Individuals can select from various exercise routines and fitness programs to suit their particular requirements. Virtual fitness programs offer various exercise modalities, such as dance, yoga, strength training, and cardiovascular routines. By alternating between activities, individuals can prevent tedium and maintain interest in their fitness regimen (Stewart et al., 2022). Virtual fitness applications frequently incorporate virtual trainers or coaches who guide users during exercises, guaranteeing correct form and technique adherence. This guidance assists users in reducing the risk of injury and optimize their exercise efficacy. Typical fitness metrics monitored by virtual fitness programs include heart rate, calories expended, and exercise duration. Users can track their progress and establish objectives for growth.

VR fitness programs incorporate social functionalities that facilitate user connections with peers or the virtual community, cultivating an atmosphere of responsibility and amicable rivalry. By providing access from the convenience of one's residence, virtual fitness programs obviate the necessity of physically attending a gym or fitness class. This convenience facilitates the incorporation of physical activity into users' schedules. Participating in virtual reality (VR) exercise can additionally facilitate relaxation and stress reduction by offering users an escape from the pressures and stresses of daily life (Mokmin & Jamiat, 2020). In particular, multiplayer capabilities are available in virtual reality fitness applications, allowing users to exercise while interacting with peers or other users in a virtual environment. Virtual fitness and exercise programs can enhance the accessibility and enjoyment of physical activity for diverse individuals. With the ongoing progression of technology, these programs will probably provide an increasing variety of captivating exercise experiences, thereby positively contributing to physical well-being and overall health (Ramasamy, 2022; Srinivasulu, 2022).

Advocating for positive lifestyle choices and encouraging maintenance through immersive experiences, frequently enabled by technologies such as Augmented Reality (AR) and Virtual Reality (VR), represents an innovative and productive strategy. These immersive experiences motivate individuals to adopt healthier behaviours and practices by utilizing AR and VR's interactive and engaging qualities. They may do so through the following means: fostering healthful behaviours. Augmented reality (AR) applications can deliver real-time nutritional information through smartphone camera scans of food products. Promoting healthier eating practices can be facilitated by users making informed decisions regarding their dietary intake (Carroll et al., 2021; Riegler et al., 2021; Rizzo et al., 2021). Virtual reality (VR) provides gamers with immersive fitness programs that elevate the exercise experience to a motivating level. Users can enjoy themselves while engaging in physical activity, which promotes consistent routines. Virtual reality (VR) can transport users to simulated outdoor environments, including dancing, cycling, or trekking. It may inspire people to engage in more excellent physical activity in the actual world. Augmented reality (AR) applications have the potential to promote outdoor activities and walking through the integration of step tracking and a competitive element. As a result, an active lifestyle is encouraged. Virtual reality can be utilized in addiction and smoke cessation therapies. By providing a controlled environment in which individuals can confront their triggers and appetites, immersive experiences can facilitate behavioural change (Tsamitros et al., 2021). Exposure therapy utilizes virtual reality to treat phobias, anxiety disorders, and post-traumatic stress disorder. By subjecting users to their anxieties within a secure and regulated virtual setting, the therapeutic process is rendered more tolerable. Individuals can use VR relaxation applications and immersive mindfulness experiences to alleviate anxiety and tension. Individuals can restore emotional equilibrium and relax in serene virtual environments (Segawa et al., 2020). AR and VR are capable of simulating the repercussions of detrimental behaviours, including smoking and excessive alcohol consumption. It may effectively dissuade and promote the adoption of healthier alternatives.

The necessity of sustainability and environmental issues can be brought to light through VR. Users can be educated about climate change, conservation, and eco-friendly behaviours through immersive experiences. Augmented reality applications can deliver up-to-the-minute data about nutrition, blood sugar levels, and insulin management. This intervention aids individuals diagnosed with diabetes in efficiently managing their condition. VR can be utilized to educate individuals on the causes, management, and prevention of chronic diseases. By employing immersive narrative techniques, intricate medical information can be more understandable and captivating. AR medication reminders and educational content regarding the significance of adhering to prescribed medications can be implemented through augmented reality (AR) applications, thereby enhancing patient compliance. AR Recipe and Culinary Assistance: By superimposing digital information onto culinary processes, AR applications can assist users in preparing meals that are healthier and more informed. Augmented reality applications can improve their overall health by prompting users to maintain adequate hydration. By accommodating individuals with various cultural backgrounds and abilities, AR and VR applications can be more accessible and inclusive to a broader demographic (Ronaghi, 2022; Harvie, 2021).

AR and VR-generated immersive experiences can captivate, enlighten, and motivate individuals to embrace and maintain health-promoting behaviours. Technology platforms that offer engaging and interactive material encompassing diverse facets of health and wellness have the potential to impact behaviour modification and public health advocacy significantly.

IMPROVING PSYCHOLOGICAL WELL-BEING

Anxiety and phobia treatment via Virtual Reality (VR) is a novel and productive method for assisting people in surmounting their fears and controlling anxiety disorders. This therapeutic approach establishes interactive and regulated environments where patients can safely and supervisedly confront their anxieties by utilizing immersive VR technology. Exposure therapy is a subset of VR therapy in which patients are systematically introduced to their particular anxieties or phobias. For anxiety disorders, exposure therapy is a widely recognized and evidence-based treatment. VR therapy involves the complete immersion of individuals in a virtual environment that accurately simulates the circumstances or stimuli that elicit fear or anxiety. Over time, this controlled exposure assists in desensitizing patients to their anxieties. A significant benefit of virtual reality (VR) therapy is the capacity to generate individualized scenarios that correspond to each patient's particular fears or anxieties. By customizing the virtual environment to the patient's specifications, therapists can enhance the effectiveness and relevance of the experience. Exposure therapy is more genuine and engaging than conventional methods due to the immersive characteristics of virtual reality (Albakri et al., 2022; Ronaghi, 2022).

VR therapy's high level of interactivity and immersion induces in patients the sensation that they are in the feared environment, which may result in improved treatment outcomes. Comparable to in-vivo exposure therapy, VR therapy can be administered in the patient's residence or the therapist's office, providing a more private and pleasant environment. It is particularly beneficial for those who experience embarrassment or self-consciousness due to their anxieties. Therapists can regulate the extent of exposure in a feasible manner for the patient, escalating the intensity incrementally as the patient gains comfort. During VR therapy, practitioners can observe and track the patient's physiological reactions (including skin conductance and pulse rate) in real time. Utilizing this information permits modifying treatment following the patient's distress level (Albakri et al., 2022; Goel, 2023).

Patients can be linked with specialized therapists and treatment options that may not be available locally through VR therapy. Individuals residing in remote regions or facing restrictive availability of mental health services may find this resource especially beneficial. Frequently, VR therapy improves patients' ability to retain and generalize the treatment. There is a tendency for individuals to retain and implement knowledge acquired in the virtual environment when confronted with real-world circumstances. Virtual reality (VR) therapy has demonstrated efficacy in addressing anxiety and phobias across a range of conditions, including social anxiety disorder, post-traumatic stress disorder (PTSD), generalized anxiety disorder, and specific phobias (e.g., fear of flying, heights, insects). It provides a secure and regulated approach to assist people in facing and regulating their anxieties, ultimately resulting in enhanced psychological health. It is anticipated that as technology progresses, virtual reality (VR) therapy will gain further efficacy as a treatment modality for anxiety-related disorders (Albakri et al., 2022; Tarrant et al., 2018).

There has been a growing trend in the application of Augmented Reality (AR) and Virtual Reality (VR) to deliver relaxation and stress reduction techniques. These technologies provide individuals with immersive and captivating experiences that aid stress management and enhance mental and emotional health. Virtual reality (VR) and augmented reality (AR) can transport users to serene and peaceful virtual environments, including forests, beaches, and natural landscapes. These immersive environments facilitate relaxation and allow individuals to escape the pressures of the real world. AR and VR applications provide guided meditation and mindfulness sessions. Individuals can partake in various relaxation techniques within a virtual setting, including progressive muscle relaxation and deep-breathing exercises (Brelet & Gaffary, 2022; Kim et al., 2021).

These applications assist users in attaining a state of relaxation and mindfulness through the use of calming audiovisual signals and guided instructions. Virtual reality (VR) applications and games aim to alleviate tension via engaging gameplay. Individuals can engage in stress-relieving activities, including virtual painting, horticulture, or music composition, or interact with soothing virtual environments. Biofeedback devices are integrated into unavoidable virtual reality (VR) applications to track physiological manifestations of stress, including respiration patterns, skin conductance, and heart rate variability. Biofeedback training enables individuals to acquire self-regulation skills by providing immediate feedback regarding their tension levels. Virtual wellness programs provide wellness retreats and immersive leisure experiences from the convenience of an individual's residence. Utilizing VR, users can partake in spa therapies such as hot tubs, massages, and relaxation sessions. VR and AR applications frequently integrate soothing soundscapes, calming music, and binaural beats to alleviate tension and promote relaxation. The ability of binaural rhythms to modify brainwave patterns to induce a state of calm and relaxation is well-known. VR and AR applications facilitate progressive muscle relaxation exercises to alleviate physical tension and encourage relaxation.

Muscle tension is identified and released, resulting in mental and physical relaxation for the user. By simulating scenarios, VR and AR applications can assist users in developing resilience and practising coping mechanisms in the face of adversity and stress. These situations may encompass stressors such as public speaking or confronting typical situations that induce anxiety. By providing virtual travel experiences, VR enables users to investigate and experience locations they might not otherwise be able to visit in person. Engaging in this mode of escapism may offer an intellectual respite from the pressures of daily life. In order to foster mental and emotional well-being, VR and AR applications can direct users through visualization exercises while also delivering self-improvement messages and positive affirmations. Utilizing virtual reality (VR) and augmented reality (AR) in these particular contexts offers users convenient and captivating resources to alleviate tension, attain a state of relaxation, and enhance their holistic psychological and emotional state of being.

Cognitive training and mental wellness initiatives, frequently supported by digital technologies such as Augmented Reality (AR) and Virtual Reality (VR), provide various experiences and tools to enhance mental health, support overall mental wellness, and promote cognitive well-being. The following are several methods by which these technologies promote mental health and cognitive development: Cognitive rehabilitation employs virtual reality to aid in the recovery of memory and cognitive functions following injuries or as a component of the treatment regimen for neurodegenerative disorders such as dementia. VR applications offer individuals a secure and regulated setting to develop and refine their cognitive abilities, including memory, attention, and problem-solving. The purpose of VR and AR experiences is to promote mental health by cultivating positive emotions, enhancing mood, and bolstering resilience. These programs have the potential to mitigate or prevent mental health conditions such as anxiety and depression. Engaging in interactive and immersive experiences has the potential to foster mindfulness, facilitate emotional regulation, and alleviate tension. Virtual reality (VR) applications can assist users in practising cognitive-behavioural interventions, exposure therapy, relaxation techniques, and stress management. Individuals can confront their anxieties in a controlled environment through VR's immersive capabilities (Brugada-Ramentol et al., 2022).

VR is utilized to create immersive environments that, in addition to exposure therapy, progressively acquaint users with their particular phobias, thereby assisting them in confronting and conquering these fears. It offers individuals a secure and encouraging setting to confront and overcome their anxieties. VR can simulate social situations, allowing those with social anxiety to develop and hone their social skills in a secure and controlled environment. Communication, public speaking, and interpersonal abilities can be developed through virtual practice. Attention disorders, such as ADHD, may be facilitated through the use of VR cognitive training programs that enhance executive functioning, concentration, and attention span. Engaging in interactive virtual reality exercises presents individuals with a cognitive challenge (Ramasamy, 2021).

Virtual and augmented reality can provide users with scenarios that enable them to develop emotional resilience and hone coping mechanisms in the face of adversity. Users have the opportunity to gain practical experience and acquire the skills necessary to handle challenging circumstances within a regulated virtual environment. VR and AR applications provide guided experiences and immersive environments that aid in tension reduction, mindfulness, and relaxation. These experiences facilitate relaxation, tension reduction, and mental health enhancement. VR and AR applications promote healthy self-perception and mental well-being by constantly displaying self-improvement messages and positive affirmations. These communications permit users to interact with them in an interactive and immersive fashion. Reducing stigma, increasing awareness, and educating individuals about mental health issues through VR and AR experiences is possible.

These programs for mental wellness and cognitive training, frequently powered by VR and AR technologies, contribute significantly to promoting mental health, enhancing cognitive well-being, and supporting overall mental wellness. They provide interactive and easily obtainable resources to assist people in cultivating resilience, enhancing cognitive abilities, controlling anxiety, and establishing constructive coping mechanisms. It is anticipated that as technology progresses, these programs will grow in scope and provide even more inventive approaches to promoting mental health and well-being.

ENHANCING SOCIAL WELL-BEING

Augmented Reality (AR) and Virtual Reality (VR) are bringing about a paradigm shift in human interaction and communication by presenting inventive approaches to augment social engagements and interpersonal connections. Virtual reality generates immersive environments in which individuals can interact and meet. These digital communities enable users to establish connections with family, acquaintances, or strangers from around the globe. Users can cultivate a sense of connection and presence by participating in activities, engaging in games, or simply socializing in a shared virtual environment.

Individuals can use AR and VR technologies to generate digital avatars that represent them in virtual spaces. Individual users can modify these avatars to reflect their unique tastes and dispositions. Avatar-based communication enhances the personalization and engagement of social interactions by allowing users to express themselves in distinctive ways. Virtual reality (VR) platforms allow family and friends to congregate in digital environments and participate in shared activities, transcending geographical barriers. Promoting social cohesion and proximity, virtual hangouts may consist of activities such as viewing movies, attending virtual parties, collaborating on projects, or playing games.

AR improves remote work and teleconferencing by superimposing digital information onto the physical environment. This augmented communication can increase the interactivity and expression of video conferences. It increases social connection and collaboration among remote employees, thereby boosting coordination and productivity. Virtual reality (VR) language learning applications generate immersive environments that enable users to interact with speakers of various languages and practice their language skills. These experiences foster the development of global communication skills, social inclusion, and cross-cultural understanding. VR permits the organization of virtual conferences, events, and gatherings where participants can network and engage in conversation. These virtual events facilitate connections and experiences among individuals who share similar interests. Collaborative augmented and virtual reality tools enable users to engage in design duties, team brainstorming, or artistic endeavours within virtual environments. VR collaboration facilitates effective communication and innovation, especially for geographically dispersed or remote teams. Customizable virtual reality environments can simulate a variety of social contexts, including cafes, offices, and lounges (Patel, 2022).

By customizing AR and VR to accommodate individuals with disabilities, social interactions can be made more accessible and inclusive for those of varying abilities and requirements. AR and VR facilitate virtual classrooms, lectures, and training programs in educational and training environments. These immersive educational experiences facilitate student-teacher social interaction. Social VR experiences and VR gaming platforms offer users and gamers the opportunity to collaborate, compete, and interact with both acquaintances and strangers within a virtual gaming setting. Social networking and online dating platforms have incorporated augmented reality and virtual reality, enabling users to meet and interact with potential partners or engage with individuals who share similar interests in an immersive environment. By utilizing augmented reality (AR) and virtual reality (VR) for social interactions and communication, many prospects arise to collaborate, establish connections, and cultivate relationships within immersive and captivating virtual environments. These technologies can transcend geographical barriers, foster social connections, and elevate the calibre of social exchanges, thereby positively contributing to social welfare. The digital age has witnessed the proliferation of virtual communities and social support networks, thriving due to Augmented Reality (AR) and Virtual Reality (VR) innovations. Virtual reality (VR) platforms and environments facilitate the forming interest-based communities and virtual social organizations. These organizations facilitate gathering members with shared hobbies, interests, or passions. Users can establish meaningful relationships with others who share their interests by socializing and discussing topics of interest. VR and AR technologies can facilitate virtual support groups for people who are grappling with mental health challenges. Virtual support groups provide individuals with a secure and confidential environment to solicit guidance, compassion, and motivation (Dechsling et al., 2021; Scavarelli et al., 2020).

Social VR platforms and multiplayer VR games facilitate the formation of gaming communities. Individual gamers can collaborate, compete, and interact with others who share their passions. These communities facilitate social interaction among gamers, allowing them to develop friendships, exchange experiences, and participate in their preferred recreational activity. Job training and collaboration tools enabled by augmented reality allow individuals to establish connections with mentors, colleagues, and professional communities. These networks facilitate career advancement, provide access to pertinent resources, and enable individuals to remain informed about industry trends. AR and VR platforms facilitate the formation of communities committed to social causes, advocacy, and activism. Virtual conferences, conventions, and events are organized using AR and VR technologies. These assemblies offer a forum for establishing connections with colleagues and professionals, exchanging information, and networking. Virtual events provide an equivalent level of engagement and presence as in-person gatherings.

To provide peer support for individuals who are confronted with obstacles such as addiction recovery, chronic illness, or life transitions, virtual communities are established. These networks offer an environment devoid of judgment, where members can candidly share their personal experiences, solicit guidance, and discover motivation from others who have been through comparable trials. Virtual parenting and family support communities can be created using AR and VR, where parents can receive emotional support from others in similar circumstances, exchange parental advice, and discuss obstacles. Particularly beneficial are these communities for parents who are experiencing feelings of isolation or in need of guidance. Academic establishments establish alumni networks and virtual student communities through AR and VR. Students and alums can connect, share experiences, and access resources for professional and personal development via these platforms. AR and VR, language learning applications, facilitate the convergence of enthusiastic individuals about cultural immersion and language exchange. These digital communities promote intercultural comprehension and facilitate language acquisition. AR and VR-enabled social support networks and virtual communities provide a wide range of opportunities for people to connect, share experiences, seek assistance, and interact with others with similar interests and concerns, irrespective of their location.

A highly effective approach to cultivating greater empathy and advancing comprehension among communities and individuals is employing immersive experiences facilitated by Augmented Reality (AR) and Virtual Reality (VR) technologies. The subsequent examples illustrate how AR and VR accomplish these objectives. Virtual reality (VR) can engross users in scenarios that offer an authentic firsthand account of the struggles and obstacles encountered by people of diverse cultural backgrounds, worldviews, or particular life situations. This immersion facilitates the development of a more profound comprehension of alternative viewpoints. By simulating the daily lives of refugees, people with disabilities, and members of impoverished communities, for instance, virtual reality can foster compassion and understanding. Users can investigate various perspectives and narratives by utilizing the interactive storytelling capabilities of AR and VR applications. These experiences foster active user participation and comprehension of the experiences and narratives of others. Using narrative construction, users can adopt various characters' perspectives and influence the course of events, fostering empathy and a sense of shared experience. Through VR, users can be transported to historical events, distant cultures, and cultural heritage locations. These experiences facilitate users in thoroughly engaging with various cultures' customs, historical backgrounds, and everyday existence. Virtual cultural experiences promote cross-cultural comprehension, dispel stereotypes, and cultivate cultural appreciation. This immersive learning encourages empathy for others and fosters a more profound comprehension of complex social issues.

As an illustration, VR simulations have the potential to impart knowledge regarding historical events, the plight of marginalized communities, and the repercussions of prejudice and discrimination. Virtual reality can provide simulations that offer users a transient experience of various physical conditions or disabilities. These experiences aid in comprehending the daily obstacles and challenges faced by individuals with disabilities. This comprehension has the potential to foster greater empathy and advocate for practices that are accessible and inclusive. The use of AR and VR in peacebuilding and conflict resolution is possible. These technological advancements facilitate virtual dialogues and negotiations among members of opposing factions, thereby promoting reciprocal comprehension and compassion. Conflict scenarios can be simulated in virtual reality, allowing participants to investigate the viewpoints and experiences of all parties. Healthcare personnel are instructed in empathy and patient-centred care via virtual reality. By exposing medical professionals to scenarios from the patient's point of view, these training programs enhance their capacity for empathy and permit the delivery of more effective care. Virtual reality (VR) applications teach mindfulness and compassion, aiding users in developing self-awareness, emotional regulation, and empathy. By developing their self-compassion and empathy in virtual environments, users can better prepare themselves for interactions in the real world. AR and VR can facilitate experiential learning in sociology, psychology, and history. By enabling students to fully engage in social experiments or historical events, these technologies foster a more profound comprehension of human behaviour and societal concerns. In corporate environments, diversity and inclusion training is conducted via VR. By participating in simulated scenarios, employees can foster empathy and comprehension regarding the experiences of coworkers hailing from diverse backgrounds and the diversity of the workplace. Through augmented reality (AR) and virtual reality (VR) technologies, individuals can partake in immersive experiences that foster empathy and comprehension. It can provide them with valuable insights into the lives and viewpoints of others, ultimately contributing to the cultivation of increased compassion, tolerance, and social harmony. These experiences can foster open-mindedness, facilitate positive social change, and reconcile gaps in comprehension.

CASE STUDIES

Globally, stroke is the primary cause of permanent disability. Rehabilitation of the body is critical for stroke victims to regain motor functions. Augmented Reality (AR) presents an innovative strategy for enhancing the efficacy of rehabilitation by imbuing patients with motivation and engagement. To aid in the recovery of stroke patients, an augmented reality (AR) physical rehabilitation program was devised in this case study. The program comprised the subsequent essential elements. AR technology was employed to generate individualized exercises that catered to every patient's specific requirements and constraints. These exercises aimed to enhance coordination, balance, and motor abilities. By providing the patient with real-time feedback on their movements, augmented reality spectacles assisted them in performing exercises with the proper form and range of motion. The patient was guided through each exercise by implementing visual and auditory feedback. Through gamification, the rehabilitation program transformed exercises into engaging activities. Providing patients the ability to track their progress, earn incentives, and compete with one another or other patients would motivate and enhance the experience. The AR system would enable therapists to monitor their patients' progress remotely. They can modify the difficulty levels in exercises, monitor progress, and deliver prompt feedback and assistance. The AR-based rehabilitation program produced a multitude of favourable results. The patients' increased engagement and motivation in rehabilitation led to greater adherence to the exercise regimen. Motor skill and mobility improvements were more rapid and substantial in patients who utilized the augmented reality system than those who adhered to conventional rehabilitation techniques. By enabling clinicians to assist more patients via remote monitoring, accessibility to high-quality rehabilitation care was enhanced. As a result of the AR system's efficacy, the aggregate cost of healthcare and rehabilitation for stroke patients was diminished. This case study illustrates how augmented reality (AR) technology can revolutionize physical rehabilitation for stroke patients by enhancing engagement, efficacy, and accessibility.

Treatment of Post-Traumatic Stress Disorder (PTSD) can present considerable difficulty due to its intricate nature. Virtual Reality (VR) therapy has surfaced as a potentially effective method for assisting those diagnosed with PTSD in confronting and regulating their traumatic encounters. This case study focuses on the development of a virtual reality (VR) rehabilitation program intended for veterans who have suffered combat-related trauma and have PTSD. The program for VR therapy comprised the subsequent components. Virtual reality (VR) simulations replicated situations associated with distressing incidents, providing patients with a regulated setting to confront and overcome their fears and anxieties. Patients have the option to confront these situations under the supervision of a therapist progressively. The virtual reality (VR) software enabled clinicians to generate individualized scenarios corresponding to each patient's traumatic experiences. This modification increased the efficacy of the treatment. Virtual reality's immersive characteristics rendered exposure therapy more realistic and engaging than conventional approaches, resulting in more favourable treatment outcomes. Physical monitoring was incorporated into VR therapy to track the patient's exposure-related stress responses. Based on this information, clinicians were able to modify treatment accordingly. By allowing patients to gradually observe their advancements and enhancements, they would gain a sense of accomplishment and authority over their recovery. The VR therapy program for PTSD yielded several favourable outcomes: The PTSD symptoms of patients who underwent VR therapy decreased significantly, including hypervigilance, flashbacks, and nightmares. The patients articulated an elevated standard of living, diminished levels of anxiety, and enhanced social and occupational capabilities. As a result of the immersive and engaging qualities of VR therapy, treatment completion and adherence rates were significantly higher than with conventional methods. VR therapy offers patients a secure and regulated setting in which to confront their traumatic experiences, thereby reducing the likelihood of re-traumatization. By offering patients a safe and immersive environment in which to confront and manage their traumatic experiences in a supportive setting, this case study demonstrates the efficacy of virtual reality (VR) therapy in the treatment of PTSD.

Engaging in stress reduction and mindfulness practices is imperative for preserving one's mental and emotional health. Virtual Reality (VR) has been implemented in the development of stress reduction and mindfulness programs that offer consumers immersive resources to facilitate relaxation. A virtual mindfulness and stress reduction program was created to provide users with various techniques and experiences to alleviate stress and enhance mental health (Case Study). Individuals could engage in guided mindfulness and meditation sessions in VR environments. Participants engaged in body assessments, breathing exercises, and meditation in these sessions. The application provided users with access to serene virtual environments, including beaches, mountains, and forests, in which they could disconnect from the pressures of everyday existence and engage in relaxation exercises. Biofeedback devices were integrated into specific VR applications to monitor physiological stress indicators. Information in real-time that could assist users in tension and relaxation management. The program fostered mental well-being and fortitude by challenging and enhancing cognitive abilities by integrating interactive activities and exercises. Users were guided through progressive muscle relaxation techniques via VR programs to alleviate physical tension and facilitate relaxation. Individuals could partake in stress reduction objectives and challenges, such as conquering anxieties or managing stressors, within a regulated virtual setting. Users of the virtual stress reduction and mindfulness program derived numerous benefits. Participants indicated a decline in stress levels and an enhancement in serenity after participating in virtual mindfulness and stress reduction exercises. Individuals reported enhancements in their holistic psychological state, encompassing improved emotional equilibrium, disposition, and fortitude. Cognitive abilities, including memory, focus, and problem-solving, were improved due to the cognitive training exercises. VR has significantly expanded the accessibility and enjoyment of mindfulness and stress reduction practices for various users due to its immersive and engaging qualities. To customize their stress reduction program according to their requirements and preferences, users were presented with various experiences and techniques to select from. This case study demonstrates the efficacy of virtual reality (VR) in facilitating stress reduction and mindfulness by providing users with a diverse range of immersive experiences and strategies to improve their psychological and emotional state.

DISCUSSION

AR and VR offer consumers highly immersive and engaging experiences, which can increase their motivation and enjoyment of wellness practices. Enhanced levels of involvement frequently result in improved compliance with regimens and initiatives. These technologies can provide customized experiences, adapting interventions to suit each individual's specific requirements and preferences. Increased personalization has the potential to yield more favourable results in terms of mental, emotional, and physical health. Virtual and augmented reality can make wellness practices more accessible to a broader demographic. It encompasses individuals residing in remote regions or those with physical disabilities who may face constraints in accessing conventional wellness resources. Notably, this demographic responds positively to relaxation techniques and stress reduction methods. Users can seek refuge in immersive environments, alleviating daily life's pressures and potentially enhancing their mental health.

VR immersive experiences that enable users to experience alternative viewpoints or place themselves in the soles of others can foster empathy and comprehension. It has the potential to cultivate empathy, consciousness, and inclusiveness, thereby positively impacting social and emotional welfare. VR therapy has demonstrated potential in the treatment of specific phobias and post-traumatic stress disorder (PTSD), among others. VR facilitates exposure therapy in a controlled and secure environment, which contributes to its efficacy as a treatment modality. The expense of high-quality AR and VR apparatus may prevent some individuals from gaining access to these technologies.

Furthermore, using compatible hardware and high-speed internet connectivity may be mandatory, presenting obstacles for specific users. VR may induce motion sickness or distress in some users, especially in situations involving abrupt transitions in viewpoint or sudden movements. It may restrict the efficacy and duration of use for specific individuals due to the immersive qualities of AR and VR; privacy, data security, and the possibility of misuse become ethical concerns. Companies and developers must give ethical considerations precedence in their operations.

Ancestral and virtual reality (AR) and VR experiences may only be readily embraced by some users, and specific individuals may perceive the technology as daunting or unsettling, impeding its efficacy. Prolonged virtual reality (VR) utilization may result in physical inactivity, given that users frequently remain still during immersive experiences. It could impact an individual's physical health. While the short-term potential exists, research is ongoing to determine AR and VR's long-term effects on well-being, particularly mental health. Further information is required to ascertain the longevity of the advantages. Particularly in the case of highly engaging VR experiences, there is the possibility of addiction and misconduct, as with any technology. Regulators and developers are obligated to monitor these dangers and implement countermeasures. Despite the potential for AR and VR to significantly transform the promotion of well-being, they also present several obstacles and constraints that must be overcome. It is critical to exercise meticulous deliberation regarding the advantages and constraints of these technologies to guarantee their responsible and efficient utilization for the betterment of communities and individuals as a whole.

The ability of AR and VR technologies to capture and store user data raises privacy and security concerns. Organizations and developers are responsible for prioritizing the security of user information and preventing its unauthorized exploitation or disclosure. To ensure their well-being, users should be adequately advised regarding how their data is utilized and be required to give informed consent before utilizing augmented reality and virtual reality applications. Consent mechanisms and transparent data policies are essential. VR and AR experiences can induce physical and psychological side effects due to their immersive nature, including but not limited to motion nausea, eye strain, and discomfort. Maintaining user safety and comfort as a top priority is of considerable ethical significance. For well-being, users should be informed of potential adverse effects and best practices to ensure their physical and mental safety when utilizing AR and VR. The potential for excessive engagement with AR and VR technologies may result in addiction or misuse, both of which are detrimental to mental health and overall well-being. These are dangers that organizations and developers ought to be conscious of. Conscientious Design: In pursuing ethical design, it is imperative to incorporate elements that promote responsible usage, such as reminders for taking pauses and assistance for those who may develop an addiction to immersive experiences.

It should be possible for AR and VR technologies to be accessible and inclusive to a wide range of user demographics, including those of various ages, genders, abilities, and cultural backgrounds. Ignoring to consider these factors constitutes an ethical dilemma. To accommodate the requirements of all prospective users, developers ought to strive for inclusive design by incorporating attributes like customizable interfaces and accessibility alternatives. AR and VR technologies can be employed in detrimental or unscrupulous manners, including producing content that spreads misinformation, violence, or discrimination. It is the ethical duty of platforms and developers to moderate content and prevent the distribution of detrimental or offensive materials.

Educating individuals about AR and VR technologies' advantages, disadvantages, and ethical implications concerning well-being is crucial to increasing user acceptance. This information can assist users in making informed decisions regarding their usage. Developers and organizations must maintain transparency regarding the utilization, collection, and protection of data associated with AR and VR technologies. Transparency inspires user confidence. Involving prospective users in designing and developing augmented reality (AR) and virtual reality (VR) wellness applications can guarantee that the technologies fulfil their requirements and anticipations. User acceptance of AR and VR applications can be increased by ensuring they are intuitive and user-friendly. Interfaces that are complicated or challenging to use have the potential to discourage users.

When users perceive tangible, substantiated advantages of utilizing AR and VR technologies for wellness purposes—such as enhanced mental health, increased participation in wellness practices, or successful treatment results—they are more inclined to embrace these technologies. Aiding and direction to users can aid them in surmounting obstacles and acclimating to the technology. This support can assist with motion nausea, discomfort, and any other confusion regarding the application of AR and VR for wellness purposes. In augmented reality and virtual reality, social support networks and virtual communities can foster a sense of community and peer assistance among users, thereby increasing their adoption. User acceptability and ethical considerations are fundamental to AR and VR technologies' practical and responsible application in promoting well-being. Educating and involving users in the development process while prioritizing privacy, safety, diversity, and transparency can result in greater user acceptance and positive outcomes for communities and individuals.

There is considerable potential for incorporating Augmented Reality (AR) and Virtual Reality (VR) into established well-being practices to augment the efficacy of conventional approaches and elevate individuals' overall well-being. The subsequent examples illustrate how augmented and virtual reality can be incorporated into established wellness practices. VR can be incorporated into conventional therapy sessions to provide individuals with phobias, PTSD, or anxiety disorders with exposure therapy. It provides therapists with a regulated and engaging setting to direct patients through therapeutic encounters. Virtual reality (VR) can enhance mindfulness and stress reduction practices by providing immersive environments and guided meditation sessions. Users can enhance their relaxation and mental health by entering tranquil virtual environments. By integrating AR and VR into physical rehabilitation programs, exercises can be rendered more effective and engaging. Patients undergoing interactive virtual environments can perform exercises while rehabilitating from surgeries or injuries. Virtual reality can provide users with a fun and immersive way to engage in exercise regimens through virtual fitness programs. Games and competition may be integrated into these applications to encourage users to maintain an active lifestyle. Through simulation of the experiences of those afflicted with mental health conditions, AR and VR can be utilized to increase public consciousness. It increases comprehension and decreases stigma.

AR can improve health education by superimposing digital data and counselling on physical objects, furnishing users with up-to-date health-related information. Support networks and virtual communities within VR can be extensions of pre-existing support organizations. Peer support-seeking individuals can connect with others with similar interests and values through immersive environments. Social skills training can be facilitated through AR and VR, allowing those with social anxiety or communication difficulties to practice and better their interactions in virtual environments. Businesses can incorporate AR and VR into employee wellness programs. Virtual team-building exercises, stress management modules, and relaxation sessions can be implemented via VR to promote mental and emotional well-being in the workplace. VR can improve workplace relationships, foster empathy, and facilitate diversity and inclusion training. AR can increase their productivity and job satisfaction by providing employees with augmented information while they perform their duties.

Incorporating virtual reality (VR) into cognitive training programs designed for seniors can enhance memory and mental fitness. These programs may offer stimulating cognitive exercises. AR and VR can facilitate social interaction for older adults, reducing feelings of isolation and enhancing their emotional health. The utilization of augmented reality (AR) in skill development and education involves the superimposition of educational content onto tangible objects. Immersive educational experiences made possible by VR can make learning memorable and engaging. Cognitive training exercises that improve memory, attention, and problem-solving abilities can be provided by VR applications, thereby fostering cognitive health. VR programs that promote mindfulness and stress reduction can assist users in regulating their emotions and tension, thereby enhancing their emotional health. An area of tremendous potential, integrating AR and VR with established wellness practices is dynamic and ever-evolving. It is anticipated that as technology progresses and further investigation is undertaken, these technologies will continue to refine their efficacy as instruments for enhancing holistic welfare in diverse spheres.

CONCLUSION

Augmented Reality (AR) and Virtual Reality (VR) can substantially augment holistic welfare encompassing physical, mental, emotional, and social domains. These technologies provide immersive and captivating experiences that have the potential to enhance the enjoyment, efficacy, and accessibility of well-being practices. AR and VR can significantly impact the promotion of well-being by providing therapy, relaxation, and fitness tools, solutions tailored to individual needs and preferences, and encouraging empathy and understanding. There are several prospective advantages of AR and VR in promoting well-being. The increased engagement that AR and VR bring to wellness practices results in greater adherence and improved outcomes. These technologies enable customized interventions, potentially resulting in enhanced efficacy. Virtual and augmented reality can potentially expand the accessibility of wellness practices to individuals with physical or geographical constraints. Virtual reality is efficient for relaxation techniques, providing users with an escape from everyday stresses. Immersive experiences foster comprehension and empathy, thereby enhancing social and emotional welfare.

Virtual reality (VR) therapy exhibits great potential in addressing conditions such as PTSD and anxieties by providing a regulated and altogether immersive therapeutic environment. Several recommendations and factors should be considered to facilitate the widespread adoption of AR and VR to promote well-being. Establish and abide by ethical standards that place user confidentiality, data protection, openness, and safety first. Procedures for straightforward, informed assent should be established. In the context of well-being, educate and inform users regarding the advantages, disadvantages, and ethical implications of augmented reality (AR) and virtual reality (VR) technologies.

Ensure that the design of augmented reality (AR) and virtual reality (VR) applications is inclusive and accessible to a wide range of user groups by considering gender, age, ability, and cultural background, among other factors. Incorporate safety protocols, such as functionalities that promote responsible usage and assistance for individuals at risk of developing addictive tendencies. Safeguard user information and guarantee its responsible utilization following stringent privacy and data protection regulations. Provide user support to assist individuals in surmounting obstacles and efficiently adjusting to the technology.

It establishes social support networks and virtual communities that foster a sense of belonging and assistance among users' peers. Additional research is required to evaluate the long-term effects of AR and VR on physical, mental, and emotional health. To ensure that AR and VR technologies are accessible and effective for a broad spectrum of consumers, future research should incorporate diverse populations. Assess the effectiveness of augmented reality (AR) and virtual reality (VR) in various physical rehabilitation programs and mental health conditions in more extensive, diverse clinical settings.

It is imperative to consistently enhance the user experience by attending to concerns such as discomfort, motion nausea, and the learning curve. Establish and enforce stringent ethical regulations and standards to guarantee the responsible application of augmented reality (AR) and virtual reality (VR) in advancing well-being. Educators, therapists, developers, and healthcare professionals should collaborate to maximize the wellness benefits of AR and VR. AR and VR can fundamentally transform our approach to well-being by providing inventive and efficacious instruments to augment many facets of health and quality of life. Educating users, prioritizing ethical considerations, and conducting rigorous research to realize this potential is essential. Enhanced personal and community health initiatives may be rendered more engaging, inclusive, and productive through the pervasive implementation of AR and VR in promoting wellness.

REFERENCES

Albakri, G., Bouaziz, R., Alharthi, W., Kammoun, S., Al-Sarem, M., Saeed, F., & Hadwan, M. (2022d). Phobia Exposure Therapy Using Virtual and Augmented Reality: A Systematic review. *Applied Sciences (Basel, Switzerland), 12*(3), 1672. doi:10.3390/app12031672

Au, D., Sun, Y., & Wong, H. T. (2023). Editorial: Towards the well-being economy: economic, social, and environmental impact on mental wellness. *Frontiers in Psychiatry, 14*, 1228355. doi:10.3389/fpsyt.2023.1228355 PMID:37383621

Benjamin, B., Jussen, A., Rafi, A., Lux, G., & Gerken, J. (2022). A Taxonomy for Augmented and Mixed Reality Applications to Support Physical Exercises in Medical Rehabilitation—A Literature Review. *Health Care, 10*(4), 646. doi:10.3390/healthcare10040646 PMID:35455824

Brea-Gómez, B., Torres-Sánchez, I., Ortíz-Rubio, A., Calvache-Mateo, A., Cabrera-Martos, I., López-López, L., & Valenza, M. C. (2021). Virtual Reality in the Treatment of Adults with Chronic Low Back Pain: A Systematic Review and Meta-analysis of Randomized Clinical Trials. *International Journal of Environmental Research and Public Health, 18*(22), 11806. doi:10.3390/ijerph182211806 PMID:34831562

Brelet, L., & Gaffary, Y. (2022b). Stress reduction interventions: A scoping review to explore progress toward using haptic feedback in virtual reality. *Frontiers in Virtual Reality, 3*, 900970. doi:10.3389/frvir.2022.900970

Brugada-Ramentol, V., Bozorgzadeh, A., & Jalali, H. (2022). Enhance VR: A multisensory approach to cognitive training and monitoring. *Frontiers in Digital Health, 4*, 916052. Advance online publication. doi:10.3389/fdgth.2022.916052 PMID:35721794

Canali, S., Schiaffonati, V., & Aliverti, A. (2022). Challenges and recommendations for wearable devices in digital health: Data quality, interoperability, health equity, fairness. *PLOS Digital Health, 1*(10), e0000104. doi:10.1371/journal.pdig.0000104 PMID:36812619

Channa, A., Popescu, N., Skibińska, J., & Bürget, R. (2021). The Rise of Wearable Devices during the COVID-19 Pandemic: A Systematic Review. *Sensors (Basel), 21*(17), 5787. doi:10.3390/s21175787 PMID:34502679

Clarke, E. (2021). Virtual reality simulation—The future of orthopaedic training? A systematic review and narrative analysis. *Advances in Simulation (London, England), 6*(1), 2. doi:10.1186/s41077-020-00153-x PMID:33441190

Dechsling, A., Orm, S., Kalandadze, T., Sütterlin, S., Øien, R. A., Shic, F., & Nordahl-Hansen, A. (2021). Virtual and Augmented Reality in Social Skills Interventions for Individuals with Autism Spectrum Disorder: A Scoping Review. *Journal of Autism and Developmental Disorders, 52*(11), 4692–4707. doi:10.1007/s10803-021-05338-5 PMID:34783991

Doshi, R., Hiran, K. K., Gök, M., El-kenawy, E. S. M., Badr, A., & Abotaleb, M. (2023). Artificial Intelligence's Significance in Diseases with Malignant Tumours. *Mesopotamian Journal of Artificial Intelligence in Healthcare, 2023*, 35–39.

Gambella, E., Margaritini, A., Benadduci, M., Rossi, L., D'Ascoli, P., Riccardi, G. R., Pasquini, S., Civerchia, P., Pelliccioni, G., Bevilacqua, R., & Maranesi, E. (2022). An integrated intervention of computerized cognitive training and physical exercise in virtual reality for people with Alzheimer's disease: The home study protocol. *Frontiers in Neurology, 13*, 964454. doi:10.3389/fneur.2022.964454 PMID:36034306

Harvie, D. S. (2021). Immersive Education for Chronic Condition Self-Management. *Frontiers in Virtual Reality, 2*, 657761. doi:10.3389/frvir.2021.657761

Kim, H., Kim, D. J., Kim, S., Chung, W. H., Park, K., Kim, J. D. K., Kim, D., Kim, M. J., Kim, K., & Jeon, H. J. (2021d). Effect of virtual reality on stress reduction and change of physiological parameters including heart rate variability in people with high stress: An open randomized crossover trial. *Frontiers in Psychiatry, 12*, 614539. doi:10.3389/fpsyt.2021.614539 PMID:34447320

Linton, M., Dieppe, P., & Medina-Lara, A. (2016). Review of 99 self-report measures for assessing well-being in adults: Exploring dimensions of well-being and developments over time. *BMJ Open, 6*(7), e010641. doi:10.1136/bmjopen-2015-010641 PMID:27388349

Longo, U. G., Carnevale, A., Andreoli, F., Mannocchi, I., Bravi, M., Sassi, M. S. H., Santacaterina, F., Carli, M., Schena, E., & Papalia, R. (2023). Immersive virtual reality for shoulder rehabilitation: Evaluation of a physical therapy program executed with Oculus Quest 2. *BMC Musculoskeletal Disorders, 24*(1), 859. doi:10.1186/s12891-023-06861-5 PMID:37919702

Meena, G., Dhanwal, B., Mahrishi, M., & Hiran, K. K. (2021, August). Performance comparison of network intrusion detection system based on different pre-processing methods and deep neural network. In *Proceedings of the International Conference on Data Science, Machine Learning and Artificial Intelligence* (pp. 110-115). ACM. 10.1145/3484824.3484878

Mokmin, N. M., & Jamiat, N. (2020). The effectiveness of a virtual fitness trainer app in motivating and engaging students for fitness activity by applying motor learning theory. *Education and Information Technologies, 26*(2), 1847–1864. doi:10.1007/s10639-020-10337-7

Oades, L. G., & Mossman, L. H. (2017). The science of well-being and positive Psychology. In Cambridge University Press eBooks (pp. 7–23). doi:10.1017/9781316339275.003

Patel, S., Vyas, A. K., & Hiran, K. K. (2022). Infrastructure health monitoring using signal processing based on an industry 4.0 System. *Cyber-Physical Systems and Industry, 4*, 249–260.

Pinar, M. (2018). Multidimensional Well-Being and Inequality Across the European Regions with Alternative Interactions Between the Well-Being Dimensions. *Social Indicators Research, 144*(1), 31–72. doi:10.1007/s11205-018-2047-4

Proctor, C. (2014). Subjective Well-Being (SWB). Springer eBooks. doi:10.1007/978-94-007-0753-5_2905

Rajkumar, E., Gopi, A., Joshi, A. C., Thomas, A. E., Arunima, N. M., Ramya, G. S., Kulkarni, P., Rahul, P., George, A. J., John, R., & Abraham, J. (2023). Applications, benefits and challenges of telehealth in India during COVID-19 pandemic and beyond a systematic review. *BMC Health Services Research, 23*(1), 7. doi:10.1186/s12913-022-08970-8 PMID:36597088

Ramasamy, J., Doshi, R., & Hiran, K. K. (2021, August). Segmentation of brain tumor using deep learning methods: a review. In *Proceedings of the International Conference on Data Science, Machine Learning and Artificial Intelligence* (pp. 209-215). ACM. 10.1145/3484824.3484876

Ramasamy, J., Doshi, R., & Hiran, K. K. (2022, October). Detection of Brain Tumor in Medical Images Based on Feature Extraction by HOG and Machine Learning Algorithms. In *2022 International Conference on Trends in Quantum Computing and Emerging Business Technologies (TQCEBT)* (pp. 1-5). IEEE. 10.1109/TQCEBT54229.2022.10041564

Riegler, A., Riener, A., & Holzmann, C. (2021). A Systematic Review of Virtual Reality Applications for Automated Driving: 2009–2020. *Frontiers in Human Dynamics*, *3*, 689856. doi:10.3389/fhumd.2021.689856

Rizzo, A., Goodwin, G. J., De Vito, A. N., & Bell, J. D. (2021b). Recent advances in virtual reality and psychology: Introduction to the special issue. *Translational Issues in Psychological Science*, *7*(3), 213–217. doi:10.1037/tps0000316

Ronaghi, M. H. (2022). The effect of virtual reality technology and education on sustainable behaviour: A comparative quasi-experimental study. *Interactive Technology and Smart Education*. doi:10.1108/ITSE-02-2022-0025

Ruggeri, K., García-Garzón, E., Maguire, Á., Matz, S., & Huppert, F. A. (2020). Well-being is more than happiness and life satisfaction: A multidimensional analysis of 21 countries. *Health and Quality of Life Outcomes*, *18*(1), 192. doi:10.1186/s12955-020-01423-y PMID:32560725

Scavarelli, A., Arya, A., & Teather, R. J. (2020). Virtual reality and augmented reality in social learning spaces: A literature review. *Virtual Reality (Waltham Cross)*, *25*(1), 257–277. doi:10.1007/s10055-020-00444-8

Scurati, G. W., Bertoni, M., Graziosi, S., & Ferrise, F. (2021). Exploring the use of virtual reality to support environmentally sustainable behaviour: A framework to design experiences. *Sustainability (Basel)*, *13*(2), 943. doi:10.3390/su13020943

Segawa, T., Baudry, T., Bourla, A., Blanc, J., Peretti, C., Mouchabac, S., & Ferreri, F. (2020). Virtual Reality (VR) in Assessment and Treatment of Addictive Disorders: A Systematic review. *Frontiers in Neuroscience*, *13*, 1409. doi:10.3389/fnins.2019.01409 PMID:31998066

Siani, A., & Marley, S. A. (2021). Impact of the recreational use of virtual reality on physical and mental well-being during the COVID-19 lockdown. *Health and Technology*, *11*(2), 425–435. doi:10.1007/s12553-021-00528-8 PMID:33614391

Simons, G., & Baldwin, D. S. (2021). A critical review of the definition of 'well-being' for doctors and their patients in a post-COVID-19 era. *The International Journal of Social Psychiatry*, *67*(8), 984–991. doi:10.1177/00207640211032259 PMID:34240644

Srinivasulu, A.A., Gupta, A., Hiran, K., Barua, T., & Sreenivasulu, G. (2022). Omi-cron Virus Data Analytics Using Extended RNN Technique. *Int J Cancer Res Ther, 7*(3), *122* 1-3.

Stewart, T. H., Villaneuva, K., Hahn, A., Ortiz-Delatorre, J., Wolf, C., Nguyen, R., Bolter, N. D., Kern, M., & Bagley, J. R. (2022). Actual vs. perceived exertion during active virtual reality game exercise. *Frontiers in Rehabilitation Sciences*, *3*, 887740. doi:10.3389/fresc.2022.887740 PMID:36189005

Tarrant, J., Viczko, J., & Cope, H. (2018). Virtual reality for anxiety Reduction Demonstrated by Quantitative EEG: A pilot study. *Frontiers in Psychology*, *9*, 1280. doi:10.3389/fpsyg.2018.01280 PMID:30087642

Wiederhold, M. D., & Wiederhold, B. K. (2007). Virtual Reality and Interactive Simulation for Pain Distraction: Table 1. *Pain Medicine*, *8*(suppl 3), S182–S188. doi:10.1111/j.1526-4637.2007.00381.x

Zhao, M., Wang, D., & Li, J. (2021). Data management and visualization of wearable medical devices assisted by artificial intelligence. *Network Modeling and Analysis in Health Informatics and Bioinformatics*, *10*(1), 53. doi:10.1007/s13721-021-00328-0

KEY TERMS AND DEFINITIONS

Augmented Reality (AR): Technology that overlays digital information onto the real world, enhancing perception, often via smartphone apps or smart glasses.

Education: The process of acquiring knowledge and skills, often in formal settings such as schools, colleges, or online platforms.

Healthcare: The system or practice providing medical care, prevention, and treatment for physical and mental conditions.

Self-Care: Personal practices and activities undertaken to maintain and improve one's physical, mental, and emotional well-being.

Social Interactions: How individuals communicate, engage, and connect in various social contexts and settings.

Virtual Reality (VR): Immersive technology that creates a computer-generated environment, allowing users to interact and explore.

Well-being: The state of overall health, happiness, and prosperity in various aspects of life, including physical, mental, and social well-being.

Chapter 5
Multimedia Text Extraction for Healthcare Applications

B. Madhu
Dr. Ambedkar Institute of Technology, India

R. Likhitha
Dr. Ambedkar Institute of Technology, India

Prajna
Dr. Ambedkar Institute of Technology, India

ABSTRACT

Image, audio, and video are rapidly evolving multimedia data, creating a platform for the creation, exchange, and storage of information in the modern era. Multiple techniques are available for content-based image, video, and audio retrieval using image processing methods to extract text features of the data. These methods produce similar text but not the same as per the user expectation. In this chapter, the authors offer an approach that uses edge map generation and Google tesseract-based text detection in image as well as in video. The accuracy of our method is 98% for speed video extraction, 100% for image/video/audio data.

INTRODUCTION

The automatic text extraction system involves intelligent algorithms to identify and extract the textual content present in various kinds of images, video and audio. With the advent of the digital era and the availability of myriad of multimedia contents, it has become extremely important to read and interpret the texts associated with those contents. The automatic extraction of texts would not only serve to infer the semantics of those multimedia documents but also help in efficient indexing and subsequent retrieval of the same. However, the text differs in size, style, alignment etc. and low resolution of the background of complex images make the problem of text identification a complex one. Hence, the extraction of text data in images has become a challenging field of research in Image Processing. The main

DOI: 10.4018/979-8-3693-1123-3.ch005

drawback of the existing methods is texture-based or connected-component based is that they are unable to provide accurate results with great precision for the applications of text extraction. Kavyashree and Rajesh (2018) introduced text detection and analysis from background images. The applications are they have mentioned many applications of text identification and verification found such as picture indexing based on text, image searching the google based on keyword, old, required documents examination extraction of number from number plates from vehicles involved in crime etc. Doshi and Hiran (2023) and Dhir (2016) reported the concept of text extraction using video. Mishra et al. (2021), Ramasamy et al. (2021), and Thilagavathy et al. (2012) presented the concept of ANN based network for Text Extraction from Video. Applications are the natural text of video like text on banners, signs, container, CD cover, sign board, text on vehicle and caption text or text that is artificially overlaid on the video/image such as the scores in sports videos, subtitles in news video, date, and time in the video. Hiran et al. (2013) and Neogib and Balajib (2016) presented automation in the text extraction process for complex images. Text extraction process with video data is reported by Ramsamy and Doshi (2022). The method mainly concentrates on Multiframe corner point matching. Heuristic rules could be flexibly used to filter the candidate text regions according to the style of the video scene, which improved the efficiency of the algorithm and decreased the false alarm rate. A new method of document text extraction is supported by Meena et a. (2021) and Yadav and Ragot (2016). The applications of document image processing include contemporary documents like books, administrative letters and documents. Bhalekar and Bedekar (2022) and Hiran and Doshi (2013) reported generative model for Image Captions with Deep learning-based text extraction for Visually Challenged Individuals" they have specified that text extraction is useful in many social relevance applications such as video surveillance, navigation for visually challenged individuals, online education systems, medical assistance, and many more which add significant value in our daily lives. Too and Prabakar (2016) suggested the outcome of Scene Text Information from Video. The applications are extended to text in trucks, t-shirts, buildings, billboards, arbitrary text layouts, multi-scripts, artistic fonts, colours, complex and variable background. Grover et al. (2009) and Doshi et al. (2023) reported new method of text Extraction using edge information used for text searches in Images, Content based Indexing, Reading foreign language text, Archiving documents. Raju and Anita (2017) and Fagbola et al. (2022) outline the extraction of text for video key searching and assisting visually challenged people using video indexing. Jabil et al. (2016) reported artificial text extraction for pattern classification and image analysis. Jain et al. (2023) reported multiscale edge based text extraction. Text appears in scanned CD/book or video images. Video text can broadly be classified into two categories: overlay text and scene text. (Overlay text refers to those characters generated by graphic titling machines and superimposed on video frames/images, such as video captions, while scene text occurs naturally as a part of scene, such as text in information boards/signs, nameplates, food containers, etc.). Antani et al. (2000) reported text extraction of video using OCR. The text detection results from a variety of methods are fused and each single text instance. Salman et al. (2016) investigated on android application-based feature and text extraction from images. There are different applications where text extraction can be applicable for various useful applications like digital libraries, information retrieval systems, Geographical Information systems, Multimedia Systems. Further Goel et al. (2023) reported Printed Images text extraction for industries and organizations. These images can contain the data - of any language, can be of good or degraded quality, can be B&W or colored, can contain Meta data or images and so on. It also reported on an easy method of OCR text extraction. Detection of text from documents in which text is embedded in complex colored document images is a very challenging problem. There are a lot of potential users who want to extract the text from images, archiving documents etc. It aims at detecting textual regions from the document and separating it from the graphics portion. Getting information directly from applications forms and it saves a lot of time. Guo et al. (2016) proposed video text extraction for the educational and news video. Yangyu reported text Extraction based on Web Images. Since web images is an important part of the web document and have been rapidly integrated into web pages as a powerful content delivery medium. They are used for a variety of purposes, such as navigation, decoration, advertisements, logos, and informational images. The text embedded often corresponds to page headers, titles, URLs and, therefore, has a potentially high semantic value for web document analysis and understanding. One common use of this semantic value is in terms of information indexing and retrieval. Antani et al. (2000) reported Region Based and Connected Component model for the Text Extraction based on edge detectors. This problem is challenging due to the complex background, the non-uniform illumination, and the variations of text font, size, and line orientation. Digital formats make it simpler to save, retrieve, and analyse paper-based medical information, prescriptions, and reports. Electronic health records (EHRs) may be created using text extracted from scanned medical papers, and seamless data sharing between healthcare providers is made possible. Data can be extracted from medical images like Anatomical labels, patient IDs, and research details are just a few examples of the embedded text that can occasionally be found in medical images. In a medical imaging database, extracting this text from the photos can aid in the correct archiving, indexing, and retrieval of the images. There are several monitoring devices that show vital signs including heart rate, blood pressure, and oxygen levels in critical care units and other medical settings. These displays' text can be extracted to provide real-time data analysis and notifications for important changes. Critical information regarding patients' health state is frequently included in medical laboratory reports. In order to aggregate and analyse lab test information for improved patient care, text extraction from lab reports might be helpful. The proposed method performs efficient text extraction and recognition from both images and videos. Optical character recognition (OCR) is used to extract the text from images. Video text recognition is performed by converting the video input into the audio file and with the help of Google Cloud Search API it recognizes the text from the audio and writes the same in the text file. The text file can also be converted to QR code to maintain confidentiality.

PROPOSED SYSTEM

The Proposed method is based on the concept of edge mapping. An edge map is an image that shows the locations of the image's edges. The most important role in image processing systems is to generate edge maps, which are used to identify specific objects in an image and store important data about those items. The block diagram of the method is shown in Figure 1 and 2. It is divided into three modules viz. Edge map generation, Text area segmentation and Text recognition module. The input can be any type of multimedia data like Image/Audio/Video to the system and the output obtained is in the form of a text file and QR Code.

Modules/Libraries Required

- moviepy: It is required to work with audio and video files. Here we have used 'AudioFileClip' class from 'moviepy.editor' to load and manipulate audio clips from video files.
- tkinter: It is required for creating a GUI(Graphical User Interface).

Figure 1. Text extraction from image

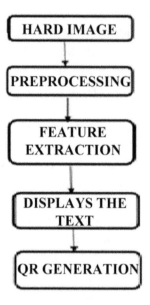

Figure 2. Text extraction from video

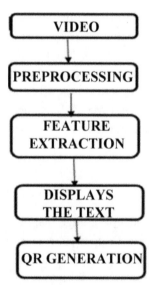

- pydub: To manipulate the audio files that are extracted.
- pytesseract: It is an OCR tool for python. It will read and recognize the text from images.
- SpeechRecognition: It is used for speech recognition tasks in our project we have included sr.AudioFile class from the library SpeechRecognition.
- wave: this module is used for reading and writing WAV files.

Figure 3. Text extraction from audio

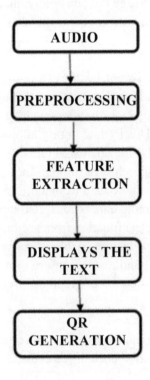

METHODOLOGIES AND TECHNIQUES

- **Preprocessing:**

Text extraction from Image: Preprocessing is the initial stage where the image is prepared and enhanced to improve the OCR accuracy. It aims to reduce noise, improve text contrast, and correct geometric distortions.

Text extraction from Video: In the preprocessing stage video is prepared and it is then converted to the audio file and save it in the wav format.

- **Processing (Recognition):**

The processing stage involves actually recognizing the text in the preprocessed image, video and audio. OCR engines use various techniques for character recognition, including traditional machine learning algorithms and deep learning models. Speech recognition use various techniques for recognizing the audio file. The primary steps in the processing stage are:

- **Text Detection:** Identifying the regions of interest in the image that potentially contain text. This step is crucial when dealing with complex images that may contain multiple elements. In audio files it detects the words used in the language.

- **Character Segmentation**: If the image contains individual characters or glyphs (e.g., handwritten text), the OCR engine may need to segment the characters to recognize them individually. In extracting the text from video, it is recognized by the audio and writes the words which are recognized.
- **Feature Extraction**: Extracting relevant features from the text regions, which are then used to represent the characters for recognition. Features may include stroke direction, edge information, or other characteristics that help distinguish different characters.
- SpeechRecognition Library (sr): This Python library allows us to recognize speech with different APIs. It is used to process the audio file and extract text.
- AudioFile and Recognizer from SpeechRecognition: These are extensions from the above library calls. AudioFile allows to read the audio data from a file and Recognizer is used to perform.
- Google Speech Recognition:The audio data is converted into text using Google's sppech recognition service using recognize_google() function from sr library.
- GUI Toolkit (Possibly tkinter): This feature enables the user to interact with a GUI to get an input in entry.get() and textarea.delete() and textarea.insert() for text manipulation in a text area. The tkinter library can be used for the creation of graphical user interface (GUI).
  - Post-processing:

After the OCR engine recognizes the characters and converts them into text, the post-processing stage is applied to improve the accuracy and coherence of the extracted text.

Techniques likely used are:

- ➤ **Tkinter:** Tkinter is a GUI library used for designing the window or user interface of the application. It allows creating buttons, input fields, and other graphical elements for user interaction with the text extraction functionalities.
- ➤ **Pytesseract:** Pytesseract is a wrapper for Tesseract OCR engine, which is a popular open-source OCR tool. It is used for reading and recognizing text in images, which is the core text extraction technique used in this project.
- ➤ **Wave:** The Wave library is used to handle audio files in WAV format. It is likely used to interface with audio files generated during the text-to-speech conversion or audio extraction from video files (e.g., MP4 to WAV).
- ➤ **Moviepy:** Moviepy is used for video processing and is employed in this project to convert video files (MP4) to audio files (WAV) to extract audio data for speech recognition.
- ➤ **PIL (Pillow):** PIL (Python Imaging Library) or Pillow is used for image processing. It provides functionalities to manipulate and enhance images, which could be relevant for pre-processing images before applying OCR techniques
  - Image to Text Extraction (imgtxt() function):

The pytesseract library is used to perform OCR (Optical Character Recognition) on the input image. It extracts text from the image using the pytesseract.image_to_string() function. The extracted text is displayed in a text area for user viewing

- Video to Text Extraction (videotxt() function):

The input video file is processed using moviepy to convert it into an audio file (WAV format). The speech_recognition library is utilized to perform speech recognition on the audio file. The function iterates through the audio in 60-second chunks, recognizing speech using the Google Web Speech API (recognize_google()), and writes the recognized text to a text file (transcription.txt).

• The GUI application allows users to select between two options:

"Image to Text Extraction" and "Video to Text Extraction." For image extraction, the user enters the file path of the image, and the application uses pytesseract to extract and display the text. For video extraction, the user enters the file name/path of the video, and the application uses moviepy and speech_recognition to extract speech from the video and display the recognized text.

RESULTS AND DISCUSSIONS

The suggested method is implemented using python in Visual Studio. There will be three options from which the user must select as shown in Figure.3.The first option for the conversion is to convert the text from an image. The image is given as an input to the process. Path name has to be specified for this conversion. The second option is to convert the text from video data. Initially the video is converted to audio then text will be displayed on the screen. The other multimedia data type is audio to text and text to audio as well as recognition of the same.

The process of text extraction from the image as well as from Video has been shown in Figure 3.

The path of an image or video need to be given as input to the process as in Figure 4. The input can be taken from the camera for the conversion process.Figure 4 and Figure 5 depicts the input as image and video respectively.

The result of the proposed method for the text extraction of an image/audio/video is 100% and for the fast speed video the detection accuracy is 98.99%.

Figure 4. User options either image to text or video to text

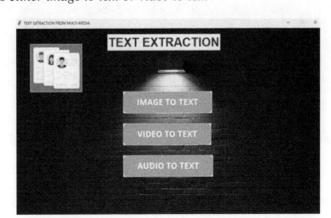

Figure 5. Image to text extraction window

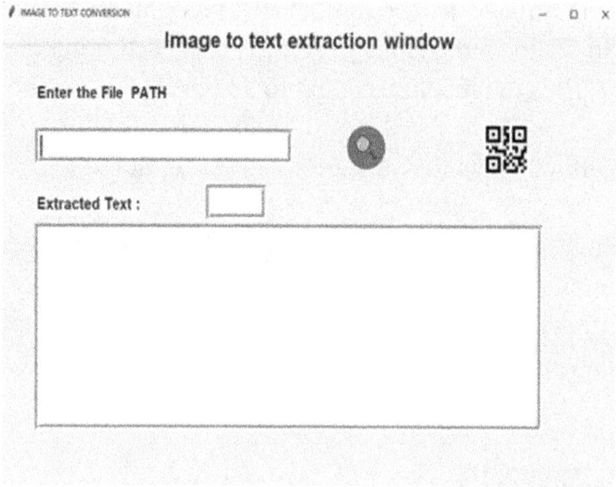

Figure 6. Video to text extraction window

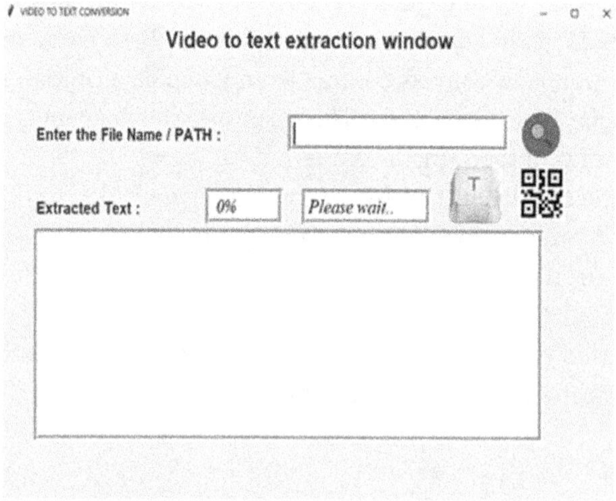

Figure 7. Audio to text extraction window, user can enter the path of audio from which text has to be extracted or user can also record the audio by click on the mic

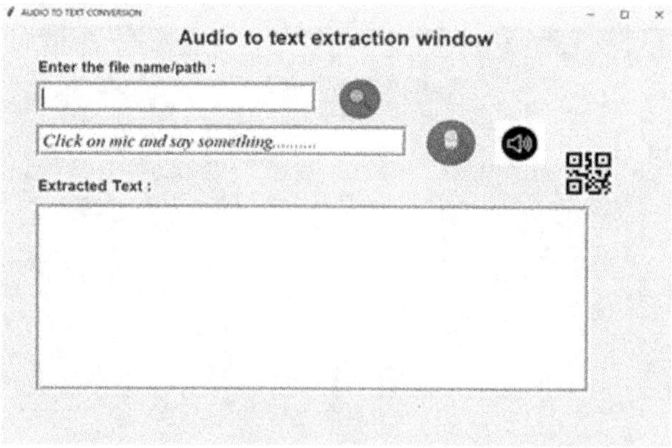

Figure 8. Path of the image has been given to extract the text and the same extracted text is displayed

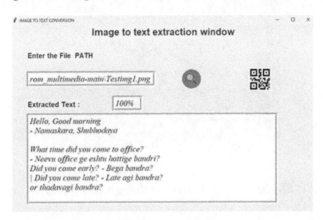

Figure 9. QR is generated to the extracted text from the image

Figure 10. Output of the scanned above QR

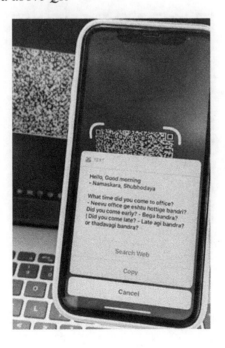

Figure 11. Test image is used to extract the text from it

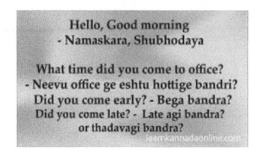

Figure 12. Path of the video has been given to extract the text and the same extracted text is displayed

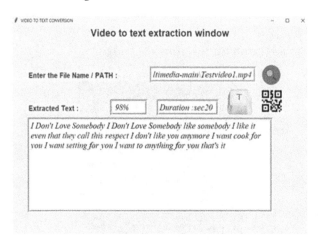

Figure 13. QR is generated to the extracted text from the video

Figure 14. Output of the Scanned QR code

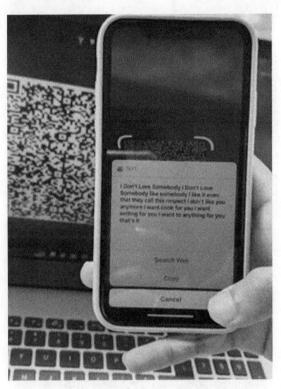

Figure 15. Video input for the extraction process

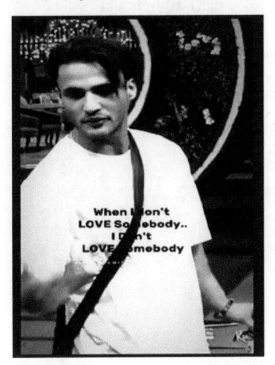

Figure 16. Path of the audio has been given to extract the text and the same extracted text is displayed

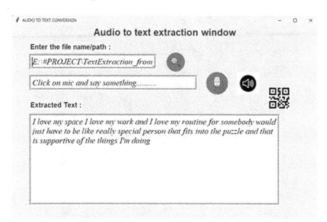

Figure 17. QR is generated to the extracted text from the audio file

Figure 18. Output of the scanned QR

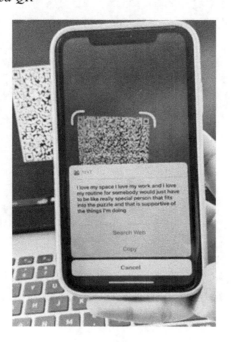

Figure 19. Audio is recorded using the mic button the same is displayed

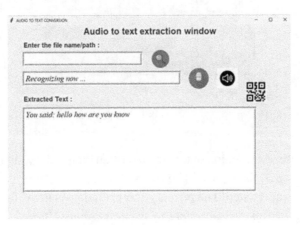

Figure 20. Result of speaker button

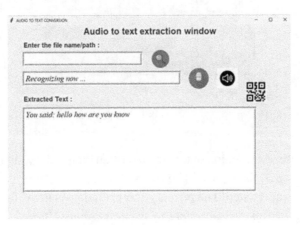

Figure 21. QR is generated to the extracted text from the recorded audio

Figure 22. Output of scanned above QR

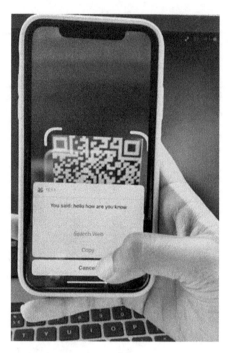

CONCLUSION

Text extraction is the process of extraction of text from written materials, visual media, or scanned PDFs. It can be used for the data analysis process. The overwhelming amount of data in healthcare make the necessary for digitization in every step. The primary source of data is in the form of scanned documents, images, and audio/video. Text extraction refers to the extraction of text from documents, images, or scanned PDFs. It is an essential part of the data analysis process and is used to gain insights from large amounts of text data. The proposed method provides an optimal solution in the conversion of multimedia data to the text for further data analysis using Edge detection and OCR. The accuracy of the suggested method is 98% for the high-speed video and 100% for the image/audio/video data.

REFERENCES

Antani, S., Crandall, D., & Kasturi, R. (2000, September). Robust extraction of text in video. In *Proceedings 15th International Conference on Pattern Recognition. ICPR-2000* (Vol. 1, pp. 831-834). IEEE.

Bhalekar, M., & Bedekar, M. (2022). D-CNN: A new model for generating image captions with text extraction using deep learning for visually challenged individuals. *Engineering, Technology & Applied Scientific Research, 12*(2), 8366–8373.

Dhir, R. (2016, March). Video Text extraction and recognition: A survey. In *2016 International Conference on Wireless Communications, Signal Processing and Networking (WiSPNET)* (pp. 1366-1373). IEEE.

Doshi, R., & Hiran, K. K. (2023). Decision Making and IoT: Bibliometric Analysis for Scopus Database. *Babylonian Journal of Internet of Things*, *2023*, 13–22.

Doshi, R., Hiran, K. K., Gök, M., El-kenawy, E. S. M., Badr, A., & Abotaleb, M. (2023). Artificial Intelligence's Significance in Diseases with Malignant Tumours. *Mesopotamian Journal of Artificial Intelligence in Healthcare*, *2023*, 35–39.

Fagbola, T. M., Fagbola, F. I., Aroba, O. J., Doshi, R., Hiran, K. K., & Thakur, S. C. (2022). Smart face masks for Covid-19 pandemic management: A concise review of emerging architectures, challenges and future research directions. *IEEE Sensors Journal*, *23*(2), 877–888.

Goel, P., Jhanwar, N., Jain, P., Khatri, S., & Hiran, K. K. (2023, August). Efficient Blood Availability for Targeted Individuals Through Cloud Computing Web Application. In *2023 International Conference on Emerging Trends in Networks and Computer Communications (ETNCC)* (pp. 1-7). IEEE.

Grover, S., Arora, K., & Mitra, S. K. (2009, December). Text extraction from document images using edge information. In *2009 Annual IEEE India Conference* (pp. 1-4). IEEE.

Guo, Z., Li, Y., Wang, Y., Liu, S., Lei, T., & Fan, Y. (2016). A method of effective text extraction for complex video scene. *Mathematical Problems in Engineering*.

Hiran, K. K., & Doshi, R. (2013). An artificial neural network approach for brain tumor detection using digital image segmentation. *Brain*, *2*(5), 227–231.

Hiran, K. K., Doshi, R., Kant, K., Ruchi, H., & Lecturer, D. S. (2013). Robust & secure digital image watermarking technique using concatenation process. *International Journal of ICT and Management*.

Jain, R. K., Hiran, K. K., & Maheshwari, R. (2023, April). Lung Cancer Detection Using Machine Learning Algorithms. In *2023 International Conference on Computational Intelligence, Communication Technology and Networking (CICTN)* (pp. 516-521). IEEE.

Jamil, A., Batool, A., Malik, Z., Mirza, A., & Siddiqi, I. (2016). Multilingual artificial text extraction and script identification from video images. *International Journal of Advanced Computer Science and Applications*, *7*(4).

Kavyashree, D., & Rajesh, T. M. (2018). Analysis on Text Detection and Extraction from Complex Background Images. *Pattern Recogn*, 37-43.

Meena, G., Dhanwal, B., Mahrishi, M., & Hiran, K. K. (2021, August). Performance comparison of network intrusion detection systems based on different pre-processing methods and deep neural network. In *Proceedings of the International Conference on Data Science, Machine Learning and Artificial Intelligence* (pp. 110-115). Academic Press.

Mishra, A., Tripathi, A., Khazanchi, D., Hiran, K. K., Vyas, A. K., & Padmanaban, S. (2021). A framework for applying artificial intelligence (AI) with Internet of NanoThings (IoNT). In *Machine Learning for Sustainable Development* (pp. 1–16). De Gruyter.

Raju, N., & Anita, H. B. (2017). Text extraction from video images. *International Journal of Applied Engineering Research: IJAER*, *12*(24), 14750–14754.

Ramasamy, J., & Doshi, R. (2022). Machine learning in cyber physical systems for healthcare: brain tumor classification from MRI using transfer learning framework. In *Real-Time Applications of Machine Learning in Cyber-Physical Systems* (pp. 65–76). IGI global.

Ramasamy, J., Doshi, R., & Hiran, K. K. (2021, August). Segmentation of brain tumor using deep learning methods: a review. In *Proceedings of the International Conference on Data Science, Machine Learning and Artificial Intelligence* (pp. 209-215). Academic Press.

SalmanG.ShanwarB.ZarkaN. (2016). *Multiscale edge-based text extraction from complex images.* doi:10.13140/RG.2.1.1197.7200

Thilagavathy, A., Aarthi, K., & Chilambuchelvan, A. (2012). Text detection and extraction from videos using ann based network. *International Journal on Soft Computing Artificial Intelligence and Applications (Commerce, Calif.)*, *1*(1).

Too, B. K., & Prabhakar, C. J. (2016). *Extraction of scene text information from video*. Academic Press.

Yadav, V., & Ragot, N. (2016, April). Text extraction in document images: highlight on using corner points. In *2016 12th IAPR Workshop on Document Analysis Systems (DAS)* (pp. 281-286). IEEE.

Chapter 6
Mental Health Treatment:
Exploring the Potential of Augmented Reality and Virtual Reality

Ranjit Singha

iD https://orcid.org/0000-0002-3541-8752

Christ University, India

Surjit Singha

iD https://orcid.org/0000-0002-5730-8677

Kristu Jayanti College (Autonomous), India

ABSTRACT

By producing immersive, individualized, and captivating therapeutic experiences, augmented reality (AR) and virtual reality (VR) may significantly transform mental health treatment. These technologies provide efficacious resolutions for exposure therapy, augmenting conventional methodologies, mitigating social disapproval, and fortifying the therapeutic alliance. Virtual and augmented reality increase the accessibility and convenience of therapy by enabling highly individualized interventions. Training for mental health professionals, rigorous research, compliance with data privacy regulations, and adherence to ethical standards are essential for responsible use. Augmented reality (AR) and virtual reality (VR) can expand the accessibility of mental health services as costs decrease, thereby ultimately enhancing the welfare of those in search of assistance and recovery. Incorporating augmented reality and virtual reality into clinical practice may make mental health treatment more engaging, effective, and individualized.

INTRODUCTION

The utilization of virtual reality (VR) and augmented reality (AR) is becoming increasingly significant in the dynamic field of healthcare and technology, as evidenced by the growing attention they receive as new instruments for addressing several dimensions of health and welfare (Sutherland et al., 2018; Xu et al., 2021). This chapter establishes the fundamental basis for our investigation into the potential transformative impact of virtual reality (VR) and augmented reality (AR) on mental health therapy.

DOI: 10.4018/979-8-3693-1123-3.ch006

Augmented Reality (AR) and Virtual Reality (VR) are two different yet interconnected technology realms that facilitate user immersion in digital surroundings or enhance their experience of the physical world. Virtual Reality (VR) is a computer-generated simulation that offers users a fully immersive and three-dimensional experience. Individuals utilize specialized headphones designed to obstruct the sensory perception of the physical environment, substituting it with a digitally synthesized realm. Virtual Reality (VR) enables users to engage with a simulated environment by utilizing many sensory inputs, including visual and auditory stimuli. This integration of sensory information facilitates a heightened state of presence and Immersion within the virtual environment (Buettner et al., 2020; Sutherland et al., 2018; Xu et al., 2021).

In contrast, Augmented Reality (AR) superimposes digital content onto the tangible environment, commonly facilitated by smartphones, headsets, or other intelligent devices. Augmented reality (AR) enhances an individual's experience by seamlessly merging computer-generated components, such as images, sounds, or data, into their immediate physical environment. According to Buettner et al. (2020), this particular technology enhances the existing physical environment rather than completely supplant it. The provision of mental health therapy is a multifaceted and crucial component of the healthcare system, encompassing a wide range of emotional, psychological, and psychiatric disorders. A notable obstacle is the enduring social disapproval associated with mental health concerns. Stigma frequently acts as a barrier for persons in their pursuit of assistance, impeding prompt implementation of intervention and treatment measures. The provision of mental health services exhibits disparities since several persons residing in geographically isolated regions or marginalized populations encounter limited availability of qualified mental health practitioners. According to Gaiha et al. (2020) and Peter et al. (2021) Sustaining continuous patient involvement and motivation during treatment can provide challenges, given that conventional therapeutic approaches may not universally connect with all individuals. Mental health practitioners frequently experience excessive workloads due to the substantial demand for their services, leading to protracted waiting periods and constrained resources. The mental health field recognizes the importance of individualization, wherein treatment approaches are ideally customized to align with each individual's specific requirements and preferences. Attaining such a degree of customization cost-efficiently poses difficulties within traditional healthcare environments (Hornstein et al., 2023; Woods et al., 2020). Given the difficulties above, this chapter establishes the foundation for a thorough investigation into the potential of augmented reality and virtual reality technologies in providing novel remedies to improve mental health interventions, enhancing the standard of care, increasing accessibility, and optimizing patient outcomes. Virtual Reality (VR) and Augmented Reality (AR) can revolutionize the mental health treatment domain through immersive and interactive features. These technologies offer novel pathways for therapeutic interventions, enhance accessibility to mental health services, and mitigate the social stigma associated with seeking assistance for mental health concerns (Pons et al., 2022; Woods et al., 2020).

To comprehensively understand the possibilities of augmented reality (AR) and virtual reality (VR) within mental health therapy, it is imperative to grasp the foundational theories and background that substantiate its utilization. This section comprehensively examines prominent theoretical frameworks and the historical progression of augmented reality (AR) and virtual reality (VR) within mental health. The Cognitive-Behavioral Theory is a fundamental framework for numerous mental health interventions, emphasizing the intricate relationship between thoughts, emotions, and behaviours. Augmented reality (AR) and virtual reality (VR) technologies have the potential to provide immersive environments that can effectively manipulate cognitive and emotional processes, hence offering novel therapeutic possibilities. Exposure therapy is a widely recognized and proven therapeutic method utilized in the treatment of anxiety disorders. Augmented reality (AR) and virtual reality (VR) technologies allow individuals to experience anxiety-inducing circumstances in a controlled environment that is both safe and closely supervised (Meena, 2021; Ramasamy, 2022).

Consequently, these technologies have proven highly effective in facilitating desensitization and reducing anxiety levels (Baus & Bouchard, 2014; Freitas et al., 2021). Presence and Immersion in virtual reality (VR) pertains to the subjective experience of "being present" in the virtual environment. Immersion encompasses the degree to which a user feels deeply engaged. A comprehensive grasp of these principles is required to develop virtual reality interventions that evoke emotional reactions and foster engagement, essential for achieving therapeutic outcomes. Over recent decades, the integration of augmented reality (AR) and virtual reality (VR) technologies has been progressively used within mental health therapy. Over time, there has been a transition in the perception of these tools from experimental to widely accepted therapeutic interventions. This shift is accompanied by an expanding body of research that provides evidence for their effectiveness, as demonstrated in studies conducted by (Ionescu et al.,2021; Rawlins et al., 2021).

The objective of this chapter is to present a thorough examination of the prospective uses of augmented reality (AR) and virtual reality (VR) within the domain of mental health therapy. This investigation encompasses a range of aspects, including but not restricted to the following. We conducted an extensive examination of the current body of research and evidence about the effectiveness of augmented reality (AR) and virtual reality (VR) in the treatment of many mental health illnesses, including anxiety disorders, phobias, post-traumatic stress disorder (PTSD), depression, and schizophrenia. The virtues and limits of various technologies as therapeutic aids were evaluated. The chapter also explored the potential of augmented reality (AR) and virtual reality (VR) in enhancing the accessibility of mental health therapy. It encompasses extending services to marginalized people, offering teletherapy alternatives, and mitigating the social stigma around help-seeking behaviours.

The investigation examined how augmented reality (AR) and virtual reality (VR) may be customized to meet individuals' specific requirements and inclinations, hence facilitating personalized therapeutic encounters. Recognizing the inherent difficulties and ethical implications entailed in using augmented reality (AR) and virtual reality (VR) within the context of mental health intervention is of utmost significance. In this discussion, we will examine matters about data privacy, informed consent, and potential negative consequences. As the ongoing development of these technologies persists, we shall conjecture on prospective trajectories within the realms of augmented reality (AR) and virtual reality (VR) for the mental health domain. The factors mentioned above encompass the incorporation of artificial intelligence, progressions in hardware technology, and the establishment of standardized treatment methods.

This chapter endeavours to comprehensively comprehend the junction between technology and healthcare by conducting a meticulous analysis of the theoretical foundations, historical backdrop, and potential ramifications of augmented reality (AR) and virtual reality (VR) in the realm of mental health therapy. Moreover, it fosters continued scholarly inquiry and investigation within this domain to unleash the complete potential of augmented reality (AR) and virtual reality (VR) in enhancing mental health and overall well-being (Ramasamy, 2021).

BENEFITS OF AR AND VR IN MENTAL HEALTH TREATMENT

The utilization of Augmented Reality (AR) and Virtual Reality (VR) has brought forth a multitude of advantages within the field of mental health treatment, fundamentally transforming the approach and implementation of therapeutic interventions. Augmented reality (AR) and virtual reality (VR) technologies can provide highly immersive and sensorially stimulating worlds that captivate the user's focus. Within the therapeutic domain, this increased level of involvement might be beneficial for individuals in sustaining their attention during counselling or psychotherapy sessions, especially when dealing with conditions such as attention deficit disorders or challenges related to concentration (Albakri et al., 2022; Zeevi, 2021). Virtual environments can evoke intense emotional reactions. Therapeutic interventions can facilitate a deeper connection between individuals and their emotions and experiences, enhancing emotional expression and processing. This approach becomes advantageous, particularly in cases involving clients who encounter difficulties in effectively expressing their emotional experiences (Dehghan et al., 2022; Li et al., 2021). Augmented reality (AR) and virtual reality (VR) applications can enhance motivation and perseverance in therapeutic exercises and schoolwork due to their interactive characteristics. According to Tao et al. (2021), the incorporation of gamification components, rewards, and progress tracking can enhance the experience of therapeutic activities by transforming them into stimulating challenges, hence mitigating the perception of these activities as burdensome tasks. This approach is particularly advantageous for persons who struggle with depressive disorders or lack motivation. Augmented reality (AR) and virtual reality (VR) technologies enable the customization of therapeutic experiences. Therapists can develop tailored virtual scenarios and exercises that align with each client's unique requirements, inclinations, and therapeutic objectives. Incorporating customization can potentially enhance the efficacy and client-centeredness of therapies (Carroll et al., 2021; Hadjipanayi et al., 2023).

Virtual reality (VR) technology has proven beneficial in the context of exposure therapy. Therapists can facilitate desensitization and anxiety reduction in patients by gradually exposing them to their fears or triggers inside a virtual world, thereby immersing them in controlled and anxiety-provoking scenarios. The immersive quality of virtual reality (VR) amplifies the efficacy of this form of exposure. Augmented reality (AR) and virtual reality (VR) technologies might enhance the multimodal experience, improving the retention of therapeutic insights and coping methods. It can be especially beneficial for persons who experience difficulties with memory, such as those diagnosed with post-traumatic stress disorder (PTSD). Virtual environments can replicate a wide range of scenarios, enabling users to explore and assess alternate perspectives and the potential implications of decision-making. The utilization of this approach holds significant potential within the context of cognitive-behavioural therapy, as it facilitates the process of restructuring maladaptive cognitive schemas and enhancing one's ability to engage in problem-solving endeavours effectively (Boeldt et al., 2019; Freitas et al., 2021; Rimer et al., 2021; Takac et al., 2021;Trappey et al., 2020).

Augmented reality (AR) and virtual reality (VR) provide a regulated and non-threatening environment for persons who face challenges in self-expression or have a traumatic background. In this context, these technologies offer a safe space for individuals to engage in self-exploration and express their emotions. It is of particular significance to address matters about anxiety, post-traumatic stress disorder (PTSD), and interpersonal interactions. Technology in therapy facilitates a collaborative environment wherein the therapist and client actively participate, establishing a foundation of rapport and trust. Integrating augmented reality (AR) and virtual reality (VR) technologies into mental health therapy can potentially enhance engagement and Immersion, hence augmenting the efficacy of therapeutic interventions. The potential of technology to provide emotionally captivating, interactive, and customized experiences can revolutionize how mental health practitioners administer therapy and facilitate individuals in attaining their treatment objectives (Carroll et al., 2021; Lan et al., 2023).

Exposure therapy is a widely recognized and efficacious method utilized in the treatment of anxiety disorders, phobias, and post-traumatic stress disorder (PTSD). Augmented (AR) and virtual (VR) environments offer a secure and regulated context for individuals to confront their anxieties or triggers. The use of controlled exposure is crucial in the gradual reduction of anxiety and phobic reactions. Patients can confront their concerns in a controlled environment, mitigating the real-world risks typically connected with such scenarios. Therapists can customize exposure situations to cater to each patient's particular requirements. This customization facilitates a step-by-step escalation in the degree of exposure, commencing with settings that elicit lower anxiety levels and advancing towards more demanding scenarios as the patient's comfort level improves. The implementation of individualized exposure therapy has a pivotal role in the efficacy of treatment (Albakri et al.,2022; Baus & Bouchard 2014).

Virtual exposure sessions can be repeated as frequently as required. This particular attribute holds significant value in strengthening and honing coping skills. In addition, augmented reality (AR) and virtual reality (VR) technology can monitor patients' progress, thereby equipping therapists with measurable data to evaluate the efficacy of the treatment and make well-informed modifications. Virtual exposure offers a high level of convenience and accessibility, as it can be accessed on-demand. Exposure therapy allows patients to participate in treatment without being dependent on real-world triggers or schedule constraints, enhancing flexibility and responsiveness as a therapeutic approach (Baus & Bouchard, 2014; Rizzo et al., 2021).

The immersive aspect of VR stimulates emotional engagement. Patients can have a heightened and authentic emotional reaction within the virtual realm, a crucial element for desensitization. This form of involvement has the potential to enhance the cognitive processing of traumatic memories and fears, making it especially pertinent in the context of post-traumatic stress disorder (PTSD) treatment. The conventional approach to exposure treatment may present difficulties for certain persons due to the discomfort experienced when confronting their concerns. Virtual exposure therapy has been found to effectively lessen the discomfort and dread commonly associated with in vivo exposure therapy. This reduction in negative emotions has been observed to lead to lower treatment drop-out rates and increased adherence to the prescribed treatment regimen. Augmented reality (AR) and virtual reality (VR) can replicate diverse surroundings and scenarios, hence rendering exposure therapy suitable for addressing a multitude of phobias and anxieties (Goel, 2023; Doshi, 2023). Virtual environments can address various concerns, such as fear of flying, heights, public speaking, or social interactions. Virtual environments can capture physiological reactions, such as heart rate and skin conductance, to assess patients' anxiety levels during exposure. This dataset enables therapists to optimize the exposure sessions and, more precisely, monitor the patient's progress. Therapists can be present in virtual environments, providing guidance to patients during exposure therapy and offering immediate support and encouragement. The strategy under consideration exhibits promise as it corresponds to the dynamic nature of mental health care, enhancing accessibility and involvement for individuals seeking therapy for their anxiety-related difficulties (Vianez et al., 2022; Veelen et al., 2021).

Augmented Reality (AR) and Virtual Reality (VR) technology have presented novel opportunities for integrating mindfulness and relaxation techniques into mental health therapy. Virtual reality (VR) can transport individuals to soothing and immersive landscapes, serene beaches, peaceful forests, or quiet mountain retreats. Virtual environments have been found to facilitate a heightened state of awareness by minimizing external disturbances and cultivating a tranquil ambience that promotes meditation and relaxation. Augmented reality (AR) and virtual reality (VR) have the potential to offer guided meditation sessions facilitated by seasoned instructors or therapists. Individuals have the option to select from a diverse range of meditation programs that are designed to cater to their particular requirements, such as the alleviation of stress, the management of anxiety, or the enhancement of sleep quality (Kim et al., 2021; Riches et al., 2023).

Individuals can personalize their mindfulness encounters in augmented reality (AR) and virtual reality (VR) by choosing specific meditation techniques, durations, and ambient environments that align with their preferences. The implementation of personalization fosters a perception of agency and motivates consistent engagement. The integration of wearable devices and sensors inside augmented reality (AR) and virtual reality (VR) settings enables the provision of instantaneous biofeedback. Individuals can observe and track their heart rate, breathing patterns, and other physiological markers, augmenting their self-awareness and promoting improved self-regulation during mindfulness and relaxation practices (Brelet & Gaffary, 2022; Hatta et al., 2022).

Virtual reality (VR) can be an educational tool for teaching stress-reduction strategies. By creating immersive simulations of stressful situations, such as a packed subway, individuals may be exposed to realistic scenarios that induce stress and anxiety. Subsequently, they can be guided through relaxation exercises aimed at helping them effectively cope with these stressors. The utilization of a practical, experiential method has the potential to yield significant efficacy in the instruction of tangible coping mechanisms. Virtual reality (VR) has the potential to function as a highly effective mechanism for diversion and pain mitigation in the context of medical procedures or dental interventions. Through the process of immersing patients in a tranquil virtual world, their attention is redirected away from feelings of discomfort, leading to a decrease in anxiety levels and an improvement in their ability to cope with the situation. Augmented reality (AR) and virtual reality (VR) technologies enable individuals to confront their phobias inside a controlled and simulated environment. Individuals have the opportunity to interact with anxiety-provoking circumstances in the presence of guided assistance, enabling them to engage in the gradual desensitization process and practice relaxing strategies. Augmented reality (AR) and virtual reality (VR) have the potential to integrate biofeedback devices capable of monitoring stress levels and delivering immediate feedback. This dataset facilitates users in recognizing their stress levels and acquiring proficiency in implementing effective relaxation strategies. According to recent studies conducted by Kim et al. (2021) and Cunningham et al. (2021), it has been found that augmented reality (AR) and virtual reality (VR) can replicate emotional states and provide guidance to individuals during emotion control exercises.

Individuals have the opportunity to engage in the identification and regulation of their emotions inside a secure and simulated setting, hence offering significant benefits for disorders such as anger management and emotional dysregulation. Virtual environments have the potential to offer a therapeutic mechanism of distancing, enabling individuals to create a psychological separation from sources of stress and anxiety. It can be especially beneficial in the context of post-traumatic stress or situations involving heightened emotional distress. Integrating augmented reality (AR) and virtual reality (VR) into mindfulness and relaxation practices presents a unique methodology for promoting overall wellness, effectively coping with stress, and improving emotional regulation.

CHALLENGES AND CONSIDERATIONS

Incorporating Augmented Reality (AR) and Virtual Reality (VR) technologies into mental health therapy signifies a notable advancement, presenting novel resolutions to enduring obstacles within the discipline. To effectively harness the promise of these technologies, it is imperative to comprehensively comprehend, tackle, and negotiate the diverse issues and concerns linked to them. The concept of informed consent is more than a mere legal obligation; it forms the fundamental basis for establishing trust and fostering a collaborative relationship between therapists and their patients. It is imperative to provide thorough elucidations regarding the utilization of technology, its prospective advantages, and the accompanying concerns. Additionally, it is crucial to outline how sensitive data will be gathered and preserved. Patients must be adequately informed and empowered to actively engage in their treatment process, possessing a comprehensive understanding of the anticipated outcomes (Bruno et al., 2022; Lan et al., 2023). Data privacy holds significant importance, particularly when considering collecting sensitive personal information. It encompasses physiological reactions and mental conditions, necessitating rigorous compliance with data privacy rules such as the General Data Privacy Regulation (GDPR) or the Health Insurance Portability and Accountability Act (HIPAA). Maintaining patient trust and adhering to regulatory standards by securely handling, storing, and, where necessary, anonymizing data is of utmost importance. Maintaining suitable boundaries between therapists and patients in virtual settings presents a distinct and noteworthy problem. Therapists must modify their approaches and set novel standards for connection and involvement. The integration of virtual space has the potential to create ambiguity between professional and personal boundaries, therefore highlighting the need for well-defined standards regarding the therapeutic connection in the digital domain (Carroll et al., 2021; Lan et al., 2023).

The prevention of technological addiction or reliance is a significant concern, as is the case with any emerging technology. To address this risk, it is crucial to establish restrictions on the utilization of technology and consistently assess the level of patient involvement. The integration of responsible usage habits should be included in treatment programs, and therapists should be equipped to address any indications of excessive dependence effectively. The issues of affordability and accessibility continue to be of paramount importance. The affordability of AR and VR devices may be a barrier to access, particularly for persons from lower socioeconomic strata, potentially restricting their usage. It is imperative to pursue endeavours aimed at cost reduction and enhanced accessibility actively to ensure that a wider demographic can reap the advantages offered by these technologies (Creed et al., 2023; Tsamitros et al., 2021). Improving the user experience relies on considering motion sickness and compatibility concerns. Ongoing progress in hardware and software is vital for mitigating discomfort and enhancing user-friendliness. Ensuring interoperability across many devices and platforms is crucial to achieving a cohesive user experience. To deliver efficacious treatment, therapists must train to use augmented reality (AR) and virtual reality (VR) technology. Providing accessible technical assistance is crucial to address any potential challenges that may develop during therapy sessions, facilitating a seamless and uninterrupted therapeutic experience (Saredakis et al., 2020; Fagbola, 2022).

Incorporating augmented reality (AR) and virtual reality (VR) technologies into conventional therapy methods requires interdisciplinary cooperation and the establishment of evidence-based practice protocols. Through collaborative efforts, mental health specialists and technology experts can effectively enhance the utilization of these technological advancements while ensuring that they do not supplant well-established methodologies. It is imperative to achieve a harmonious equilibrium between innovation and evidence-based care. Although augmented reality (AR) and virtual reality (VR) have significant potential, it is essential to acknowledge that not all patients may be prepared for or at ease with therapy that relies on technology. Therapists have a responsibility to evaluate the preparedness of each patient for augmented reality (AR) and virtual reality (VR) interventions and offer essential assistance and direction during the transition, guaranteeing that technology functions as a constructive instrument rather than a cause of unease or tension (Best et al., 2021; Scanlon et al., 2019). Adapting therapy regimens to align with augmented reality (AR) and virtual reality (VR) capabilities is crucial for achieving optimal outcomes. Therapists must be able to modify preexisting treatment materials and interventions to align them with technological advancements, customizing them to suit the unique requirements and objectives of individual patients. It is imperative to adhere strictly to ethical principles while employing augmented reality (AR) and virtual reality (VR) technologies, with particular attention to concerns around the dynamics between therapists and patients, establishing appropriate limits, safeguarding data privacy and ensuring informed permission. The ethical framework safeguards patients' rights and well-being throughout their therapeutic process (Srinivasulu, 2022; Patel, 2022).

APPLICATIONS AND CASE STUDIES

In recent times, there has been a growing utilization of Augmented Reality (AR) and Virtual Reality (VR) in many contexts of mental health therapy, yielding encouraging results. Presented below are three case studies that exemplify the utilization of Augmented Reality (AR) and Virtual Reality (VR) within diverse therapeutic contexts. Post-Traumatic Stress Disorder (PTSD) is a multifaceted and incapacitating disorder that frequently arises as a consequence of being exposed to traumatic occurrences, such as combat situations, accidents, or instances of violence. Individuals diagnosed with post-traumatic stress disorder (PTSD) frequently experience a range of symptoms, including intrusive memories, hyperarousal, and avoidance behaviours. These manifestations can profoundly influence their daily functioning and overall quality of life. Exposure therapy is a widely recognized and validated intervention for post-traumatic stress disorder (PTSD). The therapy modality under consideration entails a systematic and regulated process of gradually exposing patients to their painful memories or associated triggers. The objective is to assist individuals in addressing and assimilating these traumatic experiences, mitigating the anguish and anxiety that accompanies them. Although exposure therapy has demonstrated efficacy, its implementation can present difficulties for both patients and therapists as a result of the heightened emotional intensity involved in the treatment procedure. Virtual Reality Exposure Therapy (VRET) is considered a significant breakthrough in the field of post-traumatic stress disorder (PTSD) treatment. Utilizing virtual reality effectively harnesses its immersive attributes to establish a secure and regulated setting wherein individuals can confront their unpleasant memories. The present discourse aims to comprehensively analyze the efficacy of Virtual Reality Exposure Therapy (VRET). Virtual Reality Exposure Therapy (VRET) uses a virtual environment to immerse patients in a simulated representation of their traumatic memories or a closely analogous scenario.

The degree of Immersion enables individuals to perceive a sense of physical presence within the simulated world, hence enhancing the vividness and realism of the experience. Virtual Reality Exposure Therapy (VRET) adheres to the fundamental principles of exposure therapy, wherein individuals are systematically and incrementally exposed to stimuli that elicit anxiety or distress. Therapists possess the ability to tailor the intensity and progression of exposure following the unique requirements of each patient, facilitating the confrontation of traumatic experiences while mitigating the risk of overwhelming psychological distress. The VRET sessions are facilitated by therapists who have received specialized training. The individuals in question offer assistance in managing and navigating uncomfortable emotions that may emerge during the exposure process, including emotional support, encouragement, and coping methods. Including therapist guidance in this strategy introduces a significant element of safety and attentiveness to the procedure. Numerous studies have provided evidence supporting the considerable efficacy of Virtual Reality Exposure Therapy (VRET) as a therapeutic intervention for Post-Traumatic Stress Disorder (PTSD).

Virtual Reality Exposure Therapy (VRET) enables a systematic desensitization process, wherein individuals gradually experience a reduction in emotional reactivity towards their traumatic experiences as a result of repeated exposure. The process of desensitization results in a decrease in the level of distress and anxiety that is often linked to the recollection of specific experiences. Virtual Reality Exposure Therapy (VRET) is a therapeutic approach that facilitates the gradual exposure of patients to their fears and worries. VRET aims to teach individuals how to manage their emotional responses effectively by providing a controlled and supportive environment. Consequently, individuals undergoing treatment observe a decrease in anxiety levels and an enhancement in emotional regulation. One notable advantage of Virtual Reality Exposure Therapy (VRET) compared to conventional exposure therapy is its reduced participant attrition rate. Patients frequently report that Virtual Reality Exposure Therapy (VRET) is more captivating and less daunting, resulting in increased adherence to and completion of therapy. The distinctive benefits of Virtual Reality Exposure Therapy (VRET), including its immersive characteristics and guided exposure techniques, render it a desirable alternative for those who have Post-Traumatic Stress Disorder (PTSD). Not only does it facilitate patients in addressing their painful memories, but it also improves their general emotional well-being and quality of life. With the ongoing advancement of technology, Virtual Reality Exposure Therapy (VRET) exhibits the potential to evolve into a more readily available and efficacious intervention for Post-Traumatic Stress Disorder (PTSD), hence instilling renewed optimism among individuals who have undergone traumatic experiences (Gupta, 2022).

Social Anxiety Disorder (SAD), which is distinguished by a heightened apprehension towards social events and interactions, can have a significant impact on individuals, severely restricting their personal and occupational endeavours. Conventional therapeutic methods commonly encompass cognitive-behavioural therapy (CBT) and exposure therapy, when individuals systematically and deliberately tackle their social anxieties. Nevertheless, Augmented Reality (AR) presents a novel and exceedingly promising alternative for addressing social anxiety disorder. Augmented reality (AR) technology enables therapists to construct regulated, augmented social simulations that closely resemble real-world circumstances. Users can actively participate in computer-generated social interactions by utilizing augmented reality (AR) goggles or mobile devices. The scenarios mentioned above possess the capacity for customization and encompass a broad spectrum, from commonplace dialogues to more intricate societal circumstances. Gradual exposure is considered a fundamental component in the treatment of social anxiety. Augmented reality (AR) therapy lets patients gradually confront social obstacles in a secure, regulated, and nurturing digital setting. Therapists can modify the intensity and complexity of scenarios to cater to each patient's particular requirements. Trained therapists are essential in using augmented reality (AR) as a therapeutic modality for social anxiety. Healthcare professionals provide guidance and assistance to individuals throughout their exposure encounters, facilitating the development of adaptive coping mechanisms, the questioning of maladaptive cognitive habits, and the effective management of anxiety symptoms. Including therapist guidance in this strategy contributes to safety and attentiveness to the procedure. Augmented reality (AR) therapy is beneficial in considerably decreasing levels of anxiety experienced in real-life social situations.

Augmented reality (AR) therapy effectively promotes the development of a feeling of accomplishment and expertise. As individuals progressively surmount social obstacles, their self-esteem and self-assurance are enhanced, bolstering their value. Augmented reality therapy allows patients to engage in organized, non-threatening environments to practice and enhance their social skills. Over time, this phenomenon can result in enhanced interpersonal engagements in the physical realm and the cultivation of more efficient mechanisms for managing stress. Augmented reality (AR) therapy provides individuals with a more conducive and organized approach to engaging in social interactions. The controlled context of social encounters in a research setting mitigates the apprehension commonly associated with real-world interactions, thus fostering a heightened sense of security. Patients undergoing positive outcomes in the enhanced scenarios develop the self-assurance and abilities required to confront real-world social circumstances with diminished anxiety and increased self-confidence. Augmented reality (AR)-based treatment for social anxiety disorder (SAD) signifies a noteworthy progression in the field of mental healthcare, providing a patient-centred, empirically supported, and exceptionally immersive therapeutic method. With the ongoing advancement and increasing availability of technology, augmented reality (AR) therapy exhibits the potential to gain greater prevalence and efficacy as a means of assisting individuals in overcoming social anxiety. Consequently, this can enhance their overall well-being and engagement in social interactions.

Cognitive Behavioral Therapy (CBT) is a well-established and efficacious modality utilized in the treatment of several mental health issues, encompassing but not limited to depression, anxiety disorders, and other related ailments. The primary objective of this approach is to discern and alter detrimental cognitive processes and actions, with the ultimate goal of equipping individuals with enhanced abilities to regulate their mental well-being effectively. The use of Virtual Reality (VR) in Cognitive Behavioral Therapy (CBT) has emerged as an innovative approach in recent years, potentially enhancing the therapeutic process significantly. Virtual reality (VR) technology offers a highly immersive and interactive platform that enables patients to confront and address their concerns effectively. In the context of depression treatment, virtual reality (VR) can replicate situations linked to diminished mood, thereby establishing a lifelike and absorbing setting that effectively captivates patients at a profound level. In the context of these virtual reality simulations, individuals are provided with guidance as they engage in cognitive-behavioural therapy exercises. Qualified therapists instruct individuals to acquire the skills of recognizing and reframing negative ideas, as well as engaging in other therapeutic approaches. The exercises provided are customized to address the patient's individualized needs and specific concerns. Virtual reality (VR) situations are effective in facilitating exposure therapy and reaction prevention approaches for those with anxiety disorders. The regulated and customizable attributes of virtual reality (VR) enable patients to confront their anxieties and phobias systematically and securely. One notable benefit associated with the utilization of virtual reality (VR) in cognitive-behavioral therapy (CBT) is the increased degree of involvement it provides. The immersive qualities of virtual reality (VR) enhance the attraction and captivation of therapy, hence augmenting patients' drive to engage in the treatment process actively. Virtual reality (VR) situations have improved the recall of cognitive-behavioral therapy (CBT) abilities. Through the process of immersing patients in realistic scenarios that are designed to stimulate their specific issues, they can acquire practical experience that facilitates the application of these abilities in real-life contexts. Patients can apply their recently acquired abilities in a secure, regulated, and therapeutic virtual reality (VR) setting, facilitating a smoother transition towards implementing these skills in their everyday routines. Virtual reality (VR) directly enables patients to confront their difficulties and fears inside a controlled environment. It allows individuals to gradually become less sensitive to stimuli and develop the ability to cope with adversity, ultimately leading to a decrease in symptoms of anxiety or depression. The incorporation of virtual reality (VR) technology into cognitive-behavioral therapy (CBT) results in a therapeutic experience that is more profound in its effects. Patients express higher satisfaction levels with their treatment regimen, attributing it to increased engagement and effectiveness in addressing their needs. Virtual reality (VR) scenarios can be customized according to the specific requirements of particular patients, guaranteeing that the therapy is in harmony with their distinct challenges and objectives. Patients can adapt the abilities they learn in VR to many real-life circumstances, giving them a diverse set of tools for managing their mental health. Incorporating virtual reality (VR) technology into cognitive-behavioural therapy (CBT) signifies a noteworthy advancement in mental health intervention. With the continuous advancement and increasing accessibility of virtual reality (VR) technology, there is a promising potential for a transformative impact on therapy delivery. Virtual reality (VR)-enhanced cognitive behavioural therapy (CBT) facilitates the successful management of mental health difficulties and promotes better life satisfaction by providing immersive, engaging, and personalized experiences.

The abovementioned case exemplifies the varied and auspicious implementations of augmented reality (AR) and virtual reality (VR) within mental health therapy. These technologies offer novel approaches to address diverse mental health disorders and augment conventional therapeutic methods, thereby providing those seeking assistance and recovery with more engaging, effective, and readily available alternatives.

DISCUSSION

The utilization of Augmented Reality (AR) and Virtual Reality (VR) has emerged as influential instruments within the realm of mental health intervention. In analyzing these technologies' efficacy, acceptability, user experience, and engagement aspects, it is imperative to consider the potential constraints and prospects for their application in mental healthcare. Incorporating Augmented Reality (AR) and Virtual Reality (VR) into mental health therapy has attracted significant interest. Studies have shown evidence of their efficacy and acceptance in diverse therapeutic settings. Augmented reality (AR) and virtual reality (VR) have demonstrated significant efficacy in the context of exposure therapy for individuals with anxiety disorders, phobias, and post-traumatic stress disorder (PTSD). The regulated and immersive characteristics of these technologies allow individuals the opportunity to address their anxieties within a secure setting, resulting in a decrease in symptoms and a process of desensitization.

The utilization of augmented reality (AR) and virtual reality (VR) technologies in therapy has significantly boosted participation due to their immersive and interactive attributes. Implementing gamification, providing real-time feedback, and utilizing interactive exercises are effective strategies to stimulate the active engagement of persons in their therapy, resulting in more positive outcomes. Augmented reality (AR) and virtual reality (VR) have promising prospects for implementing individualized solutions. Therapists can customize experiences to align with individuals' unique tastes and needs, enhancing the relevance and efficacy of treatment. Virtual environments can augment conventional cognitive-behavioural therapy (CBT) by offering immersive experiences that facilitate the practice of coping mechanisms and the confrontation of negative cognitive processes. This phenomenon can result in enhanced recall of cognitive-behavioral therapy (CBT) procedures and more effective implementation of these approaches in real-world settings. The increasing acceptance of augmented reality (AR) and virtual reality (VR) in mental health therapy is evident. Numerous people perceive these technologies as captivating and less daunting than conventional therapy. The simplicity and accessibility of treatment provided by augmented reality (AR) and virtual reality (VR) are highly valued since they have the potential to mitigate stigma and overcome hurdles associated with getting help.AR and VR-based interventions frequently elicit substantial patient satisfaction, as reported by those undergoing such treatments. Individuals often experience a sense of engagement and enjoyment when utilizing technology, which has the potential to enhance their motivation and adherence to treatment strategies. The utilization of augmented reality (AR) and virtual reality (VR) has the potential to mitigate the societal stigma surrounding the act of seeking treatment for mental health concerns. Patients may experience a heightened sense of comfort while interacting with these technologies, as they can do so within the confines of their residences. Some individuals who experience discomfort with in-person or traditional exposure therapy may perceive augmented reality (AR) and virtual reality (VR) environments as more comfortable and secure alternatives. It can be especially beneficial for individuals who experience social anxiety or phobias.

Augmented reality (AR) and virtual reality (VR) present versatile therapeutic modalities, enabling therapy to be administered at a distance, mitigating geographical obstacles to accessing care. Individuals can avail themselves of therapeutic services at their leisure, a particularly advantageous option for individuals with demanding schedules. Augmented reality (AR) and virtual reality (VR) have been frequently associated with patients expressing heightened levels of engagement and active participation in their respective treatment processes. Using interactive features and personalized elements inside the technology enhances individuals' engagement and dedication to the treatment process. The efficacy and acceptability of augmented reality (AR) and virtual reality (VR) have been established in the context of mental health treatment. The technologies above can augment engagement, deliver individualized interventions, and promote accessibility, eventually enhancing the quality of care and patient outcomes. The ongoing investigation and advancement in this domain are expected to facilitate the broader integration of augmented reality (AR) and virtual reality (VR) technologies into diverse therapeutic approaches for mental health. The effectiveness of Augmented Reality (AR) and Virtual Reality (VR) mental health treatment is significantly influenced by the user experience (UX) and engagement variables. Ensuring a favourable and engaging user experience is crucial in therapy, as it contributes to the dual objectives of enhancing enjoyment and therapeutic efficacy. The following are a few pivotal aspects that influence user experience and engagement within the context of mental health treatment utilizing augmented reality (AR) and virtual reality (VR) technologies. The level of realism inside augmented reality (AR) and virtual reality (VR) settings substantially influences the level of user engagement. Incorporating highly intricate and lifelike settings can heighten the sense of Immersion experienced by individuals and elicit more profound emotional reactions. The inclusion of interactivity within therapy facilitates active user engagement. The capacity to engage with the virtual realm and manipulate various entities has the potential to enhance overall engagement. The incorporation of personalized approaches is crucial in the context of mental health interventions. Customizing the therapeutic experience to accommodate each individual's unique requirements and preferences might enhance engagement and relevance in the therapy process.

The integration of gamification components, including challenges, incentives, and progress monitoring, can enhance therapy's enjoyment and motivation levels. The incorporation of gamified features into a treatment regimen can foster a sense of accomplishment and serve as a motivating factor for users to persist in their therapeutic endeavours. Augmented reality (AR) and virtual reality (VR) environments have the potential to elicit profound emotional reactions. The establishment of an emotional connection has the potential to serve as a therapeutic mechanism, facilitating individuals in forging a more profound connection with their emotions and personal encounters. Integrating real-time input regarding performance and physiological responses, such as heart rate or skin conductance, can potentially augment the user experience. Individuals can see their progress and acquire the necessary skills to effectively manage and regulate their emotional states. Augmented reality (AR) and virtual reality (VR) have the potential to create a more conducive and secure environment for those who may encounter anxiety inside conventional therapeutic contexts. The feeling of security facilitates active participation. Augmented reality (AR) and virtual reality (VR) technologies for accessing therapy can potentially enhance participation. Individuals can participate in therapy within the confines of their surroundings, thereby mitigating logistical obstacles. The utilization of augmented reality (AR) and virtual reality (VR) technology has the potential to mitigate the societal stigma that is often attached to mental health care. Individuals may perceive These technologies as more acceptable, leading to a greater willingness to engage with them. The inclusion and support of a therapist within the virtual environment can augment the user's overall experience. Therapists can offer individuals assistance, encouragement, and a feeling of security. The novelty of augmented reality (AR) and virtual reality (VR) therapies has the potential to generate curiosity and captivate users. The novelty of the technology may enhance user engagement. The implementation of gamification, rewards, and progress tracking can enhance user motivation and persistence in the context of therapy. The perception of progress has the potential to enhance levels of involvement.

Virtual reality (VR) has the potential to serve as an effective method of diversion for those experiencing acute stress or pain, redirecting their attention away from discomfort and facilitating adaptive coping strategies. User experience and engagement are essential in mental health treatment utilizing augmented reality (AR) and virtual reality (VR) technologies. The enhancement of treatment effectiveness and improvement of patient outcomes can be achieved by creating immersive, interactive, and emotionally engaging therapy environments, taking into account individual preferences and needs. In addition, the mitigation of concerns about comfort, safety, and stigma can effectively diminish obstacles hindering the utilization of mental health services and foster active involvement from users. Although Augmented Reality (AR) and Virtual Reality (VR) have demonstrated considerable potential in mental health therapy, it is crucial to acknowledge and tackle several potential limitations and obstacles associated with their implementation.

Moreover, prospective avenues in this domain possess the capacity for substantial progress and enhancements. The present study has identified some potential limitations and areas for future research. The accessibility of AR and VR hardware can be constrained by its high cost, impeding specific individuals from obtaining it. It is imperative to exert efforts towards cost reduction and the advancement of economically viable hardware, enhancing the accessibility of augmented reality (AR) and virtual reality (VR) therapies.

Certain persons may have symptoms of motion sickness while utilizing virtual reality (VR) technology, hence imposing restrictions on its potential applications. Continued investigation and advancement are imperative to mitigate motion sickness and alleviate discomfort associated with virtual reality (VR) encounters. Ensuring the safeguarding of data privacy and effectively resolving ethical considerations, such as obtaining informed consent and maintaining appropriate boundaries between therapists and patients, is of utmost importance. There is a need to establish more stringent laws and guidelines to ensure the ethical and responsible utilization of augmented reality (AR) and virtual reality (VR) technologies within the context of treatment. The successful incorporation of augmented reality (AR) and virtual reality (VR) technologies into conventional therapeutic methods necessitates the collaboration of several disciplines, tailoring interventions to individual needs, and the development of practice standards grounded in empirical research. Establishing best practices for integration can be facilitated through ongoing collaboration between mental health specialists and technology experts. The progression of augmented reality (AR) and virtual reality (VR) hardware is anticipated to result in the development of devices characterized by reduced weight, enhanced comfort, and increased affordability. The implementation of this measure is expected to enhance user comfort and accessibility. Incorporating artificial intelligence into real-time monitoring and individualized interventions can potentially improve the effectiveness of augmented reality (AR) and virtual reality (VR) therapies. Artificial intelligence (AI) can offer personalized feedback and dynamically adjust therapeutic interventions in real-time. Establishing defined procedures and rules about using augmented reality (AR) and virtual reality (VR) in the context of mental health therapy will uphold optimal methodologies and ethical principles and safeguard data privacy. It is anticipated that the utilization of Augmented Reality (AR) and Virtual Reality (VR) will expand to encompass a broader spectrum of mental health disorders and therapeutic approaches. It encompasses various applications such as teletherapy, stress management, emotion regulation training, and other related areas.

The ongoing investigation is essential to provide a comprehensive corpus of evidence that substantiates the efficacy of augmented reality (AR) and virtual reality (VR) in mental health intervention. It encompasses many research methodologies, including clinical trials, longitudinal investigations, and outcome assessments. Maintaining strong data security and privacy measures, such as end-to-end encryption and secure patient data storage, is crucial for the ongoing acceptance and utilization of augmented reality (AR) and virtual reality (VR) in therapeutic contexts. The enhancement of the effectiveness of augmented reality (AR) and virtual reality (VR) treatments can be achieved by developing a comprehensive library consisting of specialized therapeutic content and scenarios specifically designed to cater to diverse mental health issues. The use of biofeedback devices that ensure smooth integration, enabling the provision of real-time data about physiological and emotional states, has the potential to augment the therapy process and facilitate the acquisition of self-regulation abilities by patients. Although there are certain restrictions and obstacles associated with the utilization of augmented reality (AR) and virtual reality (VR) in mental health treatment, the continuous pursuit of research, innovation, and the establishment of ethical norms can alleviate these concerns. The future trajectory of this discipline exhibits the potential to enhance accessibility to efficacious and captivating mental health interventions, ultimately lessening the overall welfare of persons in search of assistance and rehabilitation.

CONCLUSION

The potential for changing mental health therapy is excellent with the utilization of Augmented Reality (AR) and Virtual Reality (VR) technologies. The capacity to generate immersive, interactive, and individualized therapeutic encounters holds significant implications for clinical practice and accessibility enhancement. This paper explores the possibilities of augmented reality (AR) and virtual reality (VR) technologies and their consequences and provides recommendations for their incorporation into mental health treatments. The utilization of augmented reality (AR) and virtual reality (VR) has significant promise in revolutionizing the domain of mental health intervention across various dimensions. The efficacy of virtual reality (VR) technology in the context of exposure treatment, its potential to augment conventional therapeutic methods, and its capacity to render therapy more captivating and easily accessible distinguish it as a formidable instrument. The potential resides in their ability to. Augmented reality (AR) and virtual reality (VR) technologies have the potential to build immersive settings that significantly boost engagement and emotional connection, hence increasing the effectiveness of therapy. Customizing therapy to suit individual preferences and needs facilitates the implementation of more efficacious and pertinent interventions. The utilization of augmented reality (AR) and virtual reality (VR) has the potential to mitigate the social stigma surrounding mental health treatment, hence enhancing its acceptability and accessibility. Therapists can actively provide guidance and support to patients within virtual settings, thereby enhancing the strength of the therapeutic bond. The implications of augmented reality (AR) and virtual reality (VR) in clinical practice are essential. Remote therapy has the potential to enhance accessibility for those residing in remote or underserved regions, hence augmenting the convenience of receiving care. Augmented reality (AR) and virtual reality (VR) can enhance the therapeutic experience, fostering increased patient engagement and promoting their active involvement in treatment adherence. With the progression of technology and its increasing affordability, it has the potential to function as a cost-efficient substitute for conventional therapy. Augmented reality (AR) and virtual reality (VR) technologies offer the potential for tailored therapy interventions that cater to individual mental health requirements. It is imperative that mental health practitioners undergo comprehensive training in the utilization of augmented reality (AR) and virtual reality (VR) technology to deliver treatment that is both productive and ethically sound. Ongoing investigation is needed to establish a comprehensive body of evidence that substantiates the effectiveness of augmented reality (AR) and virtual reality (VR) in mental health intervention. To ensure the proper utilization of these technologies, it is imperative to adhere to rigorous data privacy legislation, obtain informed consent, and follow ethical norms. Efforts should be made to decrease the financial burden associated with augmented reality (AR) and virtual reality (VR) devices and enhance the availability of these technologies to a broader demographic. It is imperative to foster collaboration among mental health professionals, technological specialists, and researchers to advance the refinement of optimal methodologies and augment therapeutic approaches. The objective is to establish uniform norms and recommendations about using augmented reality (AR) and virtual reality (VR) technologies within the context of mental health services. Augmented reality (AR) and virtual reality (VR) have emerged as potentially transformative domains in mental health therapy. As the progression and accessibility of these technologies persist, they can offer practical, engaging therapies tailored to individual needs. By incorporating augmented reality (AR) and virtual reality (VR) technologies into clinical practice, mental health services have the potential to augment their scope and efficacy, thereby enhancing the overall well-being of persons seeking assistance and rehabilitation.

REFERENCES

Albakri, G., Bouaziz, R., Alharthi, W., Kammoun, S., Al-Sarem, M., Saeed, F., & Hadwan, M. (2022). Phobia Exposure Therapy Using Virtual and Augmented Reality: A Systematic review. *Applied Sciences (Basel, Switzerland)*, *12*(3), 1672. doi:10.3390/app12031672

Baus, O., & Bouchard, S. (2014). Moving from Virtual Reality Exposure-Based Therapy to Augmented Reality Exposure-Based Therapy: A Review. *Frontiers in Human Neuroscience*, *8*. doi:10.3389/fnhum.2014.00112 PMID:24624073

Best, P., Meireles, M., Schroeder, F., Montgomery, L., Maddock, A., Davidson, G., Galway, K., Trainor, D., Campbell, A., & Van Daele, T. (2021). Freely Available Virtual Reality Experiences as Tools to Support Mental Health Therapy: A Systematic Scoping Review and Consensus-Based Interdisciplinary Analysis. *Journal of Technology in Behavioral Science*, *7*(1), 100–114. doi:10.1007/s41347-021-00214-6 PMID:34179349

Boeldt, D., McMahon, E., McFaul, M., & Greenleaf, W. J. (2019). Using virtual reality exposure therapy to enhance treatment of anxiety disorders: Identifying areas of clinical adoption and potential obstacles. *Frontiers in Psychiatry*, *10*, 773. doi:10.3389/fpsyt.2019.00773 PMID:31708821

Brelet, L., & Gaffary, Y. (2022). Stress reduction interventions: A scoping review to explore progress toward using haptic feedback in virtual reality. *Frontiers in Virtual Reality*, *3*, 900970. Advance online publication. doi:10.3389/frvir.2022.900970

Bruno, R. R., Wolff, G., Wernly, B., Masyuk, M., Piayda, K., Leaver, S., Erkens, R., Oehler, D., Afzal, S., Heidari, H., Kelm, M., & Jung, C. (2022). Virtual and augmented reality in critical care medicine: The patient's, clinician's, and researcher's perspective. *Critical Care*, *26*(1), 326. doi:10.1186/s13054-022-04202-x PMID:36284350

Buettner, R., Baumgartl, H., Konle, T., & Haag, P. (2020). *A Review of Virtual Reality and Augmented Reality Literature in Healthcare*. IEEE Xplore. doi:10.1109/ISIEA49364.2020.9188211

Carroll, J., Hopper, L., Farrelly, A. M., Lombard-Vance, R., Bamidis, P. D., & Konstantinidis, E. I. (2021). A scoping Review of Augmented/Virtual Reality Health and Well-being Interventions for Older Adults: Redefining Immersive Virtual Reality. *Frontiers in Virtual Reality*, *2*, 655338. doi:10.3389/frvir.2021.655338

Creed, C., Al-Kalbani, M., Theil, A., Sarkar, S., & Williams, I. (2023). Inclusive AR/VR: Accessibility barriers for immersive technologies. *Universal Access in the Information Society*. Advance online publication. doi:10.1007/s10209-023-00969-0

Cunningham, A., McPolin, O., Fallis, R., Coyle, C., Best, P., & McKenna, G. (2021). A systematic review of the use of virtual reality or dental smartphone applications as interventions for management of paediatric dental anxiety. *BMC Oral Health*, *21*(1), 244. doi:10.1186/s12903-021-01602-3 PMID:33962624

Dehghan, B., Saeidimehr, S., Sayyah, M., & Rahim, F. (2022b). The Effect of Virtual Reality on Emotional Response and Symptoms Provocation in Patients with OCD: A Systematic Review and Meta-analysis. *Frontiers in Psychiatry*, *12*, 733584. doi:10.3389/fpsyt.2021.733584 PMID:35177996

Doshi, R., Hiran, K. K., Gök, M., El-kenawy, E. S. M., Badr, A., & Abotaleb, M. (2023). Artificial Intelligence's Significance in Diseases with Malignant Tumours. *Mesopotamian Journal of Artificial Intelligence in Healthcare*, *2023*, 35–39.

Fagbola, T. M., Fagbola, F. I., Aroba, O. J., Doshi, R., Hiran, K. K., & Thakur, S. C. (2022). Smart face masks for Covid-19 pandemic management: A concise review of emerging architectures, challenges and future research directions. *IEEE Sensors Journal*, *23*(2), 877–888. doi:10.1109/JSEN.2022.3225067

Freitas, R., Velosa, V. H. S., Abreu, L. T. N., Jardim, R. L., Santos, J. V., Peres, B., & Campos, P. (2021). Virtual Reality Exposure Treatment in Phobias: A Systematic Review. *The Psychiatric Quarterly*, *92*(4), 1685–1710. doi:10.1007/s11126-021-09935-6 PMID:34173160

Gaiha, S. M., Salisbury, T. T., Koschorke, M., Raman, U., & Petticrew, M. (2020e). The stigma associated with mental health problems among young people in India: A systematic review of magnitude, manifestations and recommendations. *BMC Psychiatry*, *20*(1), 538. doi:10.1186/s12888-020-02937-x PMID:33198678

Goel, P., Jhanwar, N., Jain, P., Khatri, S., & Hiran, K. K. (2023, August). Efficient Blood Availability for Targeted Individuals Through Cloud Computing Web Application. In *2023 International Conference on Emerging Trends in Networks and Computer Communications (ETNCC)* (pp. 1-7). IEEE. 10.1109/ETNCC59188.2023.10284940

Gupta, A. K., Srinivasulu, A., Hiran, K. K., Sreenivasulu, G., Rajeyyagari, S., & Subramanyam, M. (2022). Prediction of omicron virus using combined extended convolutional and recurrent neural networks technique on CT-scan images. *Interdisciplinary Perspectives on Infectious Diseases*, *2022*, 2022. doi:10.1155/2022/1525615 PMID:36562006

Hadjipanayi, C., Banakou, D., & Michael-Grigoriou, D. (2023). Art as therapy in virtual reality: A scoping review. *Frontiers in Virtual Reality*, *4*, 1065863. doi:10.3389/frvir.2023.1065863

Hatta, M. H., Sidi, H., Koon, C. S., Roos, N. C., Sharip, S., Samad, F. D. A., Xi, O. W., Das, S., & Saini, S. M. (2022). Virtual Reality (VR) Technology for Treatment of Mental Health Problems during COVID-19: A Systematic Review. *International Journal of Environmental Research and Public Health*, *19*(9), 5389. doi:10.3390/ijerph19095389 PMID:35564784

Hornstein, S., Zantvoort, K., Lueken, U., Funk, B., & Hilbert, K. (2023). Personalization strategies in digital mental health interventions: A systematic review and conceptual framework for depressive symptoms. *Frontiers in Digital Health*, *5*, 1170002. doi:10.3389/fdgth.2023.1170002 PMID:37283721

Ionescu, A., Van Daele, T., Rizzo, A., Blair, C., & Best, P. (2021). 360° Videos for Immersive Mental Health Interventions: A Systematic Review. *Journal of Technology in Behavioral Science*, *6*(4), 631–651. doi:10.1007/s41347-021-00221-7

Kim, H., Kim, D. J., Kim, S., Chung, W. H., Park, K., Kim, J. D. K., Kim, D., Kim, M. J., Kim, K., & Jeon, H. J. (2021c). Effect of virtual reality on stress reduction and change of physiological parameters including heart rate variability in people with high stress: An open randomized crossover trial. *Frontiers in Psychiatry*, *12*, 614539. doi:10.3389/fpsyt.2021.614539 PMID:34447320

Lan, L., Sikov, J., Lejeune, J., Ji, C., Brown, H. P., Bullock, K., & Spencer, A. E. (2023). A Systematic Review of Using Virtual and Augmented Reality for the Diagnosis and Treatment of Psychotic Disorders. *Current Treatment Options in Psychiatry*, *10*(2), 87–107. doi:10.1007/s40501-023-00287-5 PMID:37360960

Li, H., Dong, W., Wang, Z., Chen, N., Wu, J., Wang, G., & Jiang, T. (2021). Effect of a Virtual Reality-Based Restorative Environment on the Emotional and Cognitive Recovery of Individuals with Mild-to-Moderate Anxiety and Depression. *International Journal of Environmental Research and Public Health, 18*(17), 9053. doi:10.3390/ijerph18179053 PMID:34501643

Meena, G., Dhanwal, B., Mahrishi, M., & Hiran, K. K. (2021, August). Performance comparison of network intrusion detection system based on different pre-processing methods and deep neural network. In *Proceedings of the International Conference on Data Science, Machine Learning and Artificial Intelligence* (pp. 110-115). ACM. 10.1145/3484824.3484878

Patel, S., Vyas, A. K., & Hiran, K. K. (2022). Infrastructure health monitoring using signal processing based on an industry 4.0 System. *Cyber-Physical Systems and Industry, 4*, 249–260.

Peter, L., Schindler, S., Sander, C., Schmidt, S., Muehlan, H., McLaren, T., Tomczyk, S., Speerforck, S., & Schomerus, G. (2021). Continuum beliefs and mental illness stigma: A systematic review and meta-analysis of correlation and intervention studies. *Psychological Medicine, 51*(5), 716–726. doi:10.1017/S0033291721000854 PMID:33827725

Pons, P., Navas-Medrano, S., & Soler-Domínguez, J. L. (2022). Extended reality for mental health: Current trends and future challenges. *Frontiers of Computer Science, 4*, 1034307. Advance online publication. doi:10.3389/fcomp.2022.1034307

Ramasamy, J., Doshi, R., & Hiran, K. K. (2021, August). Segmentation of brain tumor using deep learning methods: a review. In *Proceedings of the International Conference on Data Science, Machine Learning and Artificial Intelligence* (pp. 209-215). ACM. 10.1145/3484824.3484876

Ramasamy, J., Doshi, R., & Hiran, K. K. (2022, October). Detection of Brain Tumor in Medical Images Based on Feature Extraction by HOG and Machine Learning Algorithms. In *2022 International Conference on Trends in Quantum Computing and Emerging Business Technologies (TQCEBT)* (pp. 1-5). IEEE. 10.1109/TQCEBT54229.2022.10041564

Rawlins, C. R., Veigulis, Z. P., Hebert, C. A., Curtin, C., & Osborne, T. F. (2021). Effect of immersive virtual reality on pain and anxiety at a Veterans Affairs health care facility. *Frontiers in Virtual Reality, 2*, 719681. doi:10.3389/frvir.2021.719681

Riches, S., Jeyarajaguru, P., Taylor, L., Fialho, C., Little, J. R., Ahmed, L., O'Brien, A., Van Driel, C., Veling, W., & Valmaggia, L. (2023). Virtual reality relaxation for people with mental health conditions: A systematic review. *Social Psychiatry and Psychiatric Epidemiology, 58*(7), 989–1007. doi:10.1007/s00127-022-02417-5 PMID:36658261

Rimer, E., Husby, L. V., & Solem, S. (2021). Virtual Reality Exposure Therapy for Fear of Heights: Clinicians' attitudes become more positive after trying VRET. *Frontiers in Psychology, 12*, 671871. doi:10.3389/fpsyg.2021.671871 PMID:34335386

Rizzo, A., Goodwin, G. J., De Vito, A. N., & Bell, J. D. (2021). Recent advances in virtual reality and psychology: Introduction to the special issue. *Translational Issues in Psychological Science, 7*(3), 213–217. doi:10.1037/tps0000316

Saredakis, D., Szpak, A., Birckhead, B., Keage, H. A., Rizzo, A., & Loetscher, T. (2020). Factors Associated with Virtual Reality Sickness in Head-Mounted Displays: A Systematic Review and Meta-Analysis. *Frontiers in Human Neuroscience, 14*, 96. doi:10.3389/fnhum.2020.00096 PMID:32300295

Scanlon, E., Anastopoulou, S., Conole, G., & Twiner, A. (2019). Interdisciplinary working methods: Reflections based on Technology-Enhanced Learning (TEL). *Frontiers in Education, 4*, 134. doi:10.3389/feduc.2019.00134

Sutherland, J., Bélec, J., Sheikh, A., Chepelev, L. L., Althobaity, W., Chow, B. J., Mitsouras, D., Christensen, A., Rybicki, F. J., & La Russa, D. (2018). Applying modern virtual and augmented reality technologies to medical images and models. *Journal of Digital Imaging, 32*(1), 38–53. doi:10.1007/s10278-018-0122-7 PMID:30215180

Takac, M., Collett, J., Conduit, R., & De Foe, A. (2021). A cognitive model for emotional regulation in virtual reality exposure. *Virtual Reality (Waltham Cross), 27*(1), 159–172. doi:10.1007/s10055-021-00531-4

Tao, G., Garrett, B., Taverner, T., Cordingley, E., & Sun, C. (2021). Immersive virtual reality health games: A narrative review of game design. *Journal of Neuroengineering and Rehabilitation, 18*(1), 31. doi:10.1186/s12984-020-00801-3 PMID:33573684

Trappey, A. J., Trappey, C. V., Chang, C., Kuo, R. R. T., Lin, A. P., & Nieh, C. (2020). Virtual Reality Exposure Therapy for Driving Phobia Disorder: System Design and Development. *Applied Sciences (Basel, Switzerland), 10*(14), 4860. doi:10.3390/app10144860

Tsamitros, N., Sebold, M., Gutwinski, S., & Beck, A. (2021). Virtual Reality-Based Treatment approaches in the field of substance use disorders. *Current Addiction Reports, 8*(3), 399–407. doi:10.1007/s40429-021-00377-5

Van Veelen, N., Boonekamp, R., Schoonderwoerd, T., Van Emmerik, M., Nijdam, M. J., Bruinsma, B., Geuze, E., Jones, C., & Vermetten, E. (2021). Tailored Immersion: Implementing personalized components into virtual reality for veterans with Post-Traumatic Stress Disorder. *Frontiers in Virtual Reality, 2*, 740795. doi:10.3389/frvir.2021.740795

Vianez, A., Marques, A., & Almeida, R. (2022). Virtual Reality Exposure Therapy for Armed Forces Veterans with Post-Traumatic Stress Disorder: A Systematic Review and Focus Group. *International Journal of Environmental Research and Public Health, 19*(1), 464. doi:10.3390/ijerph19010464 PMID:35010723

Woods, J., Greenfield, G., Majeed, A., & Hayhoe, B. (2020). Clinical effectiveness and cost-effectiveness of individual mental health workers colocated within primary care practices: A systematic literature review. *BMJ Open, 10*(12), e042052. doi:10.1136/bmjopen-2020-042052 PMID:33268432

Xu, X., Mangina, E., & Campbell, A. G. (2021c). HMD-Based Virtual and Augmented Reality in Medical Education: A Systematic Review. *Frontiers in Virtual Reality, 2*, 692103. doi:10.3389/frvir.2021.692103

Zeevi, L. S. (2021). Making art therapy virtual: Integrating virtual reality into art therapy with adolescents. Frontiers in Psychology. doi:10.3389/fpsyg.2021.584943

KEY TERMS AND DEFINITIONS

Accessibility: Ensuring services are reachable and usable.
Augmented Reality: Overlays digital content onto the real world, enhancing perception.
Immersive Technologies: Tech that creates profound sensory experiences.
Mental Health Treatment: Strategies to address mental health issues.
Therapeutic Interventions: Actions aimed at improving well-being.
Virtual Reality: Immersive computer-generated environment, simulating a physical presence.
Well-being: Overall health and happiness.

Chapter 7

Augmented Reality and Virtual Reality Modules for Mindfulness:
Boosting Emotional Intelligence and Mental Wellness

Bhupinder Singh
https://orcid.org/0009-0006-4779-2553
Sharda University, India

Christian Kaunert
https://orcid.org/0000-0002-4493-2235
Dublin City University, Ireland

ABSTRACT

Augmented reality (AR) and virtual reality (VR) modules are emerging as revolutionary tools for improving mindfulness, emotional intelligence, and mental health. These immersive technologies provide a one-of-a-kind and engaging platform for simulating real-life settings and guiding users through a variety of experiences aimed at regulating emotions and improving mental health. These modules can teach and reinforce mindfulness practices by immersing users in virtual worlds, allowing them to get a better awareness of their emotions, manage stress, and build emotional resilience. AR and VR modules are proving to be strong tools for personal growth and well-being, whether through guided meditation, stress reduction exercises, or interactive situations aimed at increasing empathy and self-awareness. This chapter comprehensively explores the transformational potential of AR and VR modules in building mindfulness, enhancing emotional intelligence, and contributing to overall mental well-being.

INTRODUCTION AND BACKGROUND

AR and VR modules are developing as novel methods for improving mindfulness, emotional intelligence, and general mental wellbeing. These immersive technologies provide a novel and participatory approach

DOI: 10.4018/979-8-3693-1123-3.ch007

to stress relief and training. AR and VR modules provide a secure area for users to exercise emotional control and mindfulness by immersing them in realistic, virtual worlds (Holt, 2022). These modules may include guided meditation, stress management scenarios, and interactive emotional intelligence exercises. Users have the chance to learn and practice skills that can help them better understand and regulate their emotions as they interact with these settings, ultimately leading to greater mental health and well-being. In this environment, the promise of AR and VR is exciting, adding a new dimension to how it approach mental wellness and emotional intelligence. The augmented reality modules covered here strive to improve real-world experiences by superimposing digital data on the user's actual environment. This might include guided meditations, stress-relief exercises, and interactive simulations aimed at developing emotional intelligence. VR modules create a completely immersive environment in which to practice mindfulness by simulating calm settings or regulated events. Augmented Reality (AR) and Virtual Reality (VR) integration into mindfulness practices has emerged as a viable route for improving emotional intelligence and mental wellbeing. The incorporation of biofeedback systems inside AR/VR modules provides users with real-time data on physiological reactions, assisting in the development of self-awareness and emotional control. The awareness emerges as a recurring motif. The ability to be present in the moment, to cultivate nonjudgmental awareness of one's thoughts and feelings, has far-reaching ramifications for emotional well-being. The first module of our intervention is devoted to mindfulness training, taking use of VR-AR's immersive capabilities to build virtual settings that promote introspection and relaxation. Users are urged to explore and develop their self-awareness in a dynamic and responsive digital world via guided meditations and real-time biofeedback (Liu et al., 2023).

The second module, which builds on the foundation of mindfulness, examines the complex art of emotional regulation. Recognizing the complexities of human emotions as well as the difficulties in navigating them, our simulation-based approach attempts to offer users with a controlled environment in which to practice and perfect their emotional reactions. This module's customized character is enhanced by real-time feedback and adaptive learning processes, which adjust the experience to individual needs and support the development of effective emotion management skills.

The third module extends the focus to the interpersonal realm, acknowledging the social dimensions inherent in emotional intelligence. Simulated social environments offer users opportunities to refine their communication and interpersonal skills (Singh, 2023; Meena, 2021). By immersing individuals in scenarios that mirror real-world challenges, this module seeks to bridge the gap between virtual training and practical application, promoting the transferability of acquired skills to everyday social interactions.

Objectives of the Chapter

The chapter has the following objectives to:
Examine the Current Situation

- give an overview of augmented reality (AR) and virtual reality (VR) technology as they stand now and investigate existing AR and VR applications in mental health and wellness.
- inspect the efficacy and limits of conventional mindfulness methods in addressing emotional intelligence and mental wellbeing.

AR/VR Module Design and Development

- propose design guidelines for mindfulness-enhancing AR and VR modules and discuss how psychological and therapeutic frameworks may be included into the growth process.
- improve the user experience, consider technical factors such as device requirements and user interface design.

Emotional Intelligence Impact

- observe the influence of AR and VR mindfulness courses on emotional intelligence and in order to build emotional intelligence, researchers compared the effectiveness of AR/VR modules to standard mindfulness methods.

Evaluating the Outcomes of Mental Wellness

- scrutinize the efficacy of AR/VR modules in enhancing mental wellbeing, such as stress reduction, anxiety management, and general psychological well-being.
- investigate the long-term implications of introducing augmented reality/virtual reality mindfulness into daily practices.
- consider the possible uses in a variety of demographics, such as people suffering from mental illnesses or working in high-stress industries.

Ethical Considerations and User Experience

- scan how users perceive and interact with AR/VR mindfulness programs and consider potential ethical issues like as privacy, consent, and the proper use of immersive technology in mental health.
- criteria for developers, practitioners, and users to follow in order to ensure the ethical deployment and usage of AR/VR mindfulness solutions.

This paper advances the understanding of how augmented and virtual reality may be used to improve mindfulness, emotional intelligence, and mental health. Furthermore, it lays the groundwork for future research and the development of practical applications in the sector.

Structure of the Chapter

This chapter comprehensively explores the various dimensions of Augmented Reality and Virtual Reality Modules for Mindfulness which Boosting Emotional Intelligence and Mental Wellness. Section 2 explores Cognitive and Emotional Aptitude in Comprehensive Wellness. Section 3 explains Virtual-Augmented Reality (VAR): Exploring the Role of Virtual and Augmented Reality in Mental Wellness Training. Section 4 travels Integrating Augmented Reality for Emotional Intelligence Development. Section 5 examines Simulations of Cognitive-Behavioral Therapy in a VR Environment. And, finally Section 6 lays down Conclusion and Future Scope.

Figure 1. Objectives of the chapter

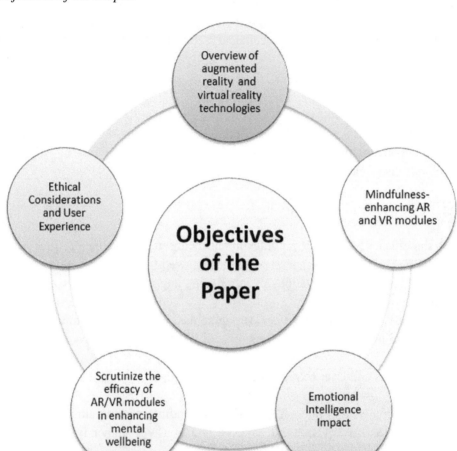

COGNITIVE AND EMOTIONAL APTITUDES IN COMPREHENSIVE WELLNESS

Central to the impact of mental-emotional intelligence on overall well-being is its role in fostering self-awareness. This self-awareness serves as a compass, guiding individuals in making decisions that align with their values and aspirations. It contributes to a more authentic and intentional way of living, fostering a sense of purpose and fulfillment that is foundational to overall well-being (Taghian et al., 2021). In the personal resilience, mental-emotional intelligence is a key factor. The ability to regulate and manage one's emotions, often termed self-regulation, is crucial in navigating the inevitable challenges and stressors of life. Individuals with good self-regulation abilities are adaptable and calm in the face of adversity, recovering from setbacks with a positive perspective. This resilience not only protects mental health, but it also leads to a more positive and optimistic attitude on life, which improves general well-being (Ray et al. 2023).

Figure 2. Structure of the chapter

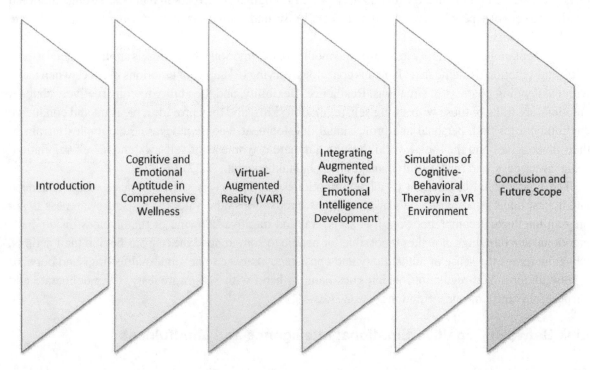

Cognitive-Emotional Acumen

Self-awareness is an important aspect of mental-emotional intelligence since it requires a deep and perceptive observation of one's own emotional states, causes, and inclinations. It is a comprehensive understanding of the fundamental causes and influences that influence one's behavior, not only the acknowledgment of feelings. High self-awareness people are more equipped to live genuine lives, integrating their actions with their values and making informed decisions based on a deep understanding of their emotional surroundings (Arpaia et al., 2021).

They can easily adjust to changing conditions, assess scenarios, and make wise decisions because to their cognitive capability. Furthermore, having a sharp cognitive sense encourages creativity and originality, enabling people to approach problems from a different angle and come up with original solutions. Emotional intelligence is a supplement to cognitive intelligence since it gives people a better awareness and comprehension of both their own and other people's feelings. Emotional intelligence

Figure 3. Cognitive and emotional aptitudes in comprehensive wellness

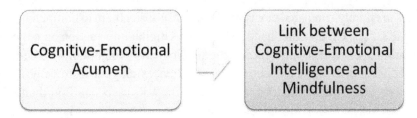

makes it easier to communicate with empathy, which strengthens interpersonal bonds. Strong emotional intelligence enables people to resolve disputes skillfully, understand social cues with ease, and cultivate healthy relationships.

Self-regulation, or the ability to control and modify one's emotional reactions, is another crucial aspect of mental-emotional intelligence. It means consciously trying to keep your emotions in check when faced with challenging or stressful situations. Resilience, flexibility, and the ability to constructively channel emotions are traits of those with strong self-regulation skills, and they provide a pleasant and conducive environment for both personal and professional development. People navigate the complex terrain of their inner selves and the social world through a dynamic synthesis of self-awareness, self-regulation, social awareness, and relationship management (Jadhakhan et al., 2022).

The fundamental component of mental-emotional intelligence is self-awareness, which is a deep and honest understanding of one's own emotions, motivations, and values. This self-awareness is not only an intellectual comprehension; it is a visceral and intuitive knowing of the nuances inside one's emotional surroundings. It makes it possible for people to comprehend the reasons behind their actions, which increases the sense of authenticity and consistency between one's internal feelings and outward representations. Self-regulation, which goes hand in hand with self-awareness, is the deliberate and purposeful control of one's emotions.

Link Between Cognitive-Emotional Intelligence and Mindfulness

The observation of thoughts and feelings without immediately passing judgment enables individuals to construct a buffer between inputs and response, encouraging a more methodical and studied approach to emotional management. The connection between mental-emotional intelligence and mindfulness extends to the social dimensions of both concepts. Social awareness, a component of mental-emotional intelligence, involves understanding and empathizing with the emotions of others. Mindfulness practices, which encourage present-moment attention and attunement, naturally enhance one's capacity for empathetic understanding (Reger, 2020). By being fully present in social interactions, individuals can pick up on non-verbal cues, accurately perceive the emotional states of others, and respond with greater sensitivity and emotional intelligence. The mindfulness practices contribute to an overall sense of well-being, complementing the goals of mental-emotional intelligence. The stress reduction techniques inherent in mindfulness not only foster emotional resilience but also contribute to a more positive emotional state. As individuals cultivate a mindful approach to their internal and external experiences, they are better equipped to navigate the complexities of life with a calm and centered demeanor.

VIRTUAL-AUGMENTED REALITY (VAR): EXPLORING THE ROLE OF VIRTUAL AND AUGMENTED REALITY IN MENTAL WELLNESS TRAINING

VR immerses users in entirely simulated environments, transporting them to computer-generated worlds that engage multiple senses. On the other hand, AR overlays digital information onto the physical world, enhancing real-world experiences by integrating digital elements (Singh, 2024). The defining features of VAR is its capacity to offer users a spectrum of experiences ranging from fully immersive virtual environments to more subtle augmentations of reality. In the VR, users can find themselves traversing fantastical landscapes, participating in simulated training scenarios, or engaging in immersive storytelling experiences. This not only has profound implications for entertainment and gaming but also extends into areas such as education, where VR can facilitate virtual field trips, historical reenactments, and hands-on training in a risk-free environment (Marvaso et al., 2022; Doshi, 2023).

AR augments real-world experiences by superimposing digital data on the user's actual environment. This has found uses in a wide range of disciplines, including navigation and gaming, as well as professional teaching and healthcare. AR navigation systems, for example, give real-time assistance by superimposing directions over the user's perspective of the physical world, while AR training apps allow users to observe and interact with three-dimensional models projected into their real-world surroundings. VAR's influence extends beyond entertainment and practical applications to human cognition and perception (Drigas et al., 2022). VAR has the ability to alter how people learn, interpret information, and interact with their environment by offering immersive and interactive experiences. VAR technologies are being investigated for therapeutic uses in the area of mental health, including exposure treatment for anxiety disorders, mindfulness training, and stress reduction simulations. Because of VAR's capacity to generate realistic and controlled settings, it is an appealing tool for giving individuals with individualized and adaptable experiences that can help to their psychological well-being.

The possibilities for the future are huge as VAR technologies evolve, with hardware getting more complex and applications growing more diversified. VAR is a monument to the ever-evolving confluence of technology and human experience, from improving how it learn and train to revolutionizing healthcare treatments and expanding our concept of digital and physical locations. It brings up new possibilities for creativity, innovation, and the exploration of immersive, interactive environments with the ability to improve our knowledge of reality and modify how it interacts with the digital and physical components of our existence (Elor & Kurniawan, 2020; Ramasamy & Doshi 2022).

The understanding of virtual and augmented reality (VAR) in the context of mental health training represents a paradigm change in how it approach and handle psychological health. VAR technologies have the potential to democratize education by providing students with immersive, interactive learning experiences. Subjects that were once confined to textbooks and lectures can now be explored through VR, making complex concepts tangible and engaging (Singh, 2023). For instance, history can be brought

Figure 4. Virtual-Augmented realities (VAR)

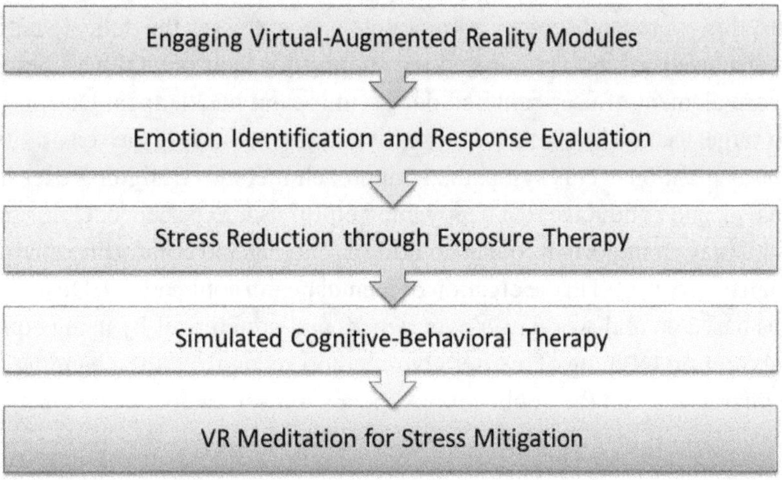

to life by immersing students in ancient civilizations, and geography can be learned by allowing them to explore global landscapes (Ebert et al., 2019).

Engaging Virtual-Augmented Reality Modules

In the education, Interactive VAR Modules redefine traditional teaching methods by transporting students from passive observers to active participants. Whether it's exploring historical events through VR time-travel experiences or dissecting three-dimensional models in AR-enhanced biology lessons, these modules immerse learners in content, fostering deeper understanding and retention. By engaging multiple senses and providing interactive elements, they cater to diverse learning styles, making education more accessible, engaging, and effective (Patangia et al., 2021; Fagbola et al., 2022).

In professional training, Interactive VAR Modules revolutionize how individuals acquire and hone skills across various industries. From virtual flight simulations for pilots to hands-on medical procedures in healthcare, these modules provide a risk-free environment for trainees to practice and refine their abilities. Real-time feedback and adaptive learning algorithms enhance the training process, tailoring the experience to individual needs and promoting a dynamic, learner-centric approach. Mental health and well-being training also benefit significantly from Interactive VAR Modules. These modules provide a platform for immersive mindfulness experiences, stress reduction simulations, and exposure therapy in a controlled and supportive environment.

The flexibility and scalability are design principles that anticipate the evolving nature of products and systems. Designers aim to create solutions that can adapt to different contexts, screen sizes, or user needs. A flexible and scalable design ensures longevity and relevance, accommodating changes and updates without compromising the overall integrity of the user experience. The design principles serve as the guiding philosophy for designers to navigate the complex terrain of creating impactful and user-centric solutions (Midha & Singh, 2023). As technology advances and user expectations evolve, these principles remain foundational, providing a timeless framework for designers to craft solutions that are not only visually appealing but also functional, accessible, and responsive to the diverse needs of users. User-centered design takes on heightened significance when applied to mental health applications, where the nuances of user experience can profoundly impact the efficacy and accessibility of these technologies. At its core, user-centered design prioritizes the needs, preferences, and experiences of the end-users throughout the entire design process (Singh, 2023; Goel, 2023). In the context of mental health applications, this approach becomes paramount, as it addresses the delicate nature of the subject matter and the diverse needs of individuals seeking support for their mental well-being.

Empathy is a core element of user-centered design in mental health apps. Designers must acquire a deep grasp of their target users' emotional and cognitive states, respecting the sensitivity and distinctiveness of mental health situations. This sympathetic approach includes designing user interfaces that are intuitive, nonintrusive, and conducive to a happy and helpful user experience. Color schemes, font, and general aesthetics all play an important role in creating a relaxing and comforting environment. Iterative user-centered design is very useful in the creation of mental health applications. Designers may adapt and improve their ideas based on real-world user experiences and preferences by using continuous feedback loops, user testing, and prototyping. This iterative method recognizes the changing nature of mental health issues and guarantees that the application responds to user feedback and changing requirements (Thompson, 2021).

As because designers must consider a wide range of users, including individuals with varying cognitive capacities, language preferences, and technical literacy, accessibility is a fundamental element in user-centered design for mental health apps. The application should be inclusive, reducing obstacles to access and ensuring that people with different requirements can browse and use the features. This might include capabilities like as voice commands, customizable text sizes, or multilingual assistance. Furthermore, user-centered design for mental health applications prioritizes privacy and security (Cotler et al., 2017). As, given the sensitive nature of mental health information, robust data protection measures must be integrated into the design, ensuring that users can trust the application to safeguard their personal information. Transparent communication about data practices and opt-in consent mechanisms contribute to building a sense of trust and reliability.

The gamification and engagement strategies are often leveraged in user-centered design for mental health applications to enhance user motivation and adherence. By incorporating elements of play, reward systems, and personalized goal-setting, designers can create experiences that encourage users to consistently engage with the application, fostering a sense of accomplishment and progress in their mental health journey. Ultimately, user-centered design in mental health applications is not just about creating a visually appealing interface; it's about crafting an empathetic and effective tool that respects the complexity of individual mental health experiences. By placing the user at the center of the design process, incorporating feedback, ensuring accessibility, and prioritizing privacy, designers can contribute to the development of applications that not only meet the diverse needs of users but also play a meaningful role in supporting mental well-being (Sharma & Singh, 2022; Ramasamy et al., 2021; Gupta et al., 2022). In this intersection of technology and mental health, user-centered design becomes a cornerstone for creating solutions that are not only functional but also compassionate and responsive to the unique challenges of mental health care.

Emotion Identification and Response Evaluation

The feedback mechanisms in emotion recognition technologies play a crucial role in closing the loop of interaction. Providing users with feedback about their emotional states not only enhances their self-awareness but also empowers them to navigate and regulate their emotions effectively. For instance, a wearable device that monitors physiological signals and provides feedback on stress levels can enable individuals to proactively manage stress by engaging in relaxation techniques or taking breaks (Cheng et al., 2019). This real-time feedback loop creates a symbiotic relationship between the user and the technology, fostering a sense of agency and control over emotional well-being. In the development and implementation of emotion recognition systems, ethical issues are critical. It is vital to protect user privacy and ensure open communication regarding data usage and storage. To create and retain user trust, it is critical to strike a balance between the benefits of emotion-aware technology and the potential for misuse or intrusion.

These exercises guided nature frequently involves vocal instructions that direct attention to breath, physiological sensations, or the surrounding environment. This vocal instruction acts as an anchor, assisting individuals in navigating the ebb and flow of their thoughts while remaining focused on the present. Breath awareness, a cornerstone of mindfulness techniques, is commonly included into mindfulness exercises (Baos et al., 2021). Guided sessions frequently urge participants to pay attention to their intake and expiration, as well as the natural rhythm of their breath. This deliberate concentration on breath acts as a portal to the present now, establishing a mental space in which people may disconnect from stresses, ruminative thoughts, and future fears. Body scan technique is widely used in guided mindfulness exercises, and participants are instructed to direct their attention systematically across different regions of the body, building awareness of physical sensations and promoting a feeling of embodied present. This exercise fosters a holistic awareness that extends beyond cognitive processes to incorporate the felt sensation of the body. This proactive approach to stress management is especially useful in fast-paced and demanding environments. of modern life (Singh, 2022; Ramasamy et al., 2022).

So, in addition to stress reduction, guided mindfulness activities help with emotional control and mental resilience. Improvements in focus, emotional balance, and cognitive flexibility have been linked to regular practice. Individuals can traverse problems with greater equanimity by cultivating a nonjudgmental awareness of thoughts and emotions, promoting a more balanced and adaptable reaction to life's ups and downs. These guided mindfulness activities act as compasses for exploring the present moment, providing an organized and accessible path to improved mental well-being. These activities, whether used for stress reduction, emotional regulation, or overall self-awareness, give people a practical and empowering way to incorporate mindfulness into their everyday lives, building a deeper connection with the richness of each moment (Miner, 2022; Srinivasulu et al., 2022).

Stress Reduction Through Exposure Therapy

The exposure therapy is not limited to external stresses; cognitive stressors are also addressed through cognitive exposures. This entails facing and overcoming stress-related maladaptive mental patterns or erroneous beliefs. Individuals may modify their cognitive reactions to stresses by methodically reviewing and reframing negative thinking processes, promoting a more adaptable and productive mentality. The long-term benefits of exposure therapy for stress reduction are substantial since people's overall health, emotional regulation, and coping skills usually improve as their stress tolerance rises. Approaching and overcoming obstacles in a systematic way helps people feel strong and confident in their abilities which helps them develop a resilient mindset that lasts outside of therapy sessions. An adaptable and dynamic technique for reducing stress is exposure therapy. This therapeutic approach exposes patients to stressors on a regular basis in a safe, encouraging environment, which promotes habituation, resilience, and adaptive coping mechanisms. Whether used for situational or cognitive pressures, exposure therapy is an essential technique for lessening the negative effects of stress on mental health and assisting people in overcoming life's challenges with more emotional equilibrium and resilience (Durnell, 2018).

Simulated Cognitive-Behavioral Therapy

The use of cutting-edge technology in the mental health field is demonstrated by the cognitive-behavioral therapy (CBT) simulations, which provide patients with a virtual treatment environment where they may participate in realistic and stimulating activities. Based on the core ideas of cognitive-behavioral therapy, these simulations offer a dynamic and realistic environment where users may learn about, explore, and apply CBT techniques to mental health issues. By using technology to mimic therapeutic environments, CBT simulations improve the accessibility of mental health therapy and increase the customization and accessibility of evidence-based practices (Singh, 2022). One of the main features of CBT simulations is their ability to replicate real-world situations within a safe virtual environment. Users can go through situations that mimic everyday challenges like stress, anxiety, or mood problems. People may hone their CBT skills in a risk-free setting, which increases their sense of competence and mastery. CBT simulations provide a safe environment for learning and experimentation, allowing users to acquire useful skills that they may apply to their everyday lives. Because CBT simulators are interactive, learning experiences may be customized and adjusted as needed. Based on their responses and selections in the simulated situations, users can get real-time feedback (Choukou et al., 2022; Patel et al., 2022). This real-time feedback system improves learning by assisting people in using cognitive behavioral therapy (CBT) procedures and assisting them in comprehending the effects of various thinking patterns and actions.

CBT simulations cater to diverse learning styles and preferences. Through the integration of multimedia elements such as audio, visuals, and interactive components, these simulations engage users on multiple sensory levels. This multi-modal approach enhances comprehension and retention of CBT concepts, making the learning experience more accessible to individuals with varying cognitive styles or preferences for different modes of information processing. CBT simulations scalability enables widespread distribution of evidence-based mental health therapies. As technology progresses, these simulations may be accessed via numerous platforms such as cellphones, tablets, and laptops, making them accessible to a diverse spectrum of people regardless of geographical location or socioeconomic level. This democratization of mental health services is especially important for overcoming hurdles to traditional therapy, such as stigma or restricted access to mental health specialists (Mer & Virdi, 2023). While CBT simulations provide novel answers, ethical questions remain critical. Protecting user privacy, obtaining informed permission, and addressing any dangers connected with simulation material are all key components of ethical development and implementation. Maintaining the integrity and efficacy of CBT simulations requires striking a balance between technical progress and ethical responsibility.

Cognitive-behavioral therapy simulations exist at the crossroads of mental health and technology, providing a transformational method to learning and applying evidence-based therapeutic practices. These simulations enable individuals to build resilience, improve coping skills, and apply CBT concepts in the context of their own life by offering a realistic and engaging platform. CBT simulations' potential to supplement mental health therapy and education remains promise as technology advances, contributing to a more accessible, engaging, and individualized environment for mental health therapies.

VR Meditation for Stress Mitigation

VR meditation's promise for stress reduction goes beyond just escapism. VR may incorporate physiological monitoring, measuring users' heart rate variability, and other stress indicators via biofeedback techniques. This real-time feedback loop adds to the customized aspect of VR meditation by allowing users to see the instant impact of their meditation practices on their physiological reactions. This biofeedback integration helps to a more educated and effective stress reduction strategy, allowing people to fine-tune their meditation practices for the best outcomes. VR meditation's accessibility further democratizes stress-reduction activities. Users can engage in guided meditations and immersive surroundings without prior meditation experience or substantial training. This accessibility is especially advantageous for people who may experience difficulties to traditional meditation, such as time restrictions, discomfort in group settings, or difficulty focusing during traditional meditation techniques (Drigas et al., 2022).

These VR meditation ethical issues center on user permission, data security, and the appropriate use of technology in mental health therapies. Individuals may engage in genuine settings that test their emotional awareness and social abilities with AR apps. For example, an AR module might simulate a workplace scenario where users need to navigate conflicts, demonstrate empathy, or provide constructive feedback. This interactive learning environment allows users to practice and refine their emotional intelligence in a controlled and supportive setting.

INTEGRATING AUGMENTED REALITY FOR EMOTIONAL INTELLIGENCE DEVELOPMENT

The implementation of Augmented Reality (AR) for emotional intelligence training signifies a transformative paradigm in the realm of skill development and interpersonal competency enhancement. Emotional intelligence, which includes self-awareness, self-regulation, empathy, and successful interpersonal communication, is often regarded as a pillar of personal and professional success. With its ability to superimpose digital information on the physical environment, augmented reality (AR) provides a dynamic and interactive platform for immersing humans in simulated circumstances, giving a unique and effective avenue for sharpening emotional intelligence abilities (D'Errico et al., 2023).

The benefits of incorporating augmented reality in emotional intelligence training stem from its capacity to generate lifelike and contextually rich environments for users to traverse. AR applications may replicate a wide range of interpersonal interactions, from workplace dynamics to social scenarios, by seamlessly merging digital aspects into the real-world environment. This contextual authenticity increases the training's applicability by allowing users to apply emotional intelligence concepts in circumstances that closely resemble the difficulties of daily life (Singh, 2022). AR emotional intelligence training's interactive aspect encourages active engagement and participation. Users are active participants in simulated events where they may practice and enhance their emotional intelligence abilities in real time, rather than passive observers. Because learners can instantly experience the repercussions of their answers within the augmented environment, this experiential learning technique improves retention and application of taught abilities.

AR's adaptability and versatility help to make emotional intelligence training projects scalable. AR applications may be adapted to certain environments, such as industries, corporate cultures, and individual preferences. AR provides a versatile tool that may be tailored to fulfill the individual emotional intelligence demands of diverse user groups, whether employed in business training programs, educational settings, or personal development projects. Real-time feedback and performance statistics are further advantages of using AR for emotional intelligence training. Within the simulated settings, the system can collect and evaluate user interactions, facial expressions, and communication styles. Individuals may obtain quick feedback on their emotional intelligence abilities using this data-driven method, allowing for targeted growth and skill development. AR analytics help to give a more informed and tailored learning experience, which aligns with the ideas of individualized and adaptive training (Hagege et al., 2023).

The ethical considerations in the implementation of AR for emotional intelligence training encompass privacy, informed consent, and responsible data usage. Clear communication about the purpose of data collection, the anonymization of user data, and the safeguarding of privacy rights are essential components of ethical AR implementation. Ensuring that users are aware of how their data will be utilized and protected is fundamental to building trust and maintaining ethical standards. The implementation of augmented reality for emotional intelligence training stands as a revolutionary step towards creating more emotionally intelligent and socially adept individuals (Jopowicz et al., 2022). By providing immersive, contextually rich simulations and real-time feedback, AR technology enhances the learning process, making emotional intelligence training more engaging, effective, and adaptable to diverse needs. As this technology continues to evolve, the integration of AR into emotional intelligence training reflects a forward-looking approach to skill development in the digital age (Marossi et al., 2023).

The versatility and accessibility of virtual therapeutic settings contribute to their capacity to address a wide range of groups. These environments, whether used in clinical settings, educational institutions, or online treatment sessions, provide a standardized and adaptable platform for providing therapeutic interventions. Because the technology can replicate a wide range of circumstances, individuals can get customized solutions suited to their own needs and difficulties (Singh, 2020).

SIMULATIONS OF COGNITIVE-BEHAVIORAL THERAPY IN A VR ENVIRONMENT

VR-based Cognitive-Behavioral Therapy (CBT) simulations represent a watershed moment in the convergence of technology and mental health therapies. Cognitive-behavioral therapy, a well-established and evidence-based treatment technique, seeks to assist clients in identifying and changing harmful thinking patterns and behaviors (Than et al., 2023). Virtual Reality (VR) integration into CBT uses immersive simulations to generate realistic and dynamic worlds in which users may engage in therapeutic exercises, role-playing situations, and skill training (Cotler, J2016). The capacity of VR-based CBT simulations to replicate different and true-to-life circumstances for therapeutic practice is one of their particular features. Users can enter virtual settings that mimic common scenarios ranging from social interactions to job problems, offering a secure and regulated environment for exposure treatment and skill development. Individuals may negotiate scenarios that closely replicate the intricacies of their daily lives, which improves the transferability of learnt abilities to real-world contexts (Chen & Ibrahim, 2023).

Traditional therapy activities are transformed into interesting and immersive learning opportunities by the interactivity of VR-based CBT simulations. Users become active participants in their therapeutic journey, whether it is confronting fears, exercising assertiveness, or navigating social settings. VR technology's feeling of presence and realism builds a stronger connection with therapeutic material, contributing to a more engaging and successful learning experience (Naylor et al., 2020). CBT simulations based on virtual reality provide a tailored and adaptable approach to mental health therapy. Based on user answers, the system may dynamically change situations, resulting in individualized therapeutic experiences that target specific issues or goals. This flexibility guarantees that people get interventions that are tailored to their specific requirements, resulting in a more personalized and successful therapy process (Liao et al., 2019).

The adaptability of VR-based CBT extends to its use in a variety of mental health disorders. VR simulations may be adapted to address a wide range of mental health issues, from anxiety and phobias to mood disorders and PTSD. Individuals with social anxiety, for example, can practice and perfect their social abilities in virtual social settings, whilst those with specific phobias can undergo exposure treatment in a controlled and immersive environment (Maçorano, 2020). Virtual reality-based Cognitive-Behavioral Therapy simulations are a game changer in the evolution of mental health therapies (Quintero, 2019). These simulations provide a dynamic, engaging, and individualized approach to therapy sessions by merging CBT concepts with the immersive capabilities of VR technology. As the area of VR-based mental health advances, the incorporation of CBT simulations has promise for improving accessibility and efficacy, contributing to a more creative and inclusive mental health treatment environment (Richir et al., 2022).

CONCLUSION AND FUTURE SCOPE

VR-based mental health therapies have a lot of potential for addressing mental health inequities in marginalized populations. These novel initiatives make use of technology to deliver accessible, cost-effective, and culturally appropriate mental health care. The advantage is the possibility of overcoming geographical constraints. Because of the scarcity of providers in their area, underserved groups frequently have difficulties in receiving mental health care. VR treatments can bridge this gap by giving therapy and support remotely, eliminating geographical barriers, and delivering services to those living in rural or isolated places. VR's immersive and interactive nature has the potential to increase engagement and involvement in mental health therapies. Many underprivileged areas may face stigma or cultural hurdles when it comes to mental health concerns. VR delivers a private and immersive environment in which people might feel more at ease investigating and treating their mental health challenges.

Virtual reality treatments may be adjusted to target individual cultural peculiarities and preferences in marginalized populations. Customizable material and situations may be created to resonate with people from a variety of cultural backgrounds, ensuring that interventions are both relevant and successful. VR-based therapies have the potential to minimize the price burden of mental health care, making it more accessible to people with limited financial means. This affordability is especially important for marginalized regions where access to standard mental health care may be limited due to financial restrictions.

Education and awareness are essential components of mental health therapies, and virtual reality can help provide psycho-education to neglected groups. Immersive VR experiences may distribute information about mental health, coping skills, and accessible services, contributing to mental health literacy and eliminating stigma. However, challenges exist, such as ensuring equitable access to VR technology. Not everyone in underserved communities may have ready access to the required hardware or reliable internet connections. Initiatives addressing these disparities, such as community centers or mobile VR units, could help make VR interventions more widely available. VR-based mental health interventions offer a promising avenue for addressing mental health disparities in underserved communities. By leveraging technology to provide accessible, culturally sensitive, and cost-effective interventions, VR has the potential to enhance mental health outcomes and contribute to a more equitable distribution of mental health resources.

REFERENCES

Arpaia, P., D'Errico, G., De Paolis, L. T., Moccaldi, N., & Nuccetelli, F. (2021). A narrative review of mindfulness-based interventions using virtual reality. *Mindfulness*, 1–16.

Baños, R. M., Etchemendy, E., Carrillo-Vega, A., & Botella, C. (2021). Positive psychological interventions and information and communication technologies. In *Research Anthology on Rehabilitation Practices and Therapy* (pp. 1648–1668). IGI Global.

Chen, X., & Ibrahim, Z. (2023). A Comprehensive Study of Emotional Responses in AI-Enhanced Interactive Installation Art. *Sustainability (Basel)*, *15*(22), 15830. doi:10.3390/su152215830

Cheng, V. W. S., Davenport, T., Johnson, D., Vella, K., & Hickie, I. B. (2019). Gamification in apps and technologies for improving mental health and well-being: Systematic review. *JMIR Mental Health, 6*(6), e13717. doi:10.2196/13717 PMID:31244479

Choukou, M. A., Zhu, X., Malwade, S., Dhar, E., & Abdul, S. S. (2022). Digital Health Solutions Transforming Long-Term Care and Rehabilitation. In *Healthcare Information Management Systems: Cases, Strategies, and Solutions* (pp. 301–316). Springer International Publishing. doi:10.1007/978-3-031-07912-2_19

Cotler, J. L. (2016). *The impact of online teaching and learning about emotional intelligence, Myers Briggs personality dimensions and mindfulness on personal and social awareness.* State University of New York at Albany.

Cotler, J. L., DiTursi, D., Goldstein, I., Yates, J., & Del Belso, D. (2017). A mindful approach to teaching. *Information Systems Education Journal, 15*(1), 12.

D'Errico, G., Barba, M. C., Gatto, C., Nuzzo, B. L., Nuccetelli, F., Luca, V. D., & Paolis, L. T. D. (2023, September). Measuring the Effectiveness of Virtual Reality for Stress Reduction: Psychometric Evaluation of the ERMES Project. In *International Conference on Extended Reality* (pp. 484-499). Cham: Springer Nature Switzerland. 10.1007/978-3-031-43401-3_32

Doshi, R., Hiran, K. K., Gök, M., El-kenawy, E. S. M., Badr, A., & Abotaleb, M. (2023). Artificial Intelligence's Significance in Diseases with Malignant Tumours. *Mesopotamian Journal of Artificial Intelligence in Healthcare, 2023*, 35–39.

Drigas, A., Mitsea, E., & Skianis, C. (2022). Virtual reality and metacognition training techniques for learning disabilities. *Sustainability (Basel), 14*(16), 10170. doi:10.3390/su141610170

Drigas, A., Mitsea, E., & Skianis, C. (2022). Subliminal Training Techniques for Cognitive, Emotional and Behavioral Balance. The Role of Emerging Technologies. *Technium Soc. Sci. J., 33*, 164.

Durnell, L. A. (2018). *Emotional Reaction of Experiencing Crisis in Virtual Reality (VR)/360* [Doctoral dissertation, Fielding Graduate University].

Ebert, D. D., Harrer, M., Apolinário-Hagen, J., & Baumeister, H. (2019). Digital interventions for mental disorders: key features, efficacy, and potential for artificial intelligence applications. *Frontiers in Psychiatry: Artificial Intelligence, Precision Medicine, and Other Paradigm Shifts*, 583-627.

Elor, A., & Kurniawan, S. (2020). The ultimate display for physical rehabilitation: A bridging review on immersive virtual reality. *Frontiers in Virtual Reality, 1*, 585993. doi:10.3389/frvir.2020.585993

Fagbola, T. M., Fagbola, F. I., Aroba, O. J., Doshi, R., Hiran, K. K., & Thakur, S. C. (2022). Smart face masks for Covid-19 pandemic management: A concise review of emerging architectures, challenges and future research directions. *IEEE Sensors Journal, 23*(2), 877–888. doi:10.1109/JSEN.2022.3225067

Goel, P., Jhanwar, N., Jain, P., Khatri, S., & Hiran, K. K. (2023, August). Efficient Blood Availability for Targeted Individuals Through Cloud Computing Web Application. In *2023 International Conference on Emerging Trends in Networks and Computer Communications (ETNCC)* (pp. 1-7). IEEE. 10.1109/ETNCC59188.2023.10284940

Gupta, A. K., Srinivasulu, A., Hiran, K. K., Sreenivasulu, G., Rajeyyagari, S., & Subramanyam, M. (2022). Prediction of omicron virus using combined extended convolutional and recurrent neural networks technique on CT-scan images. *Interdisciplinary Perspectives on Infectious Diseases*, *2022*, 2022. doi:10.1155/2022/1525615 PMID:36562006

Hagège, H., Ourmi, M. E., Shankland, R., Arboix-Calas, F., Leys, C., & Lubart, T. (2023). Ethics and Meditation: A New Educational Combination to Boost Verbal Creativity and Sense of Responsibility. *Journal of Intelligence*, *11*(8), 155. doi:10.3390/jintelligence11080155 PMID:37623538

Holt, S. (2022). Virtual reality, augmented reality and mixed reality: For astronaut mental health; and space tourism, education and outreach. *Acta Astronautica*.

Jadhakhan, F., Blake, H., Hett, D., & Marwaha, S. (2022). Efficacy of digital technologies aimed at enhancing emotion regulation skills: Literature review. *Frontiers in Psychiatry*, *13*, 809332. doi:10.3389/fpsyt.2022.809332 PMID:36159937

Jopowicz, A., Wiśniowska, J., & Tarnacka, B. (2022). Cognitive and physical intervention in metals' dysfunction and neurodegeneration. *Brain Sciences*, *12*(3), 345. doi:10.3390/brainsci12030345 PMID:35326301

Liao, D., Shu, L., Liang, G., Li, Y., Zhang, Y., Zhang, W., & Xu, X. (2019). Design and evaluation of affective virtual reality system based on multimodal physiological signals and self-assessment manikin. *IEEE Journal of Electromagnetics, RF and Microwaves in Medicine and Biology*, *4*(3), 216–224. doi:10.1109/JERM.2019.2948767

Liu, K., Madrigal, E., Chung, J. S., Parekh, M., Kalahar, C. S., Nguyen, D., & Harris, O. A. (2023). Preliminary Study of Virtual-reality-guided Meditation for Veterans with Stress and Chronic Pain. *Alternative Therapies in Health and Medicine*, *29*(6). PMID:34559692

Maçorano, R. D. N. A. (2020). *Exploratory Psychometric Validation and Efficacy Assessment Study of Social Phobia Treatment based on Augmented and Virtual Reality Serious Games and Biofeedback* [Doctoral dissertation, Universidade de Lisboa (Portugal)].

Marossi, C., Mariani, V., Arenas, A., Brondino, M., de Carvalho, C. V., Costa, P., & Pasini, M. (2023, July). Mindfulness Lessons in a Virtual Natural Environment to Cope with Work-Related Stress. In *International Conference in Methodologies and intelligent Systems for Techhnology Enhanced Learning* (pp. 227-238). Cham: Springer Nature Switzerland. 10.1007/978-3-031-41226-4_24

Marvaso, G., Pepa, M., Volpe, S., Mastroleo, F., Zaffaroni, M., Vincini, M. G., & Jereczek-Fossa, B. A. (2022). Virtual and Augmented Reality as a Novel Opportunity to Unleash the Power of Radiotherapy in the Digital Era: A Scoping Review. *Applied Sciences (Basel, Switzerland)*, *12*(22), 11308. doi:10.3390/app122211308

Meena, G., Dhanwal, B., Mahrishi, M., & Hiran, K. K. (2021, August). Performance comparison of network intrusion detection system based on different pre-processing methods and deep neural network. In *Proceedings of the International Conference on Data Science, Machine Learning and Artificial Intelligence* (pp. 110-115). ACM. 10.1145/3484824.3484878

Mer, A., & Virdi, A. S. (2023). Navigating the paradigm shift in HRM practices through the lens of artificial intelligence: A post-pandemic perspective. *The Adoption and Effect of Artificial Intelligence on Human Resources Management, Part A*, 123-154.

Midha, S., & Singh, K. (2023). Happiness-Enhancing Strategies Among Indians. In *Religious and Spiritual Practices in India: A Positive Psychological Perspective* (pp. 341–368). Springer Nature Singapore. doi:10.1007/978-981-99-2397-7_15

Miner, N. (2022). *Stairway to Heaven: Breathing Mindfulness into Virtual Reality* [Doctoral dissertation, Northeastern University].

Naylor, M., Ridout, B., & Campbell, A. (2020). A scoping review identifying the need for quality research on the use of virtual reality in workplace settings for stress management. *Cyberpsychology, Behavior, and Social Networking*, *23*(8), 506–518. doi:10.1089/cyber.2019.0287 PMID:32486836

Patangia, B., Sankruthyayana, R. G., Sathiyaseelan, A., & Balasundaram, S. (2021). How could Mindfulness Help? A Perspective on the Applications of Mindfulness in Enhancing Tomorrow's Workplace. *i-Manager's. Journal of Management*, *16*(3), 52.

Patel, S., Vyas, A. K., & Hiran, K. K. (2022). Infrastructure health monitoring using signal processing based on an industry 4.0 System. *Cyber-Physical Systems and Industry*, *4*, 249–260.

Quintero, L. (2019). *Facilitating Technology-based Mental Health Interventions with Mobile Virtual Reality and Wearable Smartwatches* [Doctoral dissertation, Department of Computer and Systems Sciences, Stockholm University].

Ramasamy, J., & Doshi, R. (2022). Machine learning in cyber physical systems for healthcare: brain tumor classification from MRI using transfer learning framework. In *Real-Time Applications of Machine Learning in Cyber-Physical Systems* (pp. 65–76). IGI global. doi:10.4018/978-1-7998-9308-0.ch005

Ramasamy, J., Doshi, R., & Hiran, K. K. (2021, August). Segmentation of brain tumor using deep learning methods: a review. In *Proceedings of the International Conference on Data Science, Machine Learning and Artificial Intelligence* (pp. 209-215). ACM. 10.1145/3484824.3484876

Ramasamy, J., Doshi, R., & Hiran, K. K. (2022, October). Detection of Brain Tumor in Medical Images Based on Feature Extraction by HOG and Machine Learning Algorithms. In *2022 International Conference on Trends in Quantum Computing and Emerging Business Technologies (TQCEBT)* (pp. 1-5). IEEE. 10.1109/TQCEBT54229.2022.10041564

Ray, J., Kumar, S., Pandey, S., & Akram, S. V. (2023, June). The Role of Augmented Reality and Virtual Reality in Shaping the Future of Health Psychology. In *2023 3rd International Conference on Pervasive Computing and Social Networking (ICPCSN)* (pp. 1604-1608). IEEE. 10.1109/ICPCSN58827.2023.00268

Reger, G. M. (Ed.). (2020). *Technology and mental health: a clinician's guide to improving outcomes*. Routledge. doi:10.4324/9780429020537

Richir, S., Kadri, A., & Ribeyre, N. (2022). Virtual Reality and Augmented Reality to Fight Effectively against Pandemics. In *The Nature of Pandemics* (pp. 311–348). CRC Press. doi:10.4324/9781315170220-20

Sharma, A., & Singh, B. (2022). Measuring Impact of E-commerce on Small Scale Business: A Systematic Review. *Journal of Corporate Governance and International Business Law*, 5(1).

Singh, B. (2020). GLOBAL SCIENCE AND JURISPRUDENTIAL APPROACH CONCERNING HEALTHCARE AND ILLNESS. *Indian Journal of Health and Medical Law*, 3(1), 7–13.

Singh, B. (2022). Understanding Legal Frameworks Concerning Transgender Healthcare in the Age of Dynamism. *ELECTRONIC JOURNAL OF SOCIAL AND STRATEGIC STUDIES*, 3(1), 56–65. doi:10.47362/EJSSS.2022.3104

Singh, B. (2022). Relevance of Agriculture-Nutrition Linkage for Human Healthcare: A Conceptual Legal Framework of Implication and Pathways. *Justice and Law Bulletin*, 1(1), 44–49.

Singh, B. (2022). COVID-19 Pandemic and Public Healthcare: Endless Downward Spiral or Solution via Rapid Legal and Health Services Implementation with Patient Monitoring Program. *Justice and Law Bulletin*, 1(1), 1–7.

Singh, B. (2023). Tele-Health Monitoring Lensing Deep Neural Learning Structure: Ambient Patient Wellness via Wearable Devices for Real-Time Alerts and Interventions. *Indian Journal of Health and Medical Law*, 6(2), 12–16.

Singh, B. (2023). Blockchain Technology in Renovating Healthcare: Legal and Future Perspectives. In Revolutionizing Healthcare Through Artificial Intelligence and Internet of Things Applications (pp. 177-186). IGI Global.

Singh, B. (2023). Federated Learning for Envision Future Trajectory Smart Transport System for Climate Preservation and Smart Green Planet: Insights into Global Governance and SDG-9 (Industry, Innovation and Infrastructure). *National Journal of Environmental Law*, 6(2), 6–17.

Singh, B. (2024). Legal Dynamics Lensing Metaverse Crafted for Videogame Industry and E-Sports: Phenomenological Exploration Catalyst Complexity and Future. *Journal of Intellectual Property Rights Law*, 7(1), 8–14.

Taghian, A., Abo-Zahhad, M., Sayed, M. S., & Abdel-Malek, A. (2021, December). Virtual, Augmented Reality, and Wearable Devices for Biomedical Applications: A Review. In *2021 9th International Japan-Africa Conference on Electronics, Communications, and Computations (JAC-ECC)* (pp. 93-98). IEEE.

Than, N. N. (2023). *Journey to Wellbeing: Seeing Beyond the Mind's Eye Through Story in a Virtual Therapeutic Space* [Doctoral dissertation, New York University Tandon School of Engineering].

Thompson, A. H. (2021). A Holistic Approach to Employee Functioning: Assessing the Impact of a Virtual-Reality Mindfulness Intervention at Work. Radovic, A., & Badawy, S. M. (2020). Technology use for adolescent health and wellness. *Pediatrics*, 145(Supplement_2), S186–S194.

Chapter 8
Mindful Movement:
VR–Enhanced Yoga and Exercise for Well–Being

Ranjit Singha
(iD) https://orcid.org/0000-0002-3541-8752
Christ University, India

Surjit Singha
(iD) https://orcid.org/0000-0002-5730-8677
Kristu Jayanti College (Autonomous), India

ABSTRACT

Investigating virtual reality (VR)-enhanced meditative movement reveals a promising strategy for improving mental and physical health. Virtual reality technology offers immersive, individualized experiences that effectively reduce tension, manage anxiety, and control pain, making it a valuable addition to conventional therapies. Research also demonstrates its efficacy in boosting motivation, maintaining an exercise regimen, and reducing stress. VR is an essential tool for treating mental health conditions such as anxiety and PTSD in clinical settings, with the potential to serve diverse populations. The significance of VR-enhanced mindful movement for overall well-being rests in its holistic approach, personalized experiences, and potential to revolutionize how individuals approach mental and physical health. With the ultimate goal of integrating VR into healthcare practices to enhance lives, a call to action includes additional research, ethical guidelines, accessibility efforts, and keeping abreast of emerging developments.

INTRODUCTION

In today's fast-paced digital age, the increased stress levels, anxiety, and emotional dissonance caused by the unrelenting demands of modern life and many technological distractions have made mental health an issue of the utmost importance. Meditative movement practices like yoga and exercise have gained popularity in response to these contemporary challenges. Mindful movement combines physical activity and mental awareness, including yoga, tai chi, Pilates, and moving meditation. It cultivates acute awareness

DOI: 10.4018/979-8-3693-1123-3.ch008

of the present moment, which includes the sensations of movement, respiration, and mental state (Clark et al., 2015; Russell & Arcuri, 2016). Due to its holistic approach, mindful movement is vital to mental health. The mindful movement recognizes the inextricable link between a healthy mind and a healthy body, as opposed to conventional exercise, which often focuses solely on physical fitness. (George et al., 2021; Guendelman et al., 2017) This method promotes balance and harmony that transcends the mat or the gym and permeates daily living. The remarkable capacity of mindful movement practices to promote emotional regulation and tension reduction is lauded. They provide a refuge where individuals can find relief from the relentless turmoil of their thoughts and the pressures of daily life. These practices have demonstrated their efficacy in reducing the symptoms of anxiety, depression, and post-traumatic stress disorder, establishing them as indispensable instruments for promoting mental health (Call et al., 2013; Lo et al., 2021; Doshi et al., 2023).

Deliberate movement improves cognitive function and concentration. It fosters mental clarity and creativity by honing attention. Increased awareness of the body's signals and sensations enables a profound connection between the physical and mental selves (Clark et al., 2015). Significantly, deliberate movement contributes to physical health as well as mental health. Regular practice improves strength, flexibility, cardiovascular health, and its positive effects on mental health (Oman, 2023; Clark et al., 2015; Fagbola et al., 2022). Frequently, mindful movement occurs in communal environments, fostering a sense of support and belonging. This community aspect can be instrumental in combating feelings of isolation and loneliness, which can significantly impact mental health (Oman, 2023; Saini et al., 2021). Mindful movement is not a short fix but a journey that lasts a lifetime. It is a practice that individuals can adapt to their changing requirements and circumstances throughout their lives. This adaptability is essential for maintaining mental health (Thiermann & Sheate, 2020).

This chapter investigates the feasibility of incorporating Virtual Reality (VR) technology into meditative movement practices. We will examine how this technology can improve the experience, efficacy, and accessibility of meditative movement, thereby contributing to the overarching objective of enhancing mental health. In recent years, Virtual Reality (VR) technology has emerged as a versatile and potent instrument, fundamentally altering how individuals engage in physical fitness and prioritize their overall health. Historically perceived as a physically demanding routine, exercise frequently lacked the immersive and engaging qualities required to sustain motivation. Siani & Marley (2021) and Winstein & Requejo (2015) state that VR has transcended its initial association with entertainment and gaming to revolutionize the exercise experience. VR transports users to captivating virtual worlds by creating immersive digital environments enhanced with 3D graphics, audio, and interactive elements. These environments vary from tranquil natural landscapes to dynamic gamified scenarios, making physical activity more engaging and enjoyable (Siani & Marley, 2021).

The incorporation of VR into exercise provides numerous benefits. It immerses users in captivating virtual environments, eliminating the monotony that can discourage regular exercise. Individualizing exercise routines according to a person's preferences and fitness level increases their effectiveness and enjoyment. Gamification elements such as earning points and completing quests motivate users to challenge themselves, transforming physical activity into a thrilling adventure. Accessing VR exercise experiences from the convenience of one's own home eliminates barriers related to time and location, democratizing fitness and making it accessible to a larger demographic.

The immersive nature of virtual reality contributes to stress reduction during exercise by providing a mental retreat from daily stressors and promoting mental health alongside physical health (Sakaki et al., 2021; Mouatt et al., 2020; Goel et al., 2023). The advent of VR technology in physical fitness represents a technological advancement and a paradigm transition in our approach to physical fitness. Its potential to make training more appealing, efficient, and accessible to many people bears promise for enhanced physical and mental health (Zhang et al., 2021; Gupta et al., 2022). This chapter will explore the specific applications of virtual reality (VR) in mindful movement practices, casting light on its transformative potential for health and overall quality of life. This chapter examines the inventive combination of Virtual Reality (VR) technology with mindful movement practices, such as yoga and exercise, and its potential to impact mental health and quality of life significantly. This investigation examines this integration's theoretical foundations, practical applications, and real-world consequences. This chapter explores how virtual reality (VR) can enhance the experience, efficacy, and accessibility of mindful movement, with a particular emphasis on strengthening mental health. This chapter's theoretical foundation is the recognition of the paramount significance of mental health in today's fast-paced, technology-driven society. The ubiquity of stress, anxiety, and emotional dissonance necessitates the development of novel treatments. Mindful movement practices, renowned for their holistic approach, have emerged as formidable instruments. These disciplines, such as yoga and exercise, emphasize the interconnectedness of the body and mind, fostering a heightened awareness of the present.

The chapter also examines the evolution of virtual reality (VR) technology, which has shifted from predominantly serving the entertainment and gaming industries to becoming a versatile tool for enhancing exercise experiences. Virtual reality utilizes immersive digital environments comprised of 3D graphics, audio, and interactive components to create captivating and engaging virtual worlds. This development represents a paradigm shift in how individuals approach physical activity, making it more appealing and sustainable. There are numerous benefits to incorporating VR technology into exercise, including enhanced immersion, personalization, motivation, and accessibility. It provides a novel method for reducing tension during physical activity by providing an escape for the mind. This dynamic field has the potential to revolutionize how individuals exercise and manage their mental health (Huang et al., 2022; Siani & Marley, 2021). This chapter examines theory and context and comprehensively explains the transformative potential of VR-enhanced mindful movement practices for improving mental health.

UNDERSTANDING MINDFUL MOVEMENT AND ITS BENEFITS

The concept of mindful movement embodies a profound union of mindfulness principles and physical activity, resulting in a holistic and harmonious approach to well-being. At its foundation, mindful movement is a philosophy and practice that encourages people to cultivate a keen and purposeful awareness of the present moment while actively engaging in various physical activities. This flexible approach applies to various movement-based disciplines, including but not limited to yoga, tai chi, Pilates, and moving meditation. The underlying principle of mindful movement is to disconnect from the continuous distractions of the modern world, the unceasing flow of thoughts, and the disconnection between the body and mind. Instead, it encourages individuals to embrace each movement and sensation with complete awareness to immerse themselves in the physical experience thoroughly. Mindful movement practices encourage participants to engage their senses, respiration, and consciousness while moving. The emphasis is not solely on the outcome or a particular fitness objective but on the journey itself. This journey requires careful attention to every movement, respiration, and sensation. It entails being entirely present in the here and now and letting go of concerns about the past or the future (Clark et al., 2015).

Integrating focused and purposeful respiration is a crucial component of mindful movement. The breath becomes a guide, synchronizing with the movement's cadence, enhancing concentration and fostering profound mindfulness. Each inhalation and exhale establishes a link between the body and the mind. The meditative movement practice transcends physical exercise and becomes a mental workout. This method encourages practitioners to investigate their inner landscape and connect with themselves deeply. It is a journey into the self in which one can find inner serenity, heightened self-awareness, and enhanced well-being. The concept of mindful movement exemplifies an exquisite synthesis of mindfulness and physical activity. It provides a means for individuals to connect with their inner selves, nurturing a profound sense of presence and awareness in every physical interaction (Kelly et al., 2022; Dollinger et al., 2021; Meena et al., 2021). It investigates the incorporation of Virtual Reality (VR) technology to enhance the mindful movement experience. Mindful movement practices offer many psychological and physiological advantages, making them valuable for enhancing overall health. First, they are effective stress-reduction techniques, eliciting a state of relaxation that reduces the production of stress hormones like cortisol. This effect induces a profound sense of peace and tranquillity, aiding individuals in coping with the stresses and anxieties of modern life. By immersing themselves in the present moment, practitioners temporarily detach themselves from the outside world's unrelenting demands, substantially reducing their stress levels.

These practices play a significant role in emotional regulation. By nurturing heightened self-awareness, individuals can navigate their emotions effectively (Zhang et al., 2019; Guendelman et al., 2017; Patel et al., 2022). The connection between physical and mental states enables practitioners to manage their feelings proactively instead of reactively, promoting emotional resilience and IQ.

Meditative movement improves cognitive function by enhancing concentration, attention, and clarity. It cultivates enhanced engagement and creativity by actively engaging the mind in monitoring physical activities and sensations. This practice improves overall cognitive abilities by strengthening the body and mind (Clark et al., 2015; Ramasamy et al., 2022). While mindful movement focuses predominantly on mental and emotional health, it significantly improves physical health. Regular exercise improves strength, flexibility, and cardiovascular health, resulting in a profound sense of wellness and vitality.

Numerous studies indicate that meditative movement practices effectively reduce anxiety and depressive symptoms. These practices provide a holistic approach to managing these emotional challenges by addressing emotional regulation, relieving tension, and enhancing overall mental and physical health. They provide vital tools for reducing the emotional burdens of anxiety and depression. Mindful movement's psychological and physiological benefits are extensive and multifaceted, including stress reduction, emotional regulation, enhanced cognitive function, improved physical health, and decreased anxiety and depression symptoms. Mindful movement practices provide a holistic approach to well-being by harmonizing the mind and body to nurture a profound sense of mental and emotional equilibrium (Dollinger et al., 2021; Zhang et al., 2022; Ramasamy et al., 2021). This chapter will explore the potential of integrating Virtual Reality (VR) technology into a meditative movement to enhance these benefits and contribute to overall mental health.

Mindful movement, a unique combination of physical activity and mindfulness principles, is essential for reducing tension and regulating emotions. This synergy between mental focus and physical activity is an effective method for enhancing emotional well-being. Mindful movement is a highly effective technique for tension reduction. It provides a secure and welcoming space for individuals to escape endless demands and pressures temporarily. Practitioners experience a profound sensation of relaxation due to their complete involvement in the present moment and each movement. This immersion in the present moment effectively reduces the production of stress hormones such as cortisol, resulting in tranquillity and peace (Sharma & Rush, 2014). Mindful movement is a mental sanctuary, relieving contemporary life's stresses and anxieties.

Moreover, mindful movement has a significant impact on emotional regulation. Individuals engage in these practices and develop a heightened awareness of their physical and mental states. This increased self-awareness enables them to identify and manage their emotions more effectively. Individuals learn to respond thoughtfully to emotional impulses rather than impulsively. It enhances emotional intelligence, fostered by mindful movement, and enables individuals to manage their emotions precisely and skillfully. The practice cultivates a deeper connection between the mind and body, allowing individuals to harmonize their emotional responses and physical sensations. This emotional resilience provides a robust means of contending with daily challenges, ultimately promoting dynamic equilibrium and well-being (Guendelman et al., 2017; Heppner et al., 2015; Ramasamy et al., 2022).

Mindful movement is a refuge for stress reduction and emotional regulation, enabling individuals to temporarily disconnect from the demands of the external world and find solace in the present. This immersion reduces tension and induces a profound sense of peace and tranquillity. Moreover, mindful movement enables individuals to navigate their emotions skillfully and precisely, nurturing emotional resilience and intelligence. Combining mindfulness and physical activity in these practices offers a holistic approach to stress and emotion management, contributing to improved mental health. This chapter will explore the potential of incorporating Virtual Reality (VR) technology into a meditative movement to enhance these stress-reduction and emotional regulation benefits.

VIRTUAL REALITY IN WELLNESS AND EXERCISE

Virtual Reality (VR) is a cutting-edge technology with expanded wellness applications. It involves the creation of immersive digital environments that simulate real-world experiences using 3D imagery, audio, and interactive components. This technology has transcended its initial function in entertainment and gaming to become a versatile instrument with transformative potential for enhancing overall health. In wellness, VR technology opens the door to improved mental, emotional, and physical health. It provides novel approaches to various aspects of wellness, such as tension reduction, emotional regulation, and physical fitness. VR experiences are particularly compelling for mental and emotional health due to their immersive nature. VR provides a retreat from the pressures and distractions of the modern world by immersing users in relaxing or captivating virtual environments. These immersive experiences can alleviate stress and promote emotional equilibrium (Lindner, 2020; Srinivasulu et al., 2022).

Virtual reality has the potential to revolutionize physical fitness engagement. Typical exercise regimens can frequently become monotonous and uninspiring. By transporting users to enthralling virtual environments, VR technology adds a thrilling and dynamic dimension to physical activity. This immersion combats the monotony of exercise, making it more pleasurable and engaging. In addition, VR offers a highly customized method of locomotion. Users can select activities tailored to their fitness objectives, such as weight loss, strength training, or stress reduction. Gamification elements of the technology, such as earning points or completing quests, encourage individuals to stretch their limits and remain engaged. VR exercise experiences can be accessed from the comfort of one's residence, removing time and location barriers. Incorporating virtual reality (VR) into wellness and exercise affects the mind-body connection. Users become engrossed in the virtual world, isolating themselves from external disturbances and enhancing their physical and mental harmony. Its heightened focus on the present moment enhances mental lucidity, creativity, and a holistic approach to well-being (Siani & Marley, 2021; Bedir & Erhan, 2021).

Virtual Reality technology is making significant strides in the wellness industry by providing innovative solutions to reduce tension, regulate emotions, and increase exercise motivation. These immersive experiences have the potential to transform how individuals approach their well-being, providing a dynamic and engaging path to a healthier and more balanced existence. Virtual Reality (VR) technology has the potential to revolutionize exercise engagement by addressing the monotony and lack of motivation that frequently discourage individuals from sustaining a regular fitness routine. By immersing users in captivating virtual environments, virtual reality eliminates the redundancy of conventional exercise. Individual fitness objectives are catered to by customizing virtual reality workouts, enhancing their effectiveness and enjoyment. Gamification elements, such as accumulating points and completing quests, transform physical activity into a thrilling adventure that motivates individuals to surpass their limits. The accessibility of virtual reality, which enables users to exercise at home, democratizes fitness and makes it accessible to a larger population.

In addition, the immersive nature of virtual reality facilitates stress reduction during exercise by providing a mental retreat from daily stresses. Virtual reality (VR) improves exercise engagement by providing immersive experiences, personalization, motivation, accessibility, and tension reduction, transforming how individuals approach fitness and wellness. (Zhang et al., 2021; Arpaa et al., 2021).

Virtual Reality (VR) technology enables immersive experiences that profoundly affect the mind-body connection. VR is renowned for its capacity to transport users to captivating virtual environments, and within these immersive settings, a unique and potent mind-body connection is formed. Virtual reality (VR) allows users to become completely immersed in the virtual world, isolating them from external distractions. The heightened focus on the present moment and physical movement within the virtual environment results in a stronger connection between body and mind. During these experiences, users are encouraged to monitor their activities, sensations, and breathing, cultivating unrivalled attentiveness. This enhanced mind-body connection extends beyond the exercise experience and influences other aspects of well-being. Virtual reality promotes mindfulness and mental clarity by encouraging individuals to be completely present. Users engage their physical and mental selves in novel and dynamic ways, fostering creativity. This holistic approach to health is a distinguishing characteristic of VR technology.

Virtual reality's immersive experiences have a transformative effect on the mind-body connection. VR contributes to a greater comprehension of one's physical and mental self by cultivating heightened awareness and mindfulness.

VIRTUAL YOGA IN ENHANCING MINDFUL MOVEMENT

By incorporating Virtual Reality (VR) technology into traditional yoga practices, a revolutionary approach to meditative movement is introduced. Traditional yoga is revered for its ability to create a profound mind-body connection, and virtual reality (VR) enhances this connection. VR-enhanced yoga sessions offer an innovative way to engage with this age-old practice by immersing practitioners in tranquil and immersive virtual environments. Virtual reality technology allows users to enter a virtual world replicating serene natural landscapes, peaceful sanctuaries, and imaginative and meditative settings. (Mouatt et al., 2020) These environments facilitate a more immersive experience, enhancing concentration and engagement. In VR-enhanced yoga, experienced instructors frequently offer a variety of virtual classes and guidance to help users align their movements, postures, and respiration with the principles of yoga. Users can tailor their sessions to their experience level and preferences, investigate various yoga styles, receive real-time alignment and form monitoring feedback. Waller et al. (2021) and Hamilton et al. (2020) note that the accessibility and convenience of VR-enhanced yoga make it more accessible to a larger population, making it a transformative instrument for overall health and well-being.

For a seamless and engaging experience, designing VR-enhanced yoga sessions requires deliberate thought. Several essential factors must be considered to make the most of this innovative approach to meditative movement. Noteworthy is the selection of virtual environments, which should elicit tranquillity and mindfulness following yoga's principles. Including tactile sensations and vibrations, haptic feedback and immersion enhance the sense of connection with the virtual environment. Real-time instruction from qualified instructors ensures adherence to yoga principles, while customization options accommodate individual preferences and objectives. (Nagarathna et al., 2021) Motion monitoring and feedback increase safety and efficiency. Accessibility and user-friendly design are essential, and various yoga practices should be provided to accommodate a variety of preferences and requirements. Considering these design considerations, VR-enhanced yoga sessions can enhance the mind-body connection and traditional yoga practice, ultimately contributing to overall health and well-being.

CASE STUDIES

Several case studies have investigated the efficacy of virtual reality yoga platforms in enhancing mindful movement and well-being. These platforms have demonstrated the revolutionary potential of virtual reality technology for traditional yoga practices.

Oculus Move is a virtual reality (VR) fitness platform that provides a selection of yoga sessions in immersive virtual environments. According to a case study conducted with Oculus Move Yoga, participants reported higher levels of engagement and motivation than in traditional in-person yoga classes. The ability to personalize sessions, receive real-time feedback, and practice in tranquil virtual environments contributed to a deeper mind-body connection and increased satisfaction.

Supernatural is a virtual reality fitness platform incorporating yoga with cardio and mindful movement. A study investigating the effects of Supernatural's virtual reality (VR) yoga sessions revealed that participants experienced reduced stress and enhanced emotional regulation. The immersive environments and guided instruction helped users feel more connected to their bodies and emotions, nurturing feelings of serenity and well-being.

FitXR is a virtual reality (VR) fitness platform that provides interactive yoga experiences. A FitXR Yoga case study revealed that users who engaged in VR-enhanced yoga reported excellent mental acuity and concentration. The gamified aspects of FitXR's yoga sessions, such as accumulating points for precise movements and completing challenges, increased motivation and engagement and strengthened the mind-body connection.

Within is a platform dedicated to creating immersive experiences, such as yoga. Participants in a study with Within Yoga VR reported enhanced tension reduction and emotional regulation. The platform's emphasis on tranquil virtual environments and mindfulness techniques enhanced the sense of calm and emotional fortitude.

These case studies demonstrate the efficacy of virtual reality yoga platforms in fostering engagement, tension reduction, emotional regulation, and a stronger mind-body connection. VR technology can potentially elevate traditional yoga practices, making them more accessible and advantageous for a more significant number of users. As VR-enhanced yoga continues to develop, it bears promise for promoting overall health and well-being.

VR-ENHANCED EXERCISE PROGRAMS FOR MENTAL WELL-BEING

Adapting traditional exercises for VR involves reimagining and enhancing established exercise regimens to make them more engaging, immersive, and conducive to mental health promotion. Users can run through picturesque virtual parks, cycle along virtual coastlines, and participate in thrilling virtual races. VR's immersive and engaging nature distracts from physical exertion, making cardio workouts pleasurable and encouraging regular exercise. Strength training exercises can be incorporated into VR by replicating a virtual gym or training environment. Users can interact with virtual weights and apparatus, with resistance tailored to their fitness level. Strength training can be more engaging and rewarding by incorporating gamified elements such as competing against virtual opponents or accomplishing challenging quests. VR can enhance mindful movement practices such as yoga by generating tranquil and immersive virtual settings. Practitioners can enhance their mind-body connection and cultivate serenity and mindfulness by performing yoga poses in picturesque virtual environments. In virtual reality, callisthenics and bodyweight exercises such as push-ups, lunges, and burpees can be gamified, with real-time feedback on form and performance to enhance effectiveness.

Dance and aerobic exercises can be adapted for virtual reality to create virtual dance studios and interactive dance activities that make exercise more enjoyable and entertaining. The key to these adaptations is to immerse users in enticing virtual environments, provide guided instruction, and design rewarding and engaging experiences. Stewart et al. (2022) and Kruse et al. (2020) assert that virtual reality (VR) technology has the potential to make conventional exercises more engaging and efficient, thereby enhancing mental health and overall health.

Developing immersive Virtual Reality (VR) exercise routines that foster mindfulness requires several essential considerations. It begins with captivating virtual environments that immerse users in tranquil, aesthetically pleasing settings. These settings are conducive to a meditative experience. Experienced instructors guide participants through routines while emphasizing the significance of concentrating on their movements, respiration, and sensations. Incorporating breathing exercises and brief meditation sessions into the VR regimen improves mindfulness and fosters a profound connection between the physical and mental selves. Sensory feedback, such as haptic sensations, enriches the immersive experience by enhancing the relationship between the user's body and the virtual environment. Gamification and interactive challenges encourage participants to maintain mindfulness throughout the routine. These can include tasks such as concentrating on particular aspects of the virtual environment or sustaining a specific pace and rhythm with their movements. Providing participants with progressively complex routines and personalization options ensures that their experience is tailored to their fitness level and mindfulness objectives. These factors contribute to a balanced and healthy lifestyle by creating a holistic mental and physical well-being approach (Zhang et al., 2021; Dollinger et al., 2021).

Measuring the effect of Virtual Reality (VR) enhanced exercise on psychological outcomes is essential for determining the efficacy of this innovative method of promoting mental health. For a comprehensive evaluation, numerous quantitative and qualitative approaches can be utilized. Psychometric assessments and standardized surveys can quantify stress, anxiety, and emotional regulation variables. Monitoring biometric data, such as heart rate variability and electrodermal activity, provides additional insight into participants' physiological responses. Self-reported experiences through interviews and open-ended questionnaires provide valuable qualitative data on mood, tension, and emotional regulation. Behavioural observations, cognitive function assessments, and neuroimaging techniques provide a greater understanding of alterations in behaviour, cognitive abilities, and neural processes. Hao et al. (2023) and Mouatt et al. (2020) have assessed the long-term effects of VR-enhanced exercise on psychological well-being. This multifaceted approach ensures a comprehensive comprehension of the psychological effects of VR technology on mental health, allowing for the refinement and optimization of these programs for the greatest possible benefit.

DESIGNING IMMERSIVE ENVIRONMENTS FOR MINDFUL MOVEMENT

Virtual Reality (VR) landscape design is a discipline that combines aesthetics, ambience, and sensory components. During mindful movement practices, the goal is to convey users to serene and visually captivating environments that foster tranquillity and inspiration. A vital element of the design is the incorporation of natural beauty. Key components include breathtaking vistas, tranquil lakes, lush forests, and pristine coastlines. (Kelly et al., 2022; Neo et al., 2021; Chandler et al., 2022).

A sound is an effective instrument for creating a soothing atmosphere. It is essential to include ambient sounds such as birdsong, the gentle rustling of foliage, and the murmurs of a peaceful stream. These aural components enhance the multi-sensory experience and heighten the feeling of presence within the virtual environment. It is essential to pay attention to visual details within the landscape. Calming hues, such as soft blues and verdant greens, promote tranquillity. The interplay of light and shadow encourages users to be fully present during mindful movement by creating an aesthetically pleasing ambience. Ensure the virtual space feels open and expansive as a fundamental design principle. This design allows unrestricted movement and investigation, avoiding clutter or overly complex scenery that could disturb the sense of serenity and inspiration (Neo et al., 2021; Chandler et al., 2021).

The inclusion of interactive landscape elements increases user engagement. During mindful movement practices, virtual objects such as stones, petals, and mild breezes provide tactile and visual stimuli, prompting users to forge a deeper connection with the environment. Creating calming and inspiring virtual landscapes in VR is ultimately about cultivating an environment that encourages contemplation, promotes an appreciation for the natural world's beauty, and instils a profound sense of peace. These transformative landscapes enhance the meditative movement experience and allow users to fully immerse themselves in their practice, forging a stronger bond with their inner selves. In Virtual Reality (VR), sensory stimuli enhance conscious movement experiences. These sensory elements engage the user's senses to produce a more immersive, transformative, and impactful experience (Uhl et al., 2023; Kwon & Iedema, 2022).

Virtual reality provides a visually rich environment, immersing users in tranquil landscapes, captivating visuals, and realistic depictions of nature. Visual stimuli, such as breathtaking vistas, gently swaying trees, and intricate details in the surrounding environment, enhance a sense of presence and promote mindfulness. The interplay of colours and light contributes to the aesthetic appeal and creates a tranquil and inspiring environment. Soundscapes in virtual reality are a powerful instrument for enhancing mindful movement experience. The ambient sounds of birdsong, the wind's murmur, and the gentle water flow provide an auditory backdrop that promotes tranquillity. These sounds complement the visuals, creating a multi-sensory environment that encourages users to be fully present and engaged in their practice. Haptic feedback or tactile sensations are essential for improving the sense of contact and connection with a virtual environment. Users can feel imperceptible vibrations or light touches in response to their interactions with the environment. This tactile feedback encourages a deeper level of immersion because users feel more physically connected to the virtual reality environment (Voinescu et al., 2020).

The kinaesthetic sense, associated with bodily movement and spatial awareness, is highly engaged in mindful movement practices. In response to the virtual environment, VR encourages users to engage in physical activities and postures. Moving one's body in the virtual world strengthens the mind-body connection and heightens awareness. Some VR experiences may include olfactory or gustatory sensations, albeit less frequently. These may consist of the aromas of nature, such as the perfume of flowers or the flavour of a calming herbal tea. (Zhang et al., 2021; Dollinger et al., 2021). Incorporating these sensory stimuli in virtual reality enhances the mindful movement experience and encourages users to be fully present and engaged in the practice. By creating a multi-sensory environment replicating nature's majesty and promoting tranquillity, virtual reality technology provides a platform for individuals to strengthen their mind-body connection and overall awareness. This sensory integration contributes to a holistic approach to mental and physical health (Zhang et al., 2021; Dollinger et al., 2021).

In Virtual Reality (VR), sensory stimuli augment meditative movement experiences. These sensory elements engage the user's senses to create an experience that is more immersive, powerful, and transformative. With its captivating landscapes and intricate details, the visual stimulation fosters a heightened awareness of the present moment and promotes mindfulness. The soundscapes promote tranquillity by combining the visuals with calming ambient noises, such as bird songs and leaves rustling. Tactile feedback through haptic sensations heightens the sense of contact and connection with the virtual environment, enhancing immersion (Dozio et al., 2021). Kinesthetic engagement motivates users to execute physical movements and postures, fostering a solid mind-body connection. Although less common, even olfactory and gustatory elements can engage multiple senses to promote mindfulness. These sensory stimuli within VR create a multi-sensory environment replicating nature's grandeur, promoting a holistic mental and physical health approach.

USER EXPERIENCE AND ENGAGEMENT

Diverse variables affect user participation in VR-enhanced meditative movement. The design and quality of virtual environments replicating tranquil natural settings with immersive landscapes are fundamental. Effective navigation of contemplative movement practices requires instruction from experienced leaders within the virtual space. Personalization, gamification, and accessibility increase user engagement by enabling them to customize their experiences to their preferences and abilities. Real-time feedback, community, progression, and interactivity maintain user engagement and motivation. In addition, the ability to monitor progress and improvements contributes to an engaging and rewarding experience. These factors make VR-enhanced mindful movement delightful and effective for promoting mental and physical health (Kelly et al., 2022).

Addressing motion sickness and discomfort issues is critical to delivering a positive user experience in VR-enhanced meditative movement practices. Combining strategies such as gradual exposure, high-quality hardware, explicit user guidelines, design considerations, and realistic feedback assists in mitigating these problems. The availability of seated and standing VR options, user training, and a responsive feedback system contribute to a more comfortable, streamlined user experience. The objective of continuously enhancing VR software based on user feedback and progressively introducing users to VR environments is to create an engaging and enjoyable mindful movement experience while minimizing discomfort and motion sickness (Zhang et al., 2021).

Improving presence and embodiment in virtual reality (VR) exercise is essential for creating an immersive and engaging mindful movement experience. Realistic sensory feedback, naturalistic movements, environments replicating the real world, and mirror neurons contribute to a more profound sense of presence. They enhance the user's connection to the virtual environment by engaging multiple senses, fostering user interactivity, and permitting customization. (Llorens et al., 2019) Progression, challenges, community and social interactions, and mindful guidance enhance an individual's understanding of embodiment and contribute to their overall well-being when using VR-enhanced exercise. These strategies make mindful movement more engaging and applicable, encouraging users to be fully present and connected to their practice.

PERSONALIZATION AND FEEDBACK IN VR-ENHANCED WELLNESS

Individualization of VR exercise experiences is essential for increasing the effectiveness and user engagement of VR-enhanced wellness programs. By allowing users to customize the VR workout's intensity, style, virtual environment, duration, and real-time feedback, these programs empower individuals to create an experience tailored to their specific needs and objectives. Beginners can begin at their tempo, while advanced users can challenge themselves, all within the most motivating virtual environment. Users can achieve a genuinely personalized wellness journey that results in more rewarding and effective mindful movement experiences if they can alter workouts to their schedules and select their preferred level of guidance. This strategy enhances user engagement and promotes adherence and general health.

VR-enhanced wellness programs require the incorporation of real-time posture and movement correction feedback. Real-time feedback assists users in maintaining proper form, minimizing injury risk, and optimizing the efficacy of their mindful movement practice. Advanced motion-tracking technology, visual cues, auditory prompts, haptic feedback, and customizable guidance are strategies for integrating real-time feedback. By providing users with these feedback mechanisms and data visualization tools, virtual reality (VR) wellness programs direct users toward correct posture and movement, enhancing their engagement and well-being. This multi-sensory feedback system empowers users to optimize their practice and promotes a safe and immersive mindful movement experience. Utilizing artificial intelligence (AI) to adapt virtual reality (VR) wellness programs based on user progress is a potent strategy for improving the efficacy of conscious movement experiences. AI can generate comprehensive user profiles that include preferences, fitness levels, and objectives. It provides dynamic content recommendations, monitors progress, and adjusts real-time exercise difficulty. AI facilitates goal-setting, provides personalized feedback and direction, and enables interaction with AI-powered virtual assistants. AI ensures that VR wellness programs remain engaging, motivating, and individualized by analyzing user data and employing predictive analytics. These AI-driven modifications optimize the VR-enhanced wellness voyage, improving users' overall health.

CLINICAL APPLICATIONS AND RESEARCH FINDINGS

In clinical settings, the effectiveness of Virtual Reality (VR)--enhanced mindful movement has demonstrated its potential as a valuable therapeutic aid for promoting mental and physical health. The VR-enhanced meditative movement has effectively reduced stress levels in clinical settings. Virtual reality's immersive and distraction-free nature enables individuals to concentrate on their movements and surroundings, promoting emotional regulation. In addition, clinical studies have investigated using VR-enhanced mindful movement as an adjunct to conventional anxiety management therapies. Virtual reality provides a secure and controlled environment where individuals can practice relaxation techniques and mindfulness, thereby reducing anxiety symptoms.

VR has been utilized for pain management in clinical contexts, effectively reducing pain perception and discomfort during medical procedures. In pediatric healthcare and various medical interventions, this strategy has been instrumental. VR-enhanced mindful movement is frequently used with conventional therapeutic methods such as cognitive-behavioural therapy (CBT) and mindfulness-based stress reduction (MBSR). Combining virtual reality (VR) technology and evidence-based psychotherapy has shown positive clinical outcomes, enhancing the therapeutic process. VR technology makes Biofeedback and sensory integration possible, providing real-time data on physiological responses. This information can be helpful in clinical contexts, as it can help individuals become aware of their bodily responses and teach them how to manage stress and anxiety effectively.

The interactive and engaging nature of VR-enhanced mindful movement improves accessibility and allure, increasing user engagement and greater adherence to therapeutic interventions in clinical settings. Despite the evident efficacy of VR-enhanced mindful movement in clinical settings, ongoing research is required to explore its full potential, refine treatment protocols, and tailor interventions to the specific requirements of different patient populations. Combining cutting-edge VR technology and mindfulness practices offers a promising method for enhancing mental and physical health in clinical applications (Zhang et al., 2021).

Numerous studies comparing conventional exercise to VR-enhanced exercise have shed light on the benefits and potential of VR for enhancing physical activity and mental health. These findings demonstrate that VR-enhanced exercise improves motivation, enjoyment, adherence, and cardiovascular health. It is suitable for strength training, mindfulness practices, and rehabilitation, providing a more engaging and interactive platform for diverse populations. Those who find traditional exercise challenging can benefit significantly from the perception of less exertion during VR workouts. Moreover, the diversity of virtual environments and social connections fostered by multiplayer VR experiences make it a promising method for promoting physical and mental health. Additional research is required to fully comprehend VR-enhanced exercise's long-term effects and broader potential in various contexts (Stewart et al., 2022; Mouatt et al., 2020).

Virtual Reality (VR) wellness programs offer immersive and custom-tailored interventions for treating various mental health conditions. These programs have shown efficacy in addressing particular mental health issues. For example, virtual reality exposure therapy has proven effective in treating anxiety disorders by enabling patients to confront and manage their fears in a safe, controlled environment. Similarly, it has demonstrated tremendous promise in treating Post-Traumatic Stress Disorder (PTSD) by providing individuals with a supportive environment to process traumatic memories. In the case of depression, VR wellness programs employ mindfulness practices and guided meditation in calming virtual environments, teaching stress reduction techniques and promoting a transition from harmful to positive thoughts and experiences (Siani & Marley, 2021).

VR serves as a diversion and coping mechanism for those recovering from substance use disorders, thereby reducing the risk of relapse. It aids in treating eating disorders by encouraging a positive body image and healthier food relationships. Moreover, VR programs assist individuals with Attention-Deficit/Hyperactivity Disorder (ADHD) by enhancing concentration and focus through engaging tasks. Virtual reality (VR) provides a structured environment for practising social interactions and communication skills for those with Autism Spectrum Disorders (ASD). In addition, VR wellness programs offer stress management via mindfulness and relaxation exercises and cognitive rehabilitation for neurological conditions such as traumatic brain injury and stroke. They can also aid in treating insomnia by providing relaxation techniques and promoting improved sleep patterns. Virtual reality offers phantom limb pain sufferers distraction and relaxation. Individuals with schizophrenia can use virtual reality to develop social skills, improve cognitive functions, and manage hallucinations and delusions (Tsamitros et al., 2021; Segawa et al., 2020).

These individualized VR wellness programs provide a secure and encouraging atmosphere for therapy, exposure, skill development, and relaxation. To validate the effectiveness of VR interventions for these conditions and to assure their compatibility with traditional treatments. However, additional research and clinical trials are required.

ETHICAL CONSIDERATIONS AND FUTURE DIRECTIONS

Integrating Virtual Reality (VR) into wellness and mental health raises critical ethical issues. Users must provide informed consent to participate in virtual reality (VR) wellness programs, thoroughly comprehend the nature of the experience and data collection and acknowledge the potential psychological impact. Privacy and data security are paramount, as VR platforms frequently collect sensitive user information, necessitating stringent data protection measures. When designing VR interventions for vulnerable populations, such as infants, the elderly, or those with mental health conditions, special attention must be paid to their safety and ease of navigation in the VR environment. To prevent the escalation of health disparities, it is crucial to bridge the digital divide and make VR wellness programs accessible to diverse demographics. To maintain the integrity of the therapeutic relationship within an immersive VR environment, professionals utilizing VR as a therapeutic tool must establish and sustain appropriate therapeutic boundaries. As virtual reality (VR) technology evolves, ethical guidelines and standards must evolve to inform professionals, researchers, and developers of emergent ethical issues and best practices.

On the other hand, privacy and data security concerns are raised by VR-enhanced exercise platforms. These platforms can collect vast amounts of data, including biometric information and user behaviour, in virtual environments, necessitating informed consent and stringent security. Users should have distinct ownership and control over their data, transparency regarding how it is utilized and adherence to data protection regulations. Personalization, advanced biofeedback mechanisms, increased accessibility, integration with telehealth, additional research, social interaction within virtual environments, and holistic wellness programs are predicted for the future of VR-enabled mindful movement. These advancements offer promising prospects for the field, paving the way for more personalized, engaging, and effective mental and physical health interventions.

CONCLUSION

Exploring Virtual Reality (VR)-enhanced mindful movement has revealed several key findings and insights. VR has the potential to provide individuals with immersive, engaging, and highly personalized experiences that promote mental and physical well-being. This technology effectively reduces stress, manages anxiety, controls pain, and is a valuable adjunct to traditional therapeutic approaches. The VR-enhanced mindful movement has also demonstrated its effectiveness in improving motivation, adherence to exercise routines, cardiovascular health, strength gains, and stress reduction. Research has shown that VR can be valuable in clinical settings, particularly for addressing mental health conditions such as anxiety, PTSD, and depression. It also offers significant potential for promoting well-being in diverse populations.

The significance of VR-enhanced mindful movement for overall well-being cannot be overstated. It offers a holistic approach to mental and physical health, harnessing the power of immersive and interactive technology to engage users and promote mindfulness. By fostering a deeper mind-body connection and offering a wide range of wellness programs, VR enhances motivation, reduces stress, and supports adherence to exercise routines. It has demonstrated its efficacy in addressing mental health conditions in clinical settings, offering individuals new healing and growth tools. Moreover, VR technology can be personalized, ensuring users can tailor their experiences to their unique needs and preferences, ultimately enhancing their overall well-being.

The promising potential of VR-enhanced mindful movement warrants a call to action for further research and integration into healthcare practices. It is essential to continue conducting rigorous scientific studies and clinical trials to validate the effectiveness of VR interventions for a wide range of mental health conditions and wellness goals. Healthcare practitioners, researchers, and policymakers should collaborate to create guidelines and ethical standards for using VR in therapy and wellness programs. Moreover, efforts should be made to enhance the accessibility of VR technology and address privacy concerns to ensure these platforms' safe and inclusive use. As VR evolves, professionals must stay informed about emerging developments and best practices. Ultimately, integrating VR-enhanced mindful movement into healthcare practices can transform how individuals approach mental and physical well-being, offering innovative, engaging, and effective interventions that can improve lives.

REFERENCES

Arpaïa, P., D'Errico, G., De Paolis, L. T., Moccaldi, N., & Nuccetelli, F. (2021). A Narrative review of Mindfulness-Based Interventions using Virtual Reality. *Mindfulness*, *13*(3), 556–571. doi:10.1007/s12671-021-01783-6

Call, D., Miron, L. R., & Orcutt, H. K. (2013). Effectiveness of brief mindfulness techniques in reducing symptoms of anxiety and stress. *Mindfulness*, *5*(6), 658–668. doi:10.1007/s12671-013-0218-6

Chandler, T., Richards, A. E., Jenny, B., Dickson, F., Huang, J., Klippel, A., Neylan, M., Wang, F., & Prober, S. M. (2021). Immersive landscapes: Modelling ecosystem reference conditions in virtual reality. *Landscape Ecology*, *37*(5), 1293–1309. doi:10.1007/s10980-021-01313-8

Chandler, T., Richards, A. E., Jenny, B., Dickson, F., Huang, J., Klippel, A., Neylan, M., Wang, F., & Prober, S. M. (2021b). Immersive landscapes: Modelling ecosystem reference conditions in virtual reality. *Landscape Ecology*, *37*(5), 1293–1309. doi:10.1007/s10980-021-01313-8

Clark, D., Schumann, F., & Mostofsky, S. H. (2015b). Mindful movement and skilled attention. *Frontiers in Human Neuroscience*, *9*. doi:10.3389/fnhum.2015.00297 PMID:26190986

Döllinger, N., Wienrich, C., & Latoschik, M. E. (2021). Challenges and Opportunities of Immersive Technologies for Mindfulness Meditation: A Systematic Review. *Frontiers in Virtual Reality*, *2*, 644683. doi:10.3389/frvir.2021.644683

Doshi, R., Hiran, K. K., Gök, M., El-kenawy, E. S. M., Badr, A., & Abotaleb, M. (2023). Artificial Intelligence's Significance in Diseases with Malignant Tumours. *Mesopotamian Journal of Artificial Intelligence in Healthcare*, *2023*, 35–39.

Dozio, N., Maggioni, E., Pittera, D., Gallace, A., & Obrist, M. (2021). May I smell your attention: Exploration of smell and sound for visuospatial attention in virtual reality. *Frontiers in Psychology*, *12*, 671470. Advance online publication. doi:10.3389/fpsyg.2021.671470 PMID:34366990

Fagbola, T. M., Fagbola, F. I., Aroba, O. J., Doshi, R., Hiran, K. K., & Thakur, S. C. (2022). Smart face masks for Covid-19 pandemic management: A concise review of emerging architectures, challenges and future research directions. *IEEE Sensors Journal*, *23*(2), 877–888. doi:10.1109/JSEN.2022.3225067

George, A. J., John, R., & Rajkumar, E. (2021c). Mindfulness-based positive psychology interventions: A systematic review. *BMC Psychology*, *9*(1), 116. doi:10.1186/s40359-021-00618-2 PMID:34362457

Goel, P., Jhanwar, N., Jain, P., Khatri, S., & Hiran, K. K. (2023, August). Efficient Blood Availability for Targeted Individuals Through Cloud Computing Web Application. In *2023 International Conference on Emerging Trends in Networks and Computer Communications (ETNCC)* (pp. 1-7). IEEE. 10.1109/ETNCC59188.2023.10284940

Guendelman, S., Medeiros, S., & Rampes, H. (2017). Mindfulness and Emotion Regulation: Insights from Neurobiological, Psychological, and Clinical Studies. *Frontiers in Psychology*, *8*. doi:10.3389/fpsyg.2017.00220 PMID:28321194

Gupta, A. K., Srinivasulu, A., Hiran, K. K., Sreenivasulu, G., Rajeyyagari, S., & Subramanyam, M. (2022). Prediction of omicron virus using combined extended convolutional and recurrent neural networks technique on CT-scan images. *Interdisciplinary Perspectives on Infectious Diseases*, *2022*, 2022. doi:10.1155/2022/1525615 PMID:36562006

Hamilton, D. E., McKechnie, J., Edgerton, E., & Wilson, C. (2020). Immersive virtual reality as a pedagogical tool in education: A systematic literature review of quantitative learning outcomes and experimental design. *Journal of Computers in Education*, *8*(1), 1–32. doi:10.1007/s40692-020-00169-2

Hao, J., Li, Y., Swanson, R. M., Chen, Z., & Siu, K. (2023). Effects of virtual reality on physical, cognitive, and psychological outcomes in cancer rehabilitation: A systematic review and meta-analysis. *Supportive Care in Cancer*, *31*(2), 112. doi:10.1007/s00520-022-07568-4 PMID:36633695

Huang, Z., Choi, D., Lai, B., Lü, Z., & Tian, H. (2022). Metaverse-based virtual reality experience and endurance performance in sports economy: Mediating role of mental health and performance anxiety. *Frontiers in Public Health, 10.* doi:10.3389/fpubh.2022.991489

Kelly, R., Seabrook, E., Foley, F., Thomas, N., Nedeljkovic, M., & Wadley, G. (2022c). Design considerations for supporting mindfulness in virtual reality. *Frontiers in Virtual Reality, 2,* 672556. doi:10.3389/frvir.2021.672556

Kruse, L., Karaosmanoglu, S., Rings, S., Ellinger, B., & Steinicke, F. (2021). Enabling immersive exercise activities for older adults: A comparison of virtual reality exergames and traditional video exercises. *Societies (Basel, Switzerland), 11*(4), 134. doi:10.3390/soc11040134

Lindner, P. (2020). Better, Virtually: The Past, Present, and Future of Virtual Reality Cognitive Behavior Therapy. *International Journal of Cognitive Therapy, 14*(1), 23–46. doi:10.1007/s41811-020-00090-7

Llorens, R. C., Latorre, J., Alcañíz, M., & Llorens, R. C. (2019). Embodiment and presence in virtual reality after stroke. A comparative study with healthy subjects. *Frontiers in Neurology, 10,* 1061. Advance online publication. doi:10.3389/fneur.2019.01061 PMID:31649608

Lo, H. H. M., Ngai, S. P., & Yam, K. (2021). Effects of Mindfulness-Based Stress Reduction on Health and Social Care Education: A Cohort-Controlled Study. *Mindfulness, 12*(8), 2050–2058. doi:10.1007/s12671-021-01663-z PMID:34127933

Meena, G., Dhanwal, B., Mahrishi, M., & Hiran, K. K. (2021, August). Performance comparison of network intrusion detection system based on different pre-processing methods and deep neural network. In *Proceedings of the International Conference on Data Science, Machine Learning and Artificial Intelligence* (pp. 110-115). ACM. 10.1145/3484824.3484878

Mouatt, B., Smith, A. E., Mellow, M. L., Parfitt, G., Smith, R., & Stanton, T. R. (2020). The use of virtual reality to influence motivation, affect, enjoyment, and engagement during exercise: A scoping review. Frontiers in Virtual Reality. doi:10.3389/frvir.2020.564664

Nagarathna, R., Ram, V., Majumdar, V., Rajesh, S., Singh, A., Patil, S., Anand, A., Judu, I., Bhaskara, S., Basa, J. R., & Nagendra, H. R. (2021). Effectiveness of a Yoga-Based Lifestyle Protocol (YLP) in preventing Diabetes in a High-Risk Indian cohort: A Multicenter Cluster-Randomized Controlled Trial (NMB-Trial). *Frontiers in Endocrinology, 12,* 664657. doi:10.3389/fendo.2021.664657 PMID:34177805

Neo, J. R. J., Won, A. S., & Shepley, M. M. (2021). Designing immersive virtual environments for human behaviour research. Frontiers in Virtual Reality, 2. doi:10.3389/frvir.2021.603750

Oman, D. (2023). Mindfulness for Global Public Health: Critical analysis and agenda. *Mindfulness.* doi:10.1007/s12671-023-02089-5

Patel, S., Vyas, A. K., & Hiran, K. K. (2022). Infrastructure health monitoring using signal processing based on an industry 4.0 System. *Cyber-Physical Systems and Industry, 4,* 249–260.

Ramasamy, J., & Doshi, R. (2022). Machine learning in cyber physical systems for healthcare: brain tumor classification from MRI using transfer learning framework. In *Real-Time Applications of Machine Learning in Cyber-Physical Systems* (pp. 65–76). IGI global. doi:10.4018/978-1-7998-9308-0.ch005

Ramasamy, J., Doshi, R., & Hiran, K. K. (2021, August). Segmentation of brain tumor using deep learning methods: a review. In *Proceedings of the International Conference on Data Science, Machine Learning and Artificial Intelligence* (pp. 209-215). ACM. 10.1145/3484824.3484876

Ramasamy, J., Doshi, R., & Hiran, K. K. (2022, October). Detection of Brain Tumor in Medical Images Based on Feature Extraction by HOG and Machine Learning Algorithms. In *2022 International Conference on Trends in Quantum Computing and Emerging Business Technologies (TQCEBT)* (pp. 1-5). IEEE. 10.1109/TQCEBT54229.2022.10041564

Russell, T., & Arcuri, S. M. (2015). A Neurophysiological and neuropsychological consideration of mindful movement: Clinical and research implications. *Frontiers in Human Neuroscience, 9*. doi:10.3389/fnhum.2015.00282 PMID:26074800

Saini, G. K., Haseeb, S. B., Taghi-Zada, Z., & Ng, J. Y. (2021). The effects of meditation on individuals facing loneliness: A scoping review. *BMC Psychology, 9*(1), 88. doi:10.1186/s40359-021-00585-8 PMID:34022961

Sakaki, K., Nouchi, R., Matsuzaki, Y., Saito, T., Dinet, J., & Kawashima, R. (2021). Benefits of VR Physical Exercise on Cognition in Older Adults with and without Mild Cognitive Decline: A Systematic Review of Randomized Controlled Trials. *Health Care, 9*(7), 883. doi:10.3390/healthcare9070883 PMID:34356259

Sharma, M., & Rush, S. E. (2014). Mindfulness-based stress reduction as a stress management intervention for healthy individuals. *Journal of Evidence-Based Complementary & Alternative Medicine, 19*(4), 271–286. doi:10.1177/2156587214543143 PMID:25053754

Srinivasulu, A. (2022). Omi-cron Virus Data Analytics Using Extended RNN Technique. *Int J Cancer Res Ther, 7*(3).

Stewart, T. H., Villaneuva, K., Hahn, A., Ortiz-Delatorre, J., Wolf, C., Nguyen, R., Bolter, N. D., Kern, M., & Bagley, J. R. (2022). Actual vs. perceived exertion during active virtual reality game exercise. *Frontiers in Rehabilitation Sciences, 3*, 887740. doi:10.3389/fresc.2022.887740 PMID:36189005

Thiermann, U. B., & Sheate, W. R. (2020). The Way Forward in Mindfulness and Sustainability: A Critical Review and Research Agenda. *Journal of Cognitive Enhancement: Towards the Integration of Theory and Practice, 5*(1), 118–139. doi:10.1007/s41465-020-00180-6

Tsamitros, N., Sebold, M., Gutwinski, S., & Beck, A. (2021). Virtual Reality-Based Treatment approaches in the field of substance use disorders. *Current Addiction Reports, 8*(3), 399–407. doi:10.1007/s40429-021-00377-5

Uhl, J. C., Regal, G., Gafert, M., Murtinger, M., & Tscheligi, M. (2023). Stress embodied: Developing multi-sensory experiences for VR police training. In Lecture Notes in Computer Science (pp. 573–583). Springer. doi:10.1007/978-3-031-42280-5_36

Voinescu, A., Fodor, L. A., Fraser, D. S., & David, D. (2020). Exploring Attention in VR: Effects of visual and Auditory modalities. In Advances in intelligent systems and computing (pp. 677–683). Springer. doi:10.1007/978-3-030-51828-8_89

Waller, M., Mistry, D., Jetly, R., & Frewen, P. A. (2021). Meditating in Virtual Reality 3: 360° video of the perceptual presence of instructor. *Mindfulness*, *12*(6), 1424–1437. doi:10.1007/s12671-021-01612-w PMID:33777253

Winstein, C. J., & Requejo, P. S. (2015). Innovative technologies for rehabilitation and health promotion: What is the evidence? *Physical Therapy*, *95*(3), 294–298. doi:10.2522/ptj.2015.95.2.294 PMID:25734191

Zhang, S., Chen, M., Yang, N., Lu, S., & Ni, S. (2021). Effectiveness of VR-based mindfulness on psychological and physiological health: A systematic review. *Current Psychology (New Brunswick, N.J.)*, *42*(6), 5033–5045. doi:10.1007/s12144-021-01777-6

ADDITIONAL READING

Cebolla, A., Herrero, R., Ventura, S., Miragall, M., Bellosta-Batalla, M., Llorens, R. C., & Baños, R. M. (2019). Putting oneself in the body of others: A pilot study on the efficacy of an embodied virtual reality system to generate Self-Compassion. *Frontiers in Psychology*, *10*, 1521. doi:10.3389/fpsyg.2019.01521 PMID:31338048

Crescentini, C., Chittaro, L., Capurso, V., Sioni, R., & Fabbro, F. (2016). Psychological and physiological responses to stressful situations in immersive virtual reality: Differences between users who practice mindfulness meditation and controls. *Computers in Human Behavior*, *59*, 304–316. doi:10.1016/j.chb.2016.02.031

Haro, M. V. N., López-Del-Hoyo, Y., Campos, D., Linehan, M. M., Hoffman, H. G., García-Palacios, A., Modrego-Alarcón, M., Borao, L., & García-Campayo, J. (2017). Meditation experts try Virtual Reality Mindfulness: A pilot study evaluating the feasibility and acceptability of Virtual Reality to facilitate mindfulness practice in people attending a Mindfulness conference. *PLoS One*, *12*(11), e0187777. doi:10.1371/journal.pone.0187777 PMID:29166665

Kelly, R., Seabrook, E., Foley, F., Thomas, N., Nedeljkovic, M., & Wadley, G. (2022). Design considerations for supporting mindfulness in virtual reality. *Frontiers in Virtual Reality*, *2*, 672556. doi:10.3389/frvir.2021.672556

Modrego-Alarcón, M., López-Del-Hoyo, Y., García-Campayo, J., Pérez-Aranda, A., Navarro-Gil, M., Beltrán-Ruiz, M., Morillo, H., Delgado-Suárez, I., Oliván-Arévalo, R., & Montero-Marín, J. (2021). Efficacy of a mindfulness-based programme with and without virtual reality support to reduce stress in university students: A randomized controlled trial. *Behaviour Research and Therapy*, *142*, 103866. doi:10.1016/j.brat.2021.103866 PMID:33957506

She, Y., Wang, Q., Liu, F., Lin, L., Yang, B., & Hu, B. (2023). An interaction design model for virtual reality mindfulness meditation using imagery-based transformation and positive feedback. *Computer Animation and Virtual Worlds*, *34*(3–4), e2184. doi:10.1002/cav.2184

Tong, X., Gromala, D., Choo, A., Amin, A., & Shaw, C. (2015). The Virtual Meditative Walk: An Immersive Virtual Environment for Pain Self-modulation Through Mindfulness-Based Stress Reduction Meditation. In R. Shumaker & S. Lackey (Eds.), Lecture Notes in Computer Science: Vol. 9179. *Virtual, Augmented and Mixed Reality. VAMR 2015*. Springer. doi:10.1007/978-3-319-21067-4_40

KEY TERMS AND DEFINITIONS

Anxiety Management: Techniques and approaches to alleviate and cope with anxiety, a common mental health condition characterized by excessive worry and fear.

Clinical Applications: Practical uses of interventions, technologies, or methodologies in a healthcare setting, often referring to therapeutic approaches for mental health issues.

Ethical Considerations: Reflection on moral principles and values in the design, implementation, and use of mental health technologies or interventions, ensuring responsible and respectful practices.

Mental Health: The state of psychological well-being, encompassing emotional, social, and cognitive aspects; crucial for overall health and functioning.

Mindful Movement: Purposeful and present-focused physical activity, such as yoga or tai chi, emphasises body and breath awareness for improved mental well-being.

Personalized Experiences: Tailoring interventions or technologies to individual preferences, needs, and characteristics, enhancing effectiveness and engagement in mental health and well-being practices.

Stress Reduction: Strategies or interventions aimed at minimizing the impact of stressors, promoting relaxation, and maintaining emotional balance for improved mental health.

Virtual Reality (VR): Immersive computer-generated environments that simulate reality, often used for entertainment, training, or therapy, providing a heightened sensory experience.

Well-Being: A holistic measure of health, encompassing physical, mental, and social dimensions, reflecting an individual's overall quality of life and satisfaction.

Chapter 9
The Neuropsychological Impact of Immersive Experiences in the Metaverse and Virtual and Augmented Reality

Laura De Clara
MetaCare Srl, Italy

ABSTRACT

Recent advances in mental healthcare technology, especially in virtual reality (VR) and augmented reality (AR), have revolutionized psychiatry and psychology. This chapter critically examines these innovations' potential in treating various mental disorders, from anxiety and depression to PTSD and ADHD. It emphasizes the controlled and customizable nature of VR environments, which empower individuals to confront fears within personalized settings. Interdisciplinary collaboration is stressed, showcasing applications in psychology, from assessment to clinical treatment. The chapter explores neuropsychological impacts, detailing how VR modulates emotions, enhances neural plasticity in stroke rehabilitation, and alters neural networks. Despite promise, challenges like treatment standardization and ethical concerns persist, demanding careful consideration. The chapter advocates for ongoing research and global interdisciplinary cooperation to fully exploit these technologies' potential in mental healthcare.

INTRODUCTION

In recent years, the development and use of new technologies in the field of mental health has had a significant impact on psychiatry and psychology (Ford et al., 2023; McIntyre et al., 2023; Tsamitros et al., 2023). The role of cybernetics in healthcare is increasingly being discussed (Caponnetto & Casu, 2022), particularly in light of the global prevalence of mental disorders, which affect approximately 29.2% of the world's population and pose significant challenges to both individuals and global healthcare systems (Wiebe et al., 2022). This has significant economic and social consequences.

DOI: 10.4018/979-8-3693-1123-3.ch009

However, despite the urgent need for treatment, available resources for mental health remain limited, accounting for approximately 10.4% of total global health expenditure (Wiebe et al., 2022). This disparity is particularly evident in underdeveloped countries, where more than 70% of people with mental disorders do not receive adequate care (Liu et al., 2022; Wiebe et al., 2022), contributing to the discrimination and exclusion faced by people with mental disorders or mental illness (Tay et al., 2023).

The advent of the COVID-19 pandemic has accelerated the adoption of new technologies, enabling rapid global digital access and use (Omboni et al., 2022), 2022a). Digital therapeutics, including virtual reality, are developing rapidly and promise to improve access to and quality of mental health care (McIntyre et al., 2023) and offer further potential for the treatment of mental disorders (Schröder et al., 2023). It is hoped that these technologies will become more accessible in the future due to reduced costs, including virtual reality-related devices (Donker et al., 2019; Wiebe et al., 2022).

Virtual reality has demonstrated its potential as a valuable tool for information dissemination, education and rehabilitation interventions (Liu et al., 2022), but it is also proving to be a powerful tool for improving the assessment and treatment of mental disorders (Bell et al., 2020; Ford et al., 2023).

Interventions in the field of mental health take place through the creation of immersive and interactive environments in a controlled context for gradual exposure to stimuli that induce emotions and sensations (Wechsler et al., 2019). Unlike in vivo or imaginative exposure therapies, virtual reality allows for precise control over the quality, intensity, duration and frequency of exposure (Emmelkamp & Meyerbröker, 2021). In addition, it offers the opportunity to better explore and understand the modifiability of 'self' and 'sense of reality', crucial concepts in mental disorders (Wiebe et al., 2022)

In this way, a synergistic interaction between mind and immersive experience is created: the simulation creates a transformative state because what the subject experiences is a state that enriches personal experience and therefore modifies personal ideas about self, personal perceptions of self, and personal beliefs.

Systematic reviews and meta-analyses show that virtual reality-based therapy is more effective than imaginative therapies and as effective as in vivo exposure therapy (Ford et al., 2023). These advances represent a significant step towards a future where mental health care is more accessible, effective, and personalised, bringing tangible benefits to those in need (Wiebe et al., 2022). Similarly, the use of virtual reality could expand beyond therapy, for example in the training of healthcare professionals, allowing them to gain hands-on experience in a safe and controlled virtual environment (Emmelkamp & Meyerbröker, 2021).

Looking to the future, there is the exciting prospect of further developments in virtual reality, such as the integration of artificial intelligence to tailor therapies to the specific needs of patients in real time (Darnall et al., 2020).

DIFFERENCE BETWEEN VIRTUAL REALITY (VR), AUGMENTED REALITY (AR), AND METAVERSE IN MENTAL HEALTH

In recent years, virtual reality (VR) and augmented reality (AR) have achieved incredible success in several industries, including medicine, research and entertainment, and have attracted considerable interest and investment (Zambelli et al., 2023).

How do these technologies work?

Augmented Reality (AR) overlays digital information onto the physical environment, allowing users to interact with both the real world and digital elements simultaneously (Petrigna & Musumeci, 2022). This technology integrates complementary types of information to enhance reality, facilitating user interaction with digital content while maintaining transparency (Xiong et al., 2021).

The user can take advantage of the reality enriched with other elements.

In contrast, virtual reality (VR) provides complete immersion in a computer-generated environment that is distinct from physical reality (Ford et al., 2023). The user is confronted with another environment, a virtual one, different and distinct from reality. The experience is complete, 3D, three-dimensional, with avatars interacting with the environment (Tsamitros et al., 2023). Avatars, reflecting different cultural and social characteristics, can interact, move and manipulate objects, offering a level of control that surpasses augmented reality (Petrigna & Musumeci, 2022).

In addition, virtual reality excels at stimulating visual interest and user engagement, fostering an entertainment effect that enhances cognitive skills and intelligence. The programmability of VR experiences allows them to be tailored to individual needs, making them versatile and applicable in various fields, including therapy and training; the possibility of rigorous and reproducible testing also makes this technology a valuable tool for scientific research (Bell et al., 2020).

Beyond VR and AR, the Metaverse represents a three-dimensional virtual world in which individuals, represented by avatars, engage in daily activities, social interactions, cultural events and economic activities, blurring the boundary between the real and virtual worlds (Petrigna & Musumeci, 2022). In the immersive dimension of the Metaverse, multiple users can interact with each other and with the environment.

Applied to mental health, the Metaverse is a place where the subject can receive therapy, or parts of therapy, by being immersed in an environment that presents controlled stimuli in which it is possible to interact with other avatars. The relationship is brought into an immersive reality.

THE TRANSFORMATIVE DIMENSION OF AUGMENTED REALITY AND IMMERSIVE REALITY

The emergence of virtual reality (VR), augmented reality (AR) and the Metaverse has marked a transformative shift in human interaction with the digital realm. These technologies offer considerable potential to reshape the human mind through immersive experiences, revolutionising the way we perceive and interact (Bell et al., 2020), both with objects and stimuli, and with people. The entire interactive and interpersonal world of human beings is involved and affected.

At the heart of these changes is the manipulable nature of these tools: the ability to create specific environments, control them and intervene in people's perceptions allows for the stimulation and manipulation of responses to stimuli and emotional responses (Bell et al., 2020), stimulating visual interest, arousal, entertainment, promoting intelligence and the development of cognitive skills. Virtual reality also influences emotions and identity, changing beliefs and attitudes. Through virtual avatars, individuals can embody different identities, strengthen empathy, and understand perspectives different from their own (Lara & Rueda, 2021). This emotional impact extends to learning, where virtual reality not only increases engagement, but also promotes positive emotions and reduces negative ones (Allcoat & von Mühlenen, 2018).

Immersiveness allows you to experience 'presence', the feeling of being physically present in a virtual world. This experience is central to the digital world and involves the prefrontal cortex, influencing emotions and behaviour (Baumgartner et al., 2008). 'Presence' encompasses two aspects: Place Illusion (PI) and Plausibility Illusion (Psi) (Freeman et al., 2017). PI is the feeling of being in another place despite being aware of virtual presence, while Psi refers to the perception that events in that place are close to reality. This sense of 'being there' can be used for therapeutic purposes (Freeman et al., 2017) by inducing physiological responses like real-life scenarios, such as increased heart rate in response to virtual stressors (Tieri et al., 2018).

In mental health treatment, achieving high levels of presence in VR environments is critical. Immersion in virtual reality can be a transformative tool for personal change, providing a dynamic social world in which individuals can share specific experiences (Riva & Serino, 2020). However, understanding the neural basis of these mechanisms is crucial for the safe and effective use of these technologies (Baumgartner et al., 2008).

Of course, it should also be considered that precisely because of the high level of presence and immersiveness, these tools can promote distance and escape from reality and relationships.

In summary, VR, AR and the Metaverse are powerful tools that reshape the human mind through immersive experiences, influencing emotions, behaviour and mental health. Exploring the neurological and psychological aspects of these technologies is key to realising their full potential and improving people's lives.

THE METAVERSE AS A NEW PERSPECTIVE

The Metaverse can be defined as a hybrid (digital/physical) environment that provides spaces for rich user interaction. In this view, the main feature of the Metaverse is a two-way connection between the virtual and physical worlds: behaviour in the physical world influences experience in the virtual world, and behaviour in the virtual world influences experience in the real world (Riva, Di Lernia, et al., 2021).

The use of Metaverse in the field of psychology is on a continuous upward trend, revealing potential areas of application in psychological assessment and treatment (Bansal et al., 2022; Petrigna & Musumeci, 2022; Usmani et al., 2022). In clinical practice, applications range from mental disorders to pain management, neurological conditions and paediatric issues (Calabrò et al., 2022; Vicario & Martino, 2022).

The use of Metaverse technology in clinical psychology will undoubtedly be a promising area of study in the near future (Cerasa et al., 2022; Riva, Di Lernia, et al., 2021), but to date there are few studies investigating its applications and effectiveness.

NEUROPSYCHOLOGICAL CORRELATES

The development of immersive technologies has led humanity into a world of immersive virtual experiences, opening the door to a new field of research that combines psychology, technology and neuroscience. The interaction between the individual and the virtual environment is no longer confined to the realm of mere sensory perception. It involves complex neurocognitive processes that profoundly affect brain activity and modulate neural circuits associated with various cognitive and emotional aspects (Mishra et al., 2021).

Brain Activation and Synaptic Modulation During Immersive Experiences

The advent of virtual reality (VR) has redefined the way we interact with the digital world.

The use of various imaging techniques has allowed researchers to study neural signals and functional responses of the brain during VR experiences (Mishra et al., 2021; Pandarinathan et al., 2018). A key aspect of this type of experience is the activation of brain areas involved in attention and emotion. Research has shown that the prefrontal cortex, which regulates emotions and attention, is significantly activated (Mishra et al., 2021) during immersion in complex virtual environments. This activation is a byproduct of the virtual experience and contributes to enhanced cognitive performance through increased attention and emotional control.

In addition, virtual reality has a profound effect on synaptic plasticity, the key mechanism of neural change and learning in the brain. Repeated exposure to virtual stimuli can strengthen neural connections, providing a fertile ground for cognitive learning and restructuring (Mishra et al., 2021). This ability to modulate neural plasticity has been exploited in therapy, where virtual reality has been used to facilitate the recovery of impaired cognitive functions or to improve these functions beyond pre-existing levels. For example, there is evidence of efficacy in stroke rehabilitation (Hao et al., 2022).

Studies in children show that virtual reality induces cortical reorganisation and promotes the activation of different neural connections: although the data are contradictory, they suggest improvements in some motor and functional skills, such as gait and balance (Coco-Martin et al., 2020).

In addition, virtual reality's effects on neural plasticity have been shown to result in increased cortical grey matter volume and improved cognitive performance. The key question remains: what exactly does virtual reality do to our brains? Studies have shown that virtual reality enables visual, tactile and auditory induced perceptions, offering unprecedented control and the ability to modulate the experience. What is certain is that neuroplasticity depends on use, and that intensive and repetitive training is crucial to promote functional changes in neural architecture (Coco-Martin et al., 2020)).

Implementation and Impact of Virtual Reality Therapy (VRET)

An important application of virtual reality in the treatment of mental health is Virtual Reality Exposure Therapy (VRET), which has been shown to be effective in several psychological pathologies. For example, functional neuroimaging studies have shown functional changes in brain areas involved in fear during VRESET sessions, including the thalamus, amygdala, and prefrontal cortex (Álvarez-Pérez et al., 2021). The efficacy of VRET is based on the inhibition of fear responses and inhibitory learning, supported by the modulation of brain activity. The normalisation of brain function induced by VRET requires multiple sessions to induce therapeutic changes in the brain, suggesting temporality and gradual neuroplasticity during virtual therapy (Landowska et al., 2018).

Immersive virtual reality currently primarily involves the senses of sight and hearing, but with technological advances it can also include touch, taste, and smell (Buetler et al., 2022).

Neuronal Plasticity and Virtual Reality-Based Rehabilitation

Of particular interest is the effect of virtual reality on neural plasticity, understood as the ability of the brain to adapt and change in response to experience (Hao et al., 2022). The type of change that occurs involves the modification of its structure, function, and connections to adapt to the stimuli to which it is exposed. Scientific research shows that the maximum development of the neural network is achieved by working on different channels, since multisensory stimulation is considered an essential component in the restructuring of the brain (Coco-Martin et al., 2020).

It is interesting to note how these therapies for the motor recovery of a limb, for example, simulate this mobilisation at the mental level, immersing the subject in a reality in which he is able to move this limb. Basically, there is an activation of the area of the brain responsible for the movement of the limb, an activation that occurs even if you cannot really move it, but only virtually.

Recent studies, such as that by Hao et al (2022), have investigated the effects of virtual reality-based rehabilitation on stroke patients. This research showed positive correlations between changes in neural plasticity and functional recovery in patients.

This means that the targeted use of virtual reality in rehabilitation not only improves cognitive and motor skills, but also stimulates physical changes in the brain, aiding the healing process (Laver et al., 2017; Tieri et al., 2018).

This confirms that virtual reality can be used as a rehabilitation tool to harness the adaptive sensorimotor potential of the nervous system (Coco-Martin et al., 2020).

Virtual Reality and Emotion

The relationship between virtual experience and human emotion is a crucial area of research in the field of virtual reality (Chirico & Gaggioli, 2023). For years, some studies have highlighted the potential of perceptual and conceptual stimuli in virtual reality to generate emotional responses, with significant implications for understanding psychological disorders (Bouchard et al., 2008; Gorini et al., 2010), but also for understanding human responses in general. The ability to influence internal responses suggests that virtual reality is a crucial factor in the modulation of emotions (Li et al., 2021), and the presence of emotional elements in virtual reality enhances the sense of immersion by emphasising the direct link between the emotional nature of virtual stimuli and the depth of the immersive experience (Gorini et al., 2010). Increased arousal when exposed to emotional stimuli in VR helps to enhance the sense of presence (Higuera-Trujillo et al., 2017).

The interplay between VR and emotions is further explored by studies such as those conducted by Rodríguez et al. (2015), which examine brain activity in different emotional states induced by a virtual environment. These studies revealed specific activations in different regions of the brain during the induction of emotions such as sadness and during emotional regulation strategies such as cognitive reappraisal.

Brain responses to emotion in virtual reality are complex and involve specific brain lateralisation. Recent research has shown a significant increase in cortical activity in the left hemisphere of the brain during exposure to 3D virtual reality, suggesting a potential hemispheric specialisation for emotional responses related to stereovision in virtual reality. This integrated picture of the intricate connections between perception, emotion and neuroscience in virtual reality paves the way for new perspectives in therapeutic applications and the design of immersive and emotionally resonant virtual experiences (Lee, 2023).

THERAPEUTIC APPLICATIONS

Virtual reality (VR) has been successfully used in the delivery of exposure-based therapeutic and rehabilitative treatments, allowing individuals to experience feared situations or contexts. Simulated environments can be customised to induce desired emotional sensations for therapeutic purposes, allowing patients to gradually learn how to cope with such situations in a controlled and safe environment (Bell et al., 2020). Evidence for the effectiveness of VR applications in the treatment of mental disorders is growing (Habak et al., 2020). This congruence between Emotional Real and Virtual Answers is essential to guarantee the effectiveness of treatments and therapies based on virtual reality (Schröder et al., 2023).

For example, there is a large body of research supporting the effectiveness of virtual reality for anxiety disorders, including phobias, obsessive-compulsive disorder, post-traumatic stress disorder, and even cognitive deficits. Other studies report encouraging results in the treatment of eating disorders, substance use disorders, psychosis, and neurodevelopmental disorders such as autism spectrum disorders and attention deficit hyperactivity disorder (Donker et al., 2019; Ford et al., 2023; Freeman et al., 2017; Lan et al., 2023; Landowska, 2022; Landowska et al., 2018; Riva & Serino, 2020; Tay et al., 2023).

In addition to therapeutic contexts, virtual reality has been successfully used in rehabilitation settings. For example, it has been used in post-stroke treatment, providing stroke survivors with a stimulating virtual environment for motor and cognitive rehabilitation of impaired functions, and in patients with acquired brain injury with potential memory deficits (Hao et al., 2022b; Laver et al., 2017; Song & Park, 2015). Virtual reality has also been used to assist people with Parkinson's disease to improve motor control and quality of life. For children with cerebral palsy, virtual reality has been integrated (Ford et al., 2023; Lan et al., 2023) into rehabilitation, facilitating the learning of new motor skills in an interactive and engaging virtual environment. Virtual reality has also been used in pain management, providing an innovative and effective treatment alternative for people with chronic pain (Ahmadpour et al., 2019; Ioannou et al., 2020; Lopez-Rodriguez et al., 2020; Rousseaux et al., 2020; Wong et al., 2022; Xie et al., 2023).

In addition to therapeutic and rehabilitative applications, VR is being used in clinical evaluation protocols. Research has shown that exposure to both real and virtual environments can elicit similar emotional responses, with greater emotional responses than simple photographs (Gorini et al., 2010). This suggests that virtual reality can be used as a valuable tool to assess patients' emotional responses accurately and comprehensively (Gorini et al., 2010).

Anxiety

The vast majority of studies on virtual reality (VR) and the treatment of mental distress have focused on anxiety disorders (Freeman et al., 2017), pathologies that are among the most prevalent mental disorders worldwide (Freeman et al., 2017; Schröder et al., 2023).

In recent years, virtual reality (VR) and virtual immersion (VI) have revolutionised the approach to the treatment of anxiety disorders, opening new perspectives in clinical therapy (Liu et al., 2022). Although considered recent, these methods date back to the 1990s, when researchers began to explore the clinical applicability of this technology (Wiebe et al., 2022). Initially, efforts focused on specific phobias, panic disorder, agoraphobia, social anxiety disorder, generalised anxiety disorder and post-traumatic stress disorder (Tsamitros et al., 2023). This variety of applications testifies to the wide range of anxiety disorders addressed by virtual reality. The main intervention technique used for anxiety disorders is exposure therapy (Freeman et al., 2017), which has shown promising results (Landowska et al., 2018; Liu et al., 2022; Tsamitros et al., 2023).

Here, patients are virtually exposed to anxiety-provoking scenarios, allowing them to face their fears in a safe and controlled environment (Landowska et al., 2018; Wiebe et al., 2022). Research conducted by Donker et al. (2019) confirms the effectiveness of this method, highlighting a significant reduction in post-exposure phobias, with sustained results over time. VRET has been shown to be as effective as traditional therapy, including imaginal and in vivo exposure (Wiebe et al., 2022), but more importantly, it can be a viable alternative for phobias when access to traditional therapy is limited (Tsamitros et al., 2023).

Virtual exposure therapy has also been shown to be as effective as in vivo exposure therapy in the treatment of specific phobias and agoraphobia with panic disorder. Challenges currently exist in standardising treatment protocols for panic disorder and agoraphobia (Wechsler et al., 2019). Differences in the duration and number of exposure sessions make comparisons between studies difficult. However, literature reviews suggest that, despite protocol differences, VRET provides significant symptom relief (Wiebe et al., 2022), although further research is needed to investigate the efficacy of these therapies in specific clinical settings. In this case, virtual reality exposure therapy for social anxiety is based on an exposure protocol that aims to reduce the unreasonable fear of negative evaluation by others. VRET for social phobia is significantly more effective than control or placebo groups, but compared to in vivo exposure, meta-analytic results are currently mixed. Studies reported by Wiebe et al (2022) showed a significant reduction in social anxiety after exposure, proving superior to wait-listed control groups. These improvements were maintained at follow-up, indicating the reliability and sustainability of the approach (Wiebe et al., 2022).

In the case of generalised anxiety disorder, which is characterised by excessive anxiety and unfounded fears, the effectiveness of virtual reality is currently the subject of further research. However, preliminary reports suggest a positive trend, particularly in terms of relaxation and mindfulness effects. These findings point to the potential of virtual reality in the treatment of this complex disorder (Wiebe et al., 2022).

In conclusion, the use of virtual and immersive reality in the treatment of anxiety disorders is a growing area of psychotherapy. However, despite the considerable progress made to date, further research is needed to fully understand the applications and limitations of this technology. Future efforts should focus on standardising treatment protocols and identifying patient populations that may benefit most from these innovative treatment approaches.

Depression

Depression, a condition characterised by persistent low mood or loss of interest or pleasure accompanied by other symptoms, has become an increasingly relevant issue in modern society (American Psychiatric Publishing, 2016). This disorder, with a significant global presence, is one of the leading causes of lost disability-corrected life years (DALYs) worldwide (Roth et al., 2021).

As a result, research into new treatments has become a priority for the scientific community: some applications, such as SuperBetter, MoodHacker and Sparx, have emerged as valuable self-management tools aimed at reducing depressive symptoms. These apps provide practical resources and strategies for managing depression in the comfort of your own home. In addition, the use of social platforms (i.e. platforms where people can share experiences) can play a crucial role in raising awareness of depression and encouraging those suffering from it to seek professional help (Latha et al., 2020; Omboni et al., 2022).

In terms of therapy, research shows significant efficacy in the treatment of depression through virtual reality psychotherapy. In particular, it has been shown that it is possible to integrate cognitive behavioural therapy (the current gold standard treatment) and virtual reality exposure therapy (VRET) with encouraging results (Baghaei et al., 2021; Ioannou et al., 2020; Lindner et al., 2019; Zeng et al., 2018)

Indeed, through virtual reality, individuals immerse themselves in contexts that alleviate symptoms, all within a safe, secure and motivating environment. However, despite significant advances, there are still few in-depth studies exploring the efficacy of virtual reality in the treatment of depression (Freeman et al., 2017).

In addition to applications and virtual reality in the treatment of depressive symptoms, new technologies have proven useful in other stages of depression management. Digital technologies can play a crucial role in screening, helping to identify cases of depression earlier and more efficiently. In addition, these technologies can support remote diagnosis and patient management, allowing for regular monitoring and personalised treatment adjustments (Omboni et al., 2022).

Post-Traumatic Stress Disorder (PTSD)

Virtual reality (VR) has emerged as a promising treatment modality for post-traumatic stress disorder (PTSD). Post-traumatic stress disorder is a complex condition that develops in individuals exposed to traumatic events and is characterised by intrusive symptoms, avoidance, and negative changes in mood and cognition (American Psychiatric Publishing, 2016). Virtual reality has been successfully used to provide gradual exposure to trauma triggers, facilitate recall of trauma-related thoughts, and promote memory processing (Tsamitros et al., 2023; Wiebe et al., 2022). Recent meta-analyses have confirmed the efficacy of exposure therapy (VRET) in the treatment of posttraumatic stress disorder, equating it to the efficacy of traditional active psychotherapy, although more research is needed to clarify its advantages over traditional therapies (Liu et al., 2022; Wiebe et al., 2022).

Eating Disorders

Eating disorders, such as anorexia nervosa, bulimia nervosa, and binge eating disorder, are a category of pathologies characterised by profound changes in thoughts, feelings and behaviours related to eating (American Psychiatric Publishing, 2016). These disorders may be associated with overweight and obesity, although the latter are not considered separate mental disorders.

Virtual reality (VR) has emerged as a promising treatment option for eating disorders and related problems. Over the past 25 years, virtual reality-based applications have been used to address several basic clinical aspects of eating disorders, including binge eating, appetite distortions, anxiety, body distortions, body and food distortions of attention, reduced food cravings, altered body image, and altered emotional regulation (Freeman et al., 2017; Riva, Malighetti, et al., 2021; Wiebe et al., 2022).

Several studies have demonstrated the efficacy of virtual food exposure in eliciting emotional responses similar to real food (which holds promise for future treatments), improvements in eating disorder-related diagnostic dimensions in terms of binge eating and laxative use, and improvements in food-related emotional responses in terms of anxiety and food craving (Riva, Malighetti, et al., 2021).

In summary, Virtual Reality offers an innovative approach to the treatment of eating disorders, addressing multiple aspects including body image management and food control. Despite the challenges and uncertainties that remain, advances in the research and development of virtual reality-based therapies offer a promising opportunity to improve the quality of life for patients with these conditions (Freeman et al., 2017).

Pain

Chronic pain is a major medical challenge, affecting more than 20% of the world's population and contributing significantly to global disability. This complex phenomenon, characterised by sensations, emotions, behaviours and cognitions, requires global management, which is often lacking in current treatment protocols (Rousseaux et al., 2020). In particular, people with chronic pain often face limited treatment options, including behavioural approaches, which not only lead to a deterioration in quality of life, but also to a significant social and emotional burden (Wong et al., 2022).

In this context, virtual reality (VR) therapy has emerged as a promising treatment option. This innovative technology provides an immersive experience in immersive three-dimensional and multi-sensory environments and has demonstrated efficacy in various acute and chronic pain conditions (Darnall et al., 2020; Mallari et al., 2019; Wong et al., 2022). Virtual reality can significantly reduce pain perception and acts as a powerful distraction tool, allowing patients to distance themselves from pain perception through immersive sensory stimuli (Wong et al., 2022).

This distraction effect is based on the principle that human attention is limited, and that distraction can consume the cognitive resources needed to process pain: by distracting the patient, they are deprived of the opportunity to process pain (Bushnell et al., 2013).

Although there are promising results, further studies are needed to better understand the neurobiological mechanisms involved: bodily illusions have been suggested as pain threshold modulators, but it is unclear whether the reported benefits are sustained in the long term (Mallari et al., 2019; Riva & Serino, 2020).

Cognitive Disorders

The application of Virtual Reality (VR) to degenerative cognitive disorders, particularly dementia, is an area of considerable interest in the context of neurorehabilitation. Neurocognitive disorders are characterised by a progressive decline in cognitive functions, including complex attention, executive function, learning, memory, language, perceptual-motor function, and social cognition. When cognitive decline occurs while daily functioning is still preserved, mild cognitive impairment (MCI) is diagnosed (American Psychiatric Publishing, 2016; Wiebe et al., 2022).

Studies in the field of virtual reality-based cognitive training have shown promising results in these pathologies, with significant improvements in cognitive domain functions compared to traditional physical and cognitive training methods. VR rehabilitation has been particularly successful in improving cognitive function and attention, executive function, episodic memory, language, visuo constructive skills, and visuospatial function and concentration (Wiebe et al., 2022).

In addition, for patients with Alzheimer's disease, for example, it can be crucial to address common symptoms such as anxiety, frustration and apathy that significantly affect their well-being. Virtual reality is proving to be a useful tool in addressing these symptoms by giving patients a sense of presence in an environment that isolates them from external factors. Interactive virtual environments can potentially relax patients, induce positive emotions, and reduce negative emotions (Frasson & Abdessalem, 2022).

Psychosis

Exploring the applications of virtual reality (VR) in psychotic disorders is a complex and diverse field of study, reflecting the intricate nature of the clinical picture of psychosis. The studies conducted to date in this area are limited and varied, reflecting the complexity and variety of symptoms present in psychotic disorders. Most of these studies have used virtual reality as a tool to explore psychotic experiences and understand their causes, with a particular focus on assessing paranoia (Freeman et al., 2017).

A key aspect of these studies has been the attempt to simulate environments and situations that may trigger or influence the onset of psychotic symptoms such as anxiety and paranoia. This controlled simulation provides a unique window into the minds of patients, allowing researchers to explore the distorted perceptions and interpretations of reality that are typical of psychosis.

In terms of treatment applications, some research has reported significant reductions in associated paranoid thoughts and tensions (Tsamitros et al., 2023).

However, it is important to note that only a few studies have shown encouraging results in the use of virtual reality as a therapeutic tool in psychotic disorders, a complex picture that requires caution and prudence in its application.

Autism

Autism is a complex condition involving a wide range of symptoms and behavioural challenges, including difficulties in social interaction, emotional expression, and communication. These challenges can vary significantly from individual to individual, making it essential to seek personalised approaches to education and therapeutic intervention.

Over the last decade, there has been a significant increase in publications on the application of Virtual Reality (VR) and Augmented Reality (AR) in autism(Parsons, 2015), in the assessment of the clinical picture and in the treatment of autism spectrum disorder (ASD) in particular (Dechsling et al., 2022; Parsons, 2015). Most studies conducted have focused on investigating and improving social and emotional skills, as well as training skills in patients with ASD. The ability to create interactive virtual environments allows complex social situations to be simulated, enabling therapists and educators to target specific social and communication behaviours (Dechsling et al., 2022; Vasiliki Bravou, n.d.).

One of the main benefits of using VR and AR in this context is the ability to adjust the level of sensory stimulation, which is particularly important for people with ASD who can often be hypersensitive or hyposensitive to sensory stimuli.

Another critical aspect of VR applications in autism is the ability to provide immediate, personalised feedback. Virtual environments can be programmed to respond to the patient's actions and reactions in real time, enabling highly individualised learning. This type of feedback is critical for the acquisition of social and communication skills, as patients with ASD often have difficulty understanding and responding appropriately to facial expressions and social cues.

Virtual reality can also be used for environmental desensitisation and training. For example, individuals with ASD who suffer from social phobias can be gradually exposed to social situations through the use of virtual scenarios, allowing them to gain confidence and skills in dealing with such situations in real life.

The scientific literature has shown promising results regarding the effectiveness of VR and AR applications in the field of autism. However, it is important to emphasise that research is still ongoing and further studies are needed to confirm and extend these findings. The personalisation of virtual therapies, the identification of best practices and the optimisation of intervention protocols are still the subject of research and development (Dechsling et al., 2022).

Attention Deficit Hyperactivity Disorder (ADHD)

In the context of virtual reality (VR), the application of technology to the assessment and treatment of attention deficit hyperactivity disorder (ADHD) in children has shown significant progress. According to the American Psychiatric Association (2016), ADHD is characterised by inattention and/or hyperactivity-impulsivity and is one of the most common childhood psychiatric disorders, which can have a significant impact in adulthood.

A review from Bashiri (2017) has highlighted that virtual reality offers several opportunities in the rehabilitation process of children with ADHD. This technology allows the creation of a safe and distraction-free virtual environment, reducing external interference and providing an effective learning environment. This has been found to be helpful in improving the cognitive and behavioural skills of children with ADHD, thus contributing to their rehabilitation (Bashiri et al., 2017).

The review by Wiebe et al. (2022) points out that virtual reality is also being used to study ADHD through specific neuropsychological tests that allow differentiation between children with ADHD and typically developing children. These tests provide healthcare professionals with a better understanding of the specific cognitive difficulties of patients, allowing for a more accurate diagnosis.

In conclusion, the use of virtual reality in the assessment and treatment of ADHD in children has shown great promise (Bashiri et al., 2017). This technology offers an innovative and personalised approach to rehabilitation, improving the cognitive and behavioural skills of children with ADHD and providing healthcare professionals with more accurate tools for diagnosis and treatment. The integration of virtual reality into the neuropsychological assessment process represents a significant step forward in the field of child psychiatry and offers new perspectives for improving the quality of life of children with ADHD.

FUTURE PROSPECTS AND CHALLENGES

Several key challenges and opportunities emerge in the context of future prospects for the use of virtual reality (VR) and immersive environments in the treatment of mental disorders. VR devices provide a virtual environment that can accurately replicate real-world experiences, allowing users to immerse themselves in controlled and personalised contexts. Recent studies show that most participants in virtual reality experiments report high levels of satisfaction with these experiences, suggesting considerable therapeutic potential (Wong et al., 2022). However, while some VR applications have shown promise, other areas are still under development, highlighting the need for further research and experimentation (Wiebe et al., 2022).

One of the main challenges in therapeutic applications of virtual reality is motion sickness, a phenomenon experienced by individuals wearing VR headsets that remains poorly understood and widely studied (Kim et al., 2018; Tsamitros et al., 2023). Motion sickness, also known as virtual reality sickness in the context of virtual reality, can manifest itself with symptoms such as nausea, dizziness or even vomiting.

This effect is closely related to the characteristics of the VR devices, the content of the proposed experiences, and individual differences between patients, and requires further investigation to minimise its impact during therapy sessions (Tsamitros et al., 2023).

A crucial aspect is the personalisation of virtual experiences to the specific needs of each patient, which requires a deep understanding of the interaction between virtual experiences and individual neural processes. At the same time, it is critical to keep the ethics and safety of virtual technologies at the forefront of discussions, while preserving patient privacy and autonomy (Bell et al., 2020).

Looking to the future, the integration of technologies such as neurofeedback and artificial intelligence offers innovative ways to personalise therapies (Bell et al., 2020). The use of avatars, the concept of presence in both the real and virtual worlds, and the social aspect of virtual interactions present challenges and opportunities that need to be explored in depth. Similarly, the issue of corporeality and the risk of escaping reality, as well as potential addictions to the cyber world, require careful analysis to understand the boundaries between therapeutic immersion and avoidance of reality.

CONCLUSION

Recent discoveries in the study of the neuropsychological correlates of virtual reality have opened new perspectives in the field of cognitive science (Nieto-Escamez et al., 2023). However, despite significant progress, some fundamental challenges require multidisciplinary investigations. One of the main obstacles is the study of brain activity during virtual immersion, which requires more sophisticated and advanced methodologies. This highlights the importance of combining approaches from cognitive neuroscience, experimental psychology and computer engineering to achieve a comprehensive understanding (Caponnetto & Casu, 2022).

The integration of artificial intelligence and machine learning can further personalise these therapies, tailoring them to individual needs. This innovative approach promises to revolutionise human-machine interaction and redefine our understanding of the human mind and brain (Caponnetto & Casu, 2022).

However, the exciting prospect of immersive virtual experiences in the treatment of complex mental disorders requires careful regulation to ensure equitable and safe access (Ford et al., 2023). Without adequate efforts to bridge the digital divide, many people may miss out on these therapies (Ford et al., 2023). It is critical to invest in long-term research to evaluate the effectiveness of virtual therapies and ensure patient safety and privacy (Bhugaonkar et al., 2022).

It is also important to emphasise that the goal of digital therapeutics is not to replace, but rather to complement, the traditional approach to psychiatry (Roth et al., 2021). Only through holistic collaboration and ongoing ethical and social engagement can researchers, clinicians, legislators and society at large ensure that psychotherapy in the Metaverse and virtual reality becomes a safe and effective resource for everyone who needs it (Ford et al., 2023). This ongoing collaboration is essential to realise the full potential of immersive virtual experiences in mental health.

REFERENCES

Ahmadpour, N., Randall, H., Choksi, H., Gao, A., Vaughan, C., & Poronnik, P. (2019). Virtual Reality interventions for acute and chronic pain management. *The International Journal of Biochemistry & Cell Biology*, *114*, 105568. doi:10.1016/j.biocel.2019.105568 PMID:31306747

Allcoat, D., & von Mühlenen, A. (2018). Learning in virtual reality: Effects on performance, emotion and engagement. *Research in Learning Technology, 26*(0). doi:10.25304/rlt.v26.2140

Álvarez-Pérez, Y., Rivero, F., Herrero, M., Viña, C., Fumero, A., Betancort, M., & Peñate, W. (2021). Changes in brain activation through cognitive-behavioral therapy with exposure to virtual reality: A neuroimaging study of specific phobia. *Journal of Clinical Medicine, 10*(16), 3505. doi:10.3390/jcm10163505 PMID:34441804

American Psychiatric Publishing. (2016). American Psychiatric Association Diagnostic and statistical manual of mental disorders, fifth edition [DSM-5®]. American Psychiatric Publishing.

Baghaei, N., Chitale, V., Hlasnik, A., Stemmet, L., Liang, H. N., & Porter, R. (2021). Virtual reality for supporting the treatment of depression and anxiety: Scoping review. In JMIR Mental Health, 8(9). doi:10.2196/29681

Bansal, G., Rajgopal, K., Chamola, V., Xiong, Z., & Niyato, D. (2022). Healthcare in Metaverse: A Survey on Current Metaverse Applications in Healthcare. *IEEE Access : Practical Innovations, Open Solutions, 10*, 119914–119946. doi:10.1109/ACCESS.2022.3219845

Bashiri, A., Ghazisaeedi, M., & Shahmorasdi, L. (2017). The opportunities of virtual reality in the rehabilitation of children with attention deficit hyperactivity disorder: A literature review. In Korean Journal of Pediatrics, 60(3). Korean Pediatric Society. doi:10.3345/kjp.2017.60.11.337

Baumgartner, T., Speck, D., Wettstein, D., Masnari, O., Beeli, G., & Jäncke, L. (2008). Feeling present in arousing virtual reality worlds: Prefrontal brain regions differentially orchestrate presence experience in adults and children. *Frontiers in Human Neuroscience, 2*(AUG). doi:10.3389/neuro.09.008.2008 PMID:18958209

Bell, I. H., Nicholas, J., Alvarez-Jimenez, M., Thompson, A., & Valmaggia, L. (2020). Virtual reality as a clinical tool in mental health research and practice. *Dialogues in Clinical Neuroscience, 22*(2), 169–177. doi:10.31887/DCNS.2020.22.2/lvalmaggia PMID:32699517

Bhugaonkar, K., Bhugaonkar, R., & Masne, N. (2022). The Trend of Metaverse and Augmented & Virtual Reality Extending to the Healthcare System. *Cureus.* doi:10.7759/cureus.29071 PMID:36258985

Bouchard, S., St-Jacques, J., Robillard, G., & Renaud, P. (2008). Anxiety increases the feeling of presence in virtual reality. *Presence (Cambridge, Mass.), 17*(4), 376–391. doi:10.1162/pres.17.4.376

Buetler, K. A., Penalver-Andres, J., Özen, Ö., Ferriroli, L., Müri, R. M., Cazzoli, D., & Marchal-Crespo, L. (2022). "Tricking the Brain" Using Immersive Virtual Reality: Modifying the Self-Perception Over Embodied Avatar Influences Motor Cortical Excitability and Action Initiation. *Frontiers in Human Neuroscience, 15*, 787487. doi:10.3389/fnhum.2021.787487 PMID:35221950

Bushnell, M. C., Čeko, M., & Low, L. A. (2013). Cognitive and emotional control of pain and its disruption in chronic pain. In Nature Reviews Neuroscience, 14(7). doi:10.1038/nrn3516

Calabrò, R. S., Cerasa, A., Ciancarelli, I., Pignolo, L., Tonin, P., Iosa, M., & Morone, G. (2022). The Arrival of the Metaverse in Neurorehabilitation: Fact, Fake or Vision? In Biomedicines, 10(10). MDPI. doi:10.3390/biomedicines10102602

Caponnetto, P., & Casu, M. (2022). Update on Cyber Health Psychology: Virtual Reality and Mobile Health Tools in Psychotherapy, Clinical Rehabilitation, and Addiction Treatment. *International Journal of Environmental Research and Public Health*, *19*(6), 3516. doi:10.3390/ijerph19063516 PMID:35329201

Cerasa, A., Gaggioli, A., Marino, F., Riva, G., & Pioggia, G. (2022). The promise of the metaverse in mental health: The new era of MEDverse. *Heliyon*, *8*(11), e11762. doi:10.1016/j.heliyon.2022.e11762 PMID:36458297

Chirico, A., & Gaggioli, A. (2023). How Real Are Virtual Emotions? In Cyberpsychology, Behavior, and Social Networking, 26(4). .editorial doi:10.1089/cyber.2023.29272.editorial

Coco-Martin, M. B., Piñero, D. P., Leal-Vega, L., Hernández-Rodríguez, C. J., Adiego, J., Molina-Martín, A., de Fez, D., & Arenillas, J. F. (2020). The Potential of Virtual Reality for Inducing Neuroplasticity in Children with Amblyopia. *Journal of Ophthalmology*, *2020*, 1–9. doi:10.1155/2020/7067846 PMID:32676202

Darnall, B. D., Krishnamurthy, P., Tsuei, J., & Minor, J. D. (2020). Self-administered skills-based virtual reality intervention for chronic pain: Randomized controlled pilot study. *JMIR Formative Research*, *4*(7), e17293. doi:10.2196/17293 PMID:32374272

Dechsling, A., Orm, S., Kalandadze, T., Sütterlin, S., Øien, R. A., Shic, F., & Nordahl-Hansen, A. (2022). Virtual and Augmented Reality in Social Skills Interventions for Individuals with Autism Spectrum Disorder: A Scoping Review. *Journal of Autism and Developmental Disorders*, *52*(11), 4692–4707. doi:10.1007/s10803-021-05338-5 PMID:34783991

Donker, T., Cornelisz, I., Van Klaveren, C., Van Straten, A., Carlbring, P., Cuijpers, P., & Van Gelder, J. L. (2019). Effectiveness of Self-guided App-Based Virtual Reality Cognitive Behavior Therapy for Acrophobia: A Randomized Clinical Trial. *JAMA Psychiatry*, *76*(7), 682–690. doi:10.1001/jamapsychiatry.2019.0219 PMID:30892564

Emmelkamp, P. M. G., & Meyerbröker, K. (2021). Annual review of clinical psychology virtual reality therapy in mental health. *Annual Review of Clinical Psychology*, *7*(17).

Ford, T. J., Buchanan, D. M., Azeez, A., Benrimoh, D. A., Kaloiani, I., Bandeira, I. D., Hunegnaw, S., Lan, L., Gholmieh, M., Buch, V., & Williams, N. R. (2023). Taking modern psychiatry into the metaverse: Integrating augmented, virtual, and mixed reality technologies into psychiatric care. *Frontiers in Digital Health*, *5*, 1146806. doi:10.3389/fdgth.2023.1146806 PMID:37035477

Frasson, C., & Abdessalem, H. (2022). Contribution of Virtual Reality Environments and Artificial Intelligence for Alzheimer. *Medical Research Archives*, *10*(9). doi:10.18103/mra.v10i9.3054

Freeman, D., Reeve, S., Robinson, A., Ehlers, A., Clark, D., Spanlang, B., & Slater, M. (2017). Virtual reality in the assessment, understanding, and treatment of mental health disorders. In Psychological Medicine, 47(). Cambridge University Press. doi:10.1017/S003329171700040X

Gorini, A., Griez, E., Petrova, A., & Riva, G. (2010). Assessment of the emotional responses produced by exposure to real food, virtual food and photographs of food in patients affected by eating disorders. *Annals of General Psychiatry*, *9*(1), 30. doi:10.1186/1744-859X-9-30 PMID:20602749

Habak, S., Bennett, J., Davies, A., Davies, M., Christensen, H., & Boydell, K. M. (2020). Edge of the present: A virtual reality tool to cultivate future thinking, positive mood and wellbeing. *International Journal of Environmental Research and Public Health, 18*(1), 140. doi:10.3390/ijerph18010140 PMID:33379156

Hao, J., Xie, H., Harp, K., Chen, Z., & Siu, K. C. (2022a). Effects of Virtual Reality Intervention on Neural Plasticity in Stroke Rehabilitation: A Systematic Review. In Archives of Physical Medicine and Rehabilitation, 103(3). doi:10.1016/j.apmr.2021.06.024

Hao, J., Xie, H., Harp, K., Chen, Z., & Siu, K.-C. (2022b). Effects of Virtual Reality Intervention on Neural Plasticity in Stroke Rehabilitation: A Systematic Review. *Archives of Physical Medicine and Rehabilitation, 103*(3), 523–541. doi:10.1016/j.apmr.2021.06.024 PMID:34352269

Higuera-Trujillo, J. L., López-Tarruella Maldonado, J., & Llinares Millán, C. (2017). Psychological and physiological human responses to simulated and real environments: A comparison between Photographs, 360° Panoramas, and Virtual Reality. *Applied Ergonomics, 65*, 398–409. doi:10.1016/j.apergo.2017.05.006 PMID:28601190

Ioannou, A., Papastavrou, E., Avraamides, M. N., & Charalambous, A. (2020). Virtual Reality and Symptoms Management of Anxiety, Depression, Fatigue, and Pain: A Systematic Review. *SAGE Open Nursing, 6*, 237796082093616. doi:10.1177/2377960820936163 PMID:33415290

Kim, H. K., Park, J., Choi, Y., & Choe, M. (2018). Virtual reality sickness questionnaire (VRSQ): Motion sickness measurement index in a virtual reality environment. *Applied Ergonomics, 69*, 66–73. doi:10.1016/j.apergo.2017.12.016 PMID:29477332

Lan, L., Sikov, J., Lejeune, J., Ji, C., Brown, H., Bullock, K., & Spencer, A. E. (2023). A Systematic Review of using Virtual and Augmented Reality for the Diagnosis and Treatment of Psychotic Disorders. In Current Treatment Options in Psychiatry, 10(2). Springer Science and Business Media Deutschland GmbH. doi:10.1007/s40501-023-00287-5

Landowska, A. (2022). Measuring prefrontal cortex response to virtual reality exposure therapy in freely moving participants. *Dissertation Abstracts International. B, The Sciences and Engineering, 83*(3-B).

Landowska, A., Roberts, D., Eachus, P., & Barrett, A. (2018). Within- and between-session prefrontal cortex response to virtual reality exposure therapy for acrophobia. *Frontiers in Human Neuroscience, 12*, 362. doi:10.3389/fnhum.2018.00362 PMID:30443209

Lara, F., & Rueda, J. (2021). Virtual Reality Not for "Being Someone" but for "Being in Someone Else's Shoes": Avoiding Misconceptions in Empathy Enhancement. *Frontiers in Psychology, 12*, 741516. doi:10.3389/fpsyg.2021.741516 PMID:34504468

Latha, K., Meena, K. S., Pravitha, M. R., Dasgupta, M., & Chaturvedi, S. K. (2020). Effective use of social media platforms for promotion of mental health awareness. *Journal of Education and Health Promotion, 9*(1), 124. doi:10.4103/jehp.jehp_90_20 PMID:32642480

Laver, K. E., Lange, B., George, S., Deutsch, J. E., Saposnik, G., & Crotty, M. (2017). Virtual reality for stroke rehabilitation. In Cochrane Database of Systematic Reviews, (11). John Wiley and Sons Ltd. doi:10.1002/14651858.CD008349.pub4

Lee, K. (2023). Counseling Psychological Understanding and Considerations of the Metaverse: A Theoretical Review. *Health Care*, *11*(18), 2490. doi:10.3390/healthcare11182490 PMID:37761687

Li, H., Dong, W., Wang, Z., Chen, N., Wu, J., Wang, G., & Jiang, T. (2021). Effect of a Virtual Reality-Based Restorative Environment on the Emotional and Cognitive Recovery of Individuals with Mild-to-Moderate Anxiety and Depression. *International Journal of Environmental Research and Public Health*, *18*(17), 9053. doi:10.3390/ijerph18179053 PMID:34501643

Lindner, P., Hamilton, W., Miloff, A., & Carlbring, P. (2019). How to Treat Depression With Low-Intensity Virtual Reality Interventions: Perspectives on Translating Cognitive Behavioral Techniques Into the Virtual Reality Modality and How to Make Anti-Depressive Use of Virtual Reality–Unique Experiences. *Frontiers in Psychiatry*, *10*, 792. doi:10.3389/fpsyt.2019.00792 PMID:31736809

Liu, Z., Ren, L., Xiao, C., Zhang, K., & Demian, P. (2022). Virtual Reality Aided Therapy towards Health 4.0: A Two-Decade Bibliometric Analysis. *International Journal of Environmental Research and Public Health*, *19*(3), 1525. doi:10.3390/ijerph19031525 PMID:35162546

Lopez-Rodriguez, M. M., Fernández-Millan, A., Ruiz-Fernández, M. D., Dobarrio-Sanz, I., & Fernández-Medina, I. M. (2020). New technologies to improve pain, anxiety and depression in children and adolescents with cancer: A systematic review. In International Journal of Environmental Research and Public Health, 17(10). doi:10.3390/ijerph17103563

Mallari, B., Spaeth, E. K., Goh, H., & Boyd, B. S. (2019). Virtual reality as an analgesic for acute and chronic pain in adults: A systematic review and meta-analysis. In *Journal of Pain Research* (Vol. 12, pp. 2053–2085). Dove Medical Press Ltd. doi:10.2147/JPR.S200498

McIntyre, R. S., Greenleaf, W., Bulaj, G., Taylor, S. T., Mitsi, G., Saliu, D., Czysz, A., Silvesti, G., Garcia, M., & Jain, R. (2023). Digital Health Technologies and Major Depressive Disorder. In *CNS Spectrums*. Cambridge University Press. doi:10.1017/S1092852923002225

Mishra, S., Kumar, A., Padmanabhan, P., & Gulyás, B. (2021). Neurophysiological correlates of cognition as revealed by virtual reality: Delving the brain with a synergistic approach. In Brain Sciences, 11(1). doi:10.3390/brainsci11010051

Nieto-Escamez, F., Cortés-Pérez, I., Obrero-Gaitán, E., & Fusco, A. (2023). Virtual Reality Applications in Neurorehabilitation: Current Panorama and Challenges. *Brain Sciences*, *13*(5), 819. doi:10.3390/brainsci13050819 PMID:37239291

Omboni, S., Padwal, R. S., Alessa, T., Benczúr, B., Green, B. B., Hubbard, I., Kario, K., Khan, N. A., Konradi, A., Logan, A. G., Lu, Y., Mars, M., McManus, R. J., Melville, S., Neumann, C. L., Parati, G., Renna, N. F., Ryvlin, P., Saner, H., & Wang, J. (2022). The worldwide impact of telemedicine during COVID-19: Current evidence and recommendations for the future. *Connected Health*. doi:10.20517/ch.2021.03 PMID:35233563

Pandarinathan, G., Mishra, S., Nedumaran, A. M., Padmanabhan, P., & Gulyás, B. (2018). The potential of cognitive neuroimaging: A way forward to the mind-machine interface. In Journal of Imaging, 4(5). MDPI Multidisciplinary Digital Publishing Institute. doi:10.3390/jimaging4050070

Parsons, S. (2015). Learning to work together: Designing a multi-user virtual reality game for social collaboration and perspective-taking for children with autism. *International Journal of Child-Computer Interaction*, *6*, 28–38. doi:10.1016/j.ijcci.2015.12.002

Petrigna, L., & Musumeci, G. (2022). The Metaverse: A New Challenge for the Healthcare System: A Scoping Review. In Journal of Functional Morphology and Kinesiology, 7(3). MDPI. doi:10.3390/jfmk7030063

Riva, G., Di Lernia, D., Sajno, E., Sansoni, M., Bartolotta, S., Serino, S., Gaggioli, A., & Wiederhold, B. K. (2021). Virtual Reality Therapy in the Metaverse: Merging VR for the Outside with VR for the Inside. *Annual Review of Cybertherapy and Telemedicine*, 19.

Riva, G., Malighetti, C., & Serino, S. (2021). Virtual reality in the treatment of eating disorders. *Clinical Psychology & Psychotherapy*, *28*(3), 477–488. doi:10.1002/cpp.2622 PMID:34048622

Riva, G., & Serino, S. (2020). Virtual reality in the assessment, understanding and treatment of mental health disorders. In Journal of Clinical Medicine, 9(11). MDPI. doi:10.3390/jcm9113434

Rodríguez, A., Rey, B., Clemente, M., Wrzesien, M., & Alcañiz, M. (2015). Assessing brain activations associated with emotional regulation during virtual reality mood induction procedures. *Expert Systems with Applications*, *42*(3), 1699–1709. doi:10.1016/j.eswa.2014.10.006

Roth, C. B., Papassotiropoulos, A., Brühl, A. B., Lang, U. E., & Huber, C. G. (2021). Psychiatry in the digital age: A blessing or a curse? In International Journal of Environmental Research and Public Health, 18(16). MDPI AG. doi:10.3390/ijerph18168302

Rousseaux, F., Bicego, A., Ledoux, D., Massion, P., Nyssen, A.-S., Faymonville, M.-E., Laureys, S., & Vanhaudenhuyse, A. (2020). Hypnosis Associated with 3D Immersive Virtual Reality Technology in the Management of Pain: A Review of the Literature</p>. *Journal of Pain Research*, *13*, 1129–1138. doi:10.2147/JPR.S231737 PMID:32547176

Schröder, D., Wrona, K. J., Müller, F., Heinemann, S., Fischer, F., & Dockweiler, C. (2023). Impact of virtual reality applications in the treatment of anxiety disorders: A systematic review and meta-analysis of randomized-controlled trials. In *Journal of Behavior Therapy and Experimental Psychiatry* (Vol. 81). Elsevier Ltd., doi:10.1016/j.jbtep.2023.101893

Song, G., & Park, E. (2015). Effect of virtual reality games on stroke patients' balance, gait, depression, and interpersonal relationships. *Journal of Physical Therapy Science*, *27*(7), 2057–2060. doi:10.1589/jpts.27.2057 PMID:26311925

Tay, J. L., Xie, H., & Sim, K. (2023). Effectiveness of Augmented and Virtual Reality-Based Interventions in Improving Knowledge, Attitudes, Empathy and Stigma Regarding People with Mental Illnesses—A Scoping Review. In Journal of Personalized Medicine, 13(1). MDPI. doi:10.3390/jpm13010112

Tieri, G., Morone, G., Paolucci, S., & Iosa, M. (2018). Virtual reality in cognitive and motor rehabilitation: facts, fiction and fallacies. In Expert Review of Medical Devices, 15(2). Taylor and Francis Ltd. doi:10.1080/17434440.2018.1425613

Tsamitros, N., Beck, A., Sebold, M., Schouler-Ocak, M., Bermpohl, F., & Gutwinski, S. (2023). The application of virtual reality in the treatment of mental disorders. *Der Nervenarzt, 94*(1), 27–33. doi:10.1007/s00115-022-01378-z PMID:36053303

Usmani, S. S., Sharath, M., & Mehendale, M. (2022). Future of mental health in the metaverse. *General Psychiatry, 35*(4), e100825. doi:10.1136/gpsych-2022-100825 PMID:36189180

Vasiliki Bravou, D. O. A. D. (n.d.). *Applications of Virtual Reality for Autism Inclusion. A review Aplicaciones de la realidad virtual para la inclusión del autism. Una revisión.*

Vicario, C. M., & Martino, G. (2022). Psychology and technology: how Virtual Reality can boost psychotherapy and neurorehabilitation. In AIMS Neuroscience, 9(4). AIMS Press. doi:10.3934/Neuroscience.2022025

Wechsler, T. F., Mühlberger, A., & Kümpers, F. (2019). Inferiority or even superiority of virtual reality exposure therapy in phobias? - A systematic review and quantitative meta-analysis on randomized controlled trials specifically comparing the efficacy of virtual reality exposure to gold standard in vivo exposure in Agoraphobia, Specific Phobia and Social Phobia. In Frontiers in Psychology, 10. Frontiers Media S.A. doi:10.3389/fpsyg.2019.01758

Wiebe, A., Kannen, K., Selaskowski, B., Mehren, A., Thöne, A. K., Pramme, L., Blumenthal, N., Li, M., Asché, L., Jonas, S., Bey, K., Schulze, M., Steffens, M., Pensel, M. C., Guth, M., Rohlfsen, F., Ekhlas, M., Lügering, H., Fileccia, H., & Braun, N. (2022). Virtual reality in the diagnostic and therapy for mental disorders: A systematic review. In Clinical Psychology Review, 98. doi:10.1016/j.cpr.2022.102213

Wong, K. P., Tse, M. M. Y., & Qin, J. (2022). Effectiveness of Virtual Reality-Based Interventions for Managing Chronic Pain on Pain Reduction, Anxiety, Depression and Mood: A Systematic Review. In Healthcare (Switzerland), 10(10). MDPI. doi:10.3390/healthcare10102047

Xie, J., Lan, P., Wang, S., Luo, Y., & Liu, G. (2023). Brain Activation Differences of Six Basic Emotions Between 2D Screen and Virtual Reality Modalities. *IEEE Transactions on Neural Systems and Rehabilitation Engineering, 31*, 700–709. doi:10.1109/TNSRE.2022.3229389 PMID:37015689

Xiong, J., Hsiang, E. L., He, Z., Zhan, T., & Wu, S. T. (2021). Augmented reality and virtual reality displays: emerging technologies and future perspectives. In Light: Science and Applications, 10(1). Springer Nature. doi:10.1038/s41377-021-00658-8

Zambelli, E., Speranza, T., & Cusimano, F. (2023). METAVERSO: L'UNIVERSO UMANO IN FORMATO DIGITALE (Alpes, Ed.).

Zeng, N., Pope, Z., Lee, J., & Gao, Z. (2018). Virtual Reality Exercise for Anxiety and Depression: A Preliminary Review of Current Research in an Emerging Field. *Journal of Clinical Medicine, 7*(3), 42. doi:10.3390/jcm7030042 PMID:29510528

Chapter 10
The Study of Cardiology Through an Augmented Reality–Based System

Gerardo Reyes Ruiz

ⓘ https://orcid.org/0000-0003-0212-2952

Centro de Estudios Superiores Navales (CESNAV), Mexico

ABSTRACT

This chapter presents an augmented reality project applied to the study of cardiology, which is crystallized through a system known as service-oriented architecture (SOA). This system serves as an innovative and efficient learning platform for students interested in cardiology because it helps them to understand abstract concepts in cardiology, which require visual and manipulable objects that are difficult to obtain, due to the large space they occupy in magnetic media or because of the difficulty of obtaining their models in physical form. This system strengthened the process of anatomical identification of the human heart and allowed a better interaction with the student, i.e., the system enhanced the use of sight, hearing, and kinesthetic, which, together, allowed a better assimilation of knowledge. The effectiveness of this system was validated using a survey of 389 students from four public universities where the following aspects were verified: 1) Significant learning; 2) Motivation; 3) Ease of use, and; 4) Performance.

INTRODUCTION

Human capital, in economies based increasingly on the level of knowledge, is the key element that enables the technological, economic, and social development of a territory (Gruzina et al., 2021). consequently, the role of human capital and its training is increasingly widely recognized; many references and projects emphasize this relationship. For its part, and as stated in the work titled "A Strategy For American Innovation: Securing Our Economic Growth And Prosperity" (National Economic Council, 2011): one of the priorities of the United States of America to ensure its economic growth and prosperity revolves around increasing support for both education and the training of intellectual human resources. Likewise, Gumbau-Albert and Maudos (2022) studied in depth the role of intangible assets in economic growth,

DOI: 10.4018/979-8-3693-1123-3.ch010

among which "knowledge capital", "human capital", "social capital" and "entrepreneurship capital" are explicitly reaffirmed. Bloom et al. (2024) point out the urgent investment in young people to obtain a considerable impact through the following aspects: 1) Education; 2) Work; 3) Health; 4) Family and 5) Civic Rights. Therefore, it can be deduced from these works that the level of knowledge is basic to enable both the generation of innovation and its adoption by third parties.

The need for better-prepared human resources with innovative and/or entrepreneurial ideas, whether generated during their studies or not, motivates the research community to respond, albeit promptly, to each of the problems generated, in turn, by these needs. Thus, Khurram et al (2007) predicted that new generations of learners must be prepared and adapt as early as possible to the challenges that new technologies will bring in the not-too-distant future. On the other hand, it is evident that the COVID-19 pandemic motivated technological advances, which have had a direct impact on all activities of daily life and education has been no exception (Godber and Atkins, 2021; Bozkurt et al., 2022; Betthäuser, Bach-Mortensen and Engzell, 2023). In the latter scenario, new strategies have been created and implemented to support the teaching-learning process, which systematically strengthens the way of teaching and learning the most current educational content (Haleem et al., 2022). Consequently, during the last decade, the concern for the study of learning design has increased significantly.

Likewise, the need for increasingly younger and better prepared human resources motivates teachers and researchers to generate new educational environments or learning techniques for these young people to assimilate the so-called new technologies as quickly and effectively as possible so that, when they need them, it will be easier for them to enter a highly competitive globalized environment (McDiarmid and Zhao, 2023; Haleem et al., 2022). In this context, it makes sense to create and provide a new way of learning for a specific group of students, in particular for young people who have the opportunity to learn an innovative and efficient technological tool in a controlled environment, such as their school (Lin and Yu, 2023). It is clear that knowledge transfer has gradually evolved and it is also logical that the process of educating has also shown changes (Rasa and Laherto, 2022; Kayapinar, 2021). Thus, the new generations of students have a lot to do with the so-called new technologies, mainly because they have grown up with them and are prepared to use them and adapt to assimilate them quickly (Szymkowiak et al., 2021; Qazi et al., 2021; Rathi et al., 2023). Undoubtedly, the challenge is for academics and developers of such technologies, since they must create new contexts and innovative, efficient, and interesting technological tools to capture the greatest possible attention of students but, above all, prepare them as soon as possible for the challenges that a globalized world holds for them in the future (ECLAC, 2021; Dziuban et al., 2018).

Under this approach to educational needs, Augmented Reality (AR) plays a transcendental and extremely important role, as the combination of physical reality with virtual resources can be displayed in the form of multimedia content (Kamińska et al., 2023; Abad-Segura et al., 2020). The multiple scenarios offered by AR are extremely proficient (Villagran-Vizcarra et al., 2023; Roopa, Prabha and Senthil, 2021), however, medicine has been little explored in this context. Medical learning also requires optimal means, both technological and otherwise, which should enable and facilitate learners in the concept of learning by doing (Hemanth, Kose, Deperlioglu, and de Albuquerque, 2020); Cheng et al., 2022). This dynamic can be achieved with interactive systems since this interaction makes knowledge reach the brain in a sensory, visual, auditory, and kinesthetic way (Li and Liu, 2022). All this is to acquire the necessary, sufficient, and current academic competencies for their adequate professional development as future physicians (Mikhailova, 2018). Likewise, the creation of accessible systems is required, i.e., that do not require accessories that are not very accessible and difficult to obtain; in other words, that are not expensive (Li and Wong, 2022). Therefore, to acquire know-how competencies, medical students must learn to perform medical procedures on living or dead people using new technologies (Mathew et al., 2023; Dodds et al., 2022). It is precisely here that new technologies become meaningful and relevant because multiple medical processes can be simulated through AR (Goo, Park, and Yoo, 2020). Developing a platform that handles AR would be a training tool for each student, whose studies are related to medicine, to evaluate his or her learning before performing any procedure with live people (Jung et al., 2022). Thus, the present work aims to create an interactive system or platform to support the learning of medical procedures and, in particular, to learn about the functioning of the human heart in a novel and efficient way.

BACKGROUND

In the last decades, new technologies based on information provision and knowledge generation have shown great results and advances in multiple labor and knowledge areas (Vicsek, 2021; Passavanti et at., 2020; Mahr and Huh, 2022). In the latter context, it has been shown that the Internet of Things (IoT) has been one of the most efficient methods for educating young people (Shammar and Zahary, 2020). The introduction of new technology-assisted learning tools such as smartphones, tablets, MOOCs, SPOCs, smart boards, laptops, online learning tools, dynamic visualizations, virtual labs, blended learning, and MashUp Technologies, among others, have altered the learning and training process worldwide (Haleem et al., 2022). These technologies are becoming increasingly accessible to people as they can gain many benefits from their use and learning such as using education-oriented applications.

Nowadays the use of new technologies, almost all based on the internet, is indispensable and, of course, all these new technologies have revolutionized the way people relate to each other, in addition, now communications are faster and more efficient (Hitzler, 2021; Andersson, 2018). Due to this technological revolution, the use of mobile devices reached a considerable level of dependency on people. Moreover, these mobile devices have become necessary, and almost indispensable, for people to interact and communicate - in a more impersonal but, above all, in a more efficient way (Harris et al.,, 2020). Of course, these mobile devices also became indispensable, especially after the COVID-19 pandemic, especially for people to shop online, which turned out to be the safest way to ensure their health (Katsumata et al., 2022; Chemnad et al., 2022). In this way, mobile devices became an extremely important medium to present some technologies innovatively and efficiently (Stocchi et al., 2022).

Consequently, and to generate an innovative educational environment of this nature, it is necessary to create a fast, direct, and efficient interaction with users (in our case students studying medicine), which can be achieved, undoubtedly, through a system based on Augmented Reality (AR) (tom Dieck et al., 2023a). This technology meets these last three needs first because it presents an immediate response -even in real time- to data transmission, however, this response will depend on the speed at which the data is transmitted. Secondly, and through the use of a mobile device, AR can interact directly and easily with people, thirdly, this technology is efficient because it can display information and features, totally specific, even in real-time (tom Dieck et al., 2023b; Habil, El-Deeb and El-Bassiouny, 2023). Therefore, these extraordinary qualities make AR an innovative and efficient technology to create/generate new uses, and forms and, in particular, to create new learning environments, which can provide people with new experiences when studying (Cao and Yu, 2023; Arulanand et al., 2020).

What is Augmented Reality?

Augmented Reality (AR) emerged in 1996, when ARQuake (Piekarski and Thomas, 2002), the first outdoor game with AR mobile devices, developed by Bruce H. Thomas, was presented. Subsequently, in 2008 the travel and tourism guide application Wikitude (2023) was released, which was made using an AR-based digital compass, orientation, and accelerometer sensors, maps, video, and informative content from Wikipedia. In 2009, ARToolkit (2023) was born, which is a platform fully oriented to generate AR. From these applications, AR has been used as the basis for numerous projects in different areas, ranging from entertainment, industry, maintenance, music, medicine, and education, among many others (El Filali and Krit, 2020). Moreover, very specific applications have been realized such as a harp that was designed for people with disabilities (Bryant and Hemsley, 2022; Ramasamy et al., 2021), which is powered by vibrations (Žilak, Car and Culjak, 2022; Ulrich, and Sandor, 2013).

In industry, through the development of AR manuals, it has been shown that the performance of workers using AR manuals is modified in a palpable improvement compared to workers using paper-based manuals (Wang et al., 2023; Eversberg and Lambrecht, 2023). This result is mainly due to the behavioral, physiological, and psychological data of the workers (Dorloh, Li and Khaday, 2023). Therefore, the use of AR in product assembly orientation has been widely recommended (Adebowale and Agumba, 2022). In addition, this technique includes information retrieval and real-time assembly and promotes error reduction in assembly (Wang and Qi, 2022), all under the cognitive workload and high skill transfer to improve tasks (El Kassis, Ayer and El Asmar, 2023). Intelligent Tutorial Systems (ITSs) have also been realized (Guo et al., 2021, Jain et al., 2023), such as the "Intelligent Augmented Reality Training for Motherboard Assembly", which helps with training for manual assembly tasks (Westerfield, Mitrovic and Billinghurst, 2015). In addition, ITS is a tool, also quite efficient, to support learning processes (Wang et al., 2023), and if ICTs are added to this dynamic then totally novel results can be obtained (Sharma and Harkishan, 2022). Therefore, AR can be a very supportive technological tool for learning, which could be verified in the system "Augmented Reality in Informal Learning Environments: A Field Experiment in a Mathematics Exhibition" (Sommerauer and Müller, 2014).

In education, AR can be used to teach molecular structures, mathematics, architecture, astronomy, and physical activities to children with disabilities (Tezer et al., 2019; Salina et al., 2023). In medicine and education, specialized projects have been developed that show AR as an efficient tool in medical learning (Parsons and MacCallum, 2021; Kurniawan, Suharjito and Witjaksono, 2018; Dhar, 2021), such as the system "An Interactive Augmented Reality System for Learning Anatomy Structure" (Chien-Huan, Chien-Hsu and Tay-Sheng, 2010), which is integrated of three activities; the first is to show the parts of the anatomical structure of the human body, the second is to allow students to identify each anatomical part of the human body, and the third is to provide an in-depth glimpse of the internal parts of the aforementioned anatomical structure (Bölek et al., 2021). On the other hand, the system "Interactive augmented reality using Scratch 2.0 to improve physical activities for children with developmental disabilities", shown by Chien-Yu and Yu-Ming (2015), uses an interactive game for body movement to improve the motor strength of children with disabilities. To conclude with AR applications, in Magic Book (Westerfield, Mitrovic and Billinghurst, 2015), which is a normal book but contains markers -usually QR codes-, the system when detecting a marker then a three-dimensional image is displayed or a video story is started (Pingxuan, 2020).

But, what is AR? It is a technology, that can be immersive, that allows virtual reality to be added to a real environment (Yawised et al., 2022; Korkut and Surer, 2023). In other words, AR can be described as an innovative technology that enables the superimposition of 2D and 3D digital objects in common real-life environments (Villagran-Vizcarra et al., 2023). These superimposed objects work through the use of mobile devices, usually, a smartphone or tablet, which have the particularity of tracking the user's position and use markers, usually QR codes -Quick Response- (Yao, Wang and Shen, 2022), which are strategically placed in real scenarios that will serve to "detonate" additional digital information (3D images, sounds, internet pages, multimedia files, among others), which will be used, in turn, to enhance reality and impress the user (Du, Liu and Wang, 2022). However, AR should not be confused with VR (Yan et al., 2022), as the latter is a computer-generated environment, which allows the user to feel immersed in the non-real objects that are generated in a fully controlled environment (Ifanov et al., 2023). VR generally requires complementary objects such as special helmets, pre-designed gloves, and headsets to assist the computer in visualizing the environment created for the user. In turn, these devices will allow the computer to generate the environment that will be displayed for users to interact in (Greengard, 2019). In addition, through VR, scenarios can be created in a room, with a 3600 perspective, where the user can be allowed to walk, jump and interact in it (McAnally et al., 2023). Thus, VR roughly refers to "immersing" oneself in a three-dimensional (3D) digital environment where sophisticated hardware and software are used (Lum et al., 2020). On the other hand, the technological differences between AR and VR are probably not so clear-cut, as both technologies mainly provide relevant information, sensory stimulation, imagination, interaction, and interaction opportunities for users and, above all, enable enhanced sensory and kinesthetic experiences through different touch points online - i.e., with the use of the internet or offline for users (Zarantonello and Schmitt, 2023). Therefore, AR and VR consistently show differences, especially in the way each contributes to the user experience during their experience/experience of using these technologies (Xiong et al., 2021; Cipresso et al., 2018).

MAIN FOCUS OF THE CHAPTER

Issues, Controversies, Problems

In a globalized world, there is currently a need for new ways of learning and, consequently, for novel technological tools that support emerging learning processes (Valverde-Berrocoso et al., 2021). New technologies help to shape innovative learning environments through which people learn or train their acquired skills in various fields of knowledge (Sailer et al., 2021). This dynamic has created an evident need for new generations to require current technological means that drive constant training (Kessler, 2018), which can be implemented in schools or be individually accessible for interested individuals to train constantly (Abuhassna et al., 2020). In this context, learning new technologies is one of the activities that are most frequently done in basic level schools, such as for learning new languages, which is mainly due to the following result: the younger the age of students learn languages other than their mother tongue then the greater the cognitive plasticity of the individual to assimilate a foreign language, especially if you have the support of a technological platform fully oriented to this objective (Pliatsikas, 2020; Birdsong, 2018).

In this increasingly competitive world, universities are playing a fundamental role in generating human resources with cutting-edge knowledge. Moreover, some universities are currently incorporating digital technologies as a support to facilitate educational processes (Okoye et al., 2023). In this context, technological elements such as computers, mobile devices, the internet, cyber cloud applications, projectors, slides, and other hardware or software resources have been the starting point for creating new learning environments. As a consequence of the above, in the last two decades, the concern for the study of learning design has increased remarkably (Fraser, 2023; Gupta et al., 2022). In this sense, the present work increases the characteristics exposed in the previous text, since the proposed platform will serve to learn processes composed of three-dimensional elements, processes in which students will learn activities that could only be done with living human bodies. Since learning can include different senses such as sight, hearing, and touch, this work proposes an interactive platform that contains elements related to these senses to make learning complete (Navab et al., 2023). Moreover, in this mentioned learning platform, students will be able to train those medical processes and repeat them as many times as they wish since the system, developed for this learning platform, will provide evaluation metrics of the processes as well as feedback from the system (Tang et al., 2022). The platform can be used as a trainer before learners perform these processes on real patients or people (Bruno et al., 2022).

In addition to the above, this new learning platform describes the design of a system as the establishment of the data structures, the general architecture of the software, and the representations of interfaces and algorithms (Kossiakoff et al., 2020). That is the process that translates requirements into software specifications. Therefore, the objective of the design phase is to make known the behavior of the proposed solution; this is conceived taking into account that the design is a pre-phase that initiates the construction of programs and/or processes of activities that are normally performed by users, which seek to be improved by adding speed, efficiency, effectiveness, savings, and visual design. The first action, which starts with the design, is the determination of the system architecture, which is nothing more than the hierarchical structure of the program modules, which is focused on how to interact between its components and the structure of the data used by them (Tilley, 2019). Thus, and for all of the above, it is considered that this book chapter is innovative from the very moment of its approach, since to date there are no works that have addressed the problems described in it. Furthermore, this chapter will likely contribute to the generation of new projects and research. For example, this work proposes the creation, in the not-too-distant future, of the implementation of holograms in the area of medicine and, more specifically, to perform surgeries.

To acquire the competencies of know-how, medical students must learn to perform medical procedures with living or dead people, and these processes can be simulated with AR. A platform that handles AR is a training medium for each student to evaluate their learning, before performing it with people. Therefore, the general objective of this work is to create a platform that can be used for learning medical procedures. In other words, the creation of a new learning platform, based on AR, will allow students in the area of medicine, particularly surgery, to obtain quality knowledge as well as a correct approach to new technologies for the timely execution of their activities in an operating room. To acquire know-how competencies, medical students must learn to perform medical procedures on living or dead people. These processes can be simulated with AR. A platform with these qualities is a training medium for each student to evaluate his or her learning, before carrying it out on people. Therefore, the general objective of this work is to show a new platform that can be used for learning medical procedures, and, to achieve this objective, we propose to test the following hypothesis:

H_0: The creation of a new and innovative learning platform, through Augmented Reality, will allow students in the area of medicine, particularly in anatomy and physiology, to obtain quality and avant-garde knowledge, as well as a correct approach to new technologies for the timely execution of their activities in an operating room.

SOLUTIONS AND RECOMMENDATIONS

Today, there are several software architectural styles. However, due to the nature of the system to be built and the one to be modeled is the "Service Oriented Architecture" (SOA) (Niknejad et al., 2020), which is an architectural paradigm for designing and developing distributed systems and has been created to provide ease and flexibility of integration with legacy systems as well as direct alignment to business processes, thus reducing implementation costs (Haorongbam, Nagpal and Sehgal, 2022). Another advantage is that it implements customer service innovation and agile adaptation in the face of change, including early reaction to competitiveness. Therefore, in this work a Service Oriented Architecture (SOA) type system is created (Niknejad et al., 2020; Mishra and Sarkar, 2022). This system is oriented to manage other modules or secondary systems, which are linked together to interact with the user who is interested in learning how the human heart works, in our case students who are in high school (HTML and JavaScript were used for the programming of these modules). In this sense, the AR is "the module" that will be seen by the student, which when "triggered/activated" will initiate the interaction showing as a result the modules that are related to each other, generally using a mobile device. This SOA system is designed using the OASIS (Outil Auteur de Simulations Interactives avec Scénarios) program (OASIS, 2023), which allows the creation and use of standard interfaces, which facilitate the services of different technologies, such as AR, and even dissimilar data formats.

On the other hand, the SketchUp Make (2023) program was used to create the 3D images, since it is a free version. Since AR is visualized with virtual objects that can be shown through the association that exists between the initial two-dimensional image with a three-dimensional one, then an image is presented on the screen of the mobile device and, gradually, it will take the shape of the three-dimensional model that we want to show the student (for the realization of this animation we used the Flash program and saved it in GIF format), which can be manipulated to visualize it from different positions and angles, giving the appearance of a real physical model. In this way, for the generation of the AR, it was necessary to program in lines of code, which is why JavaScript was used, which is also a very robust program for this type of code and where the AR-Frame libraries (2023) are essential for its implementation.

In this way, and based on the software engineering mentioned in (Kendall and Kendal, 2023) where it is exposed that for the construction of software, communication guidelines, requirements analysis, design, program construction, testing, and support are used, the work program that was established in this work was the following:

a. Analysis of the requirements of the AR system. In this phase, research was conducted on the knowledge that the student should acquire with this material, i.e., the functioning of the human heart.
b. Formulate the abstract and physical design as well as code and create the software. In this stage, the AR was constructed and designed. That is, a human heart was structured to be displayed three-dimensionally and the events were coded (the characteristics of the Main Menu that will present the AR options), which were coded with the help of JavaScript, HTML5, and with the implementation of Aframe (2023), the latter is open-source software.
c. Prepare the files, and identify and create the test data to integrate and validate the software. The AR elements were encapsulated and were used to obtain the file that can be executed on an Android or iOS-based platform, which will be enriched with the help of a web server, a webcam, high voices, or a mobile device (usually a smartphone).

Thus, the present learning platform describes the design of a system as the establishment of the data structures, the overall software architecture, and the representations of interfaces and algorithms. That is, the system process translates requirements into software specifications (Richards and Ford, 2020; Ramasamy et al., 2022; Doshi et al., 2023). The objective of the design phase is to make known the behavior of the proposed solution; this is conceived taking into account that the design is a pre-phase that initiates the construction of programs and/or processes of activities that are normally performed by users, which seek to be improved by adding speed, efficiency, effectiveness, savings, and visual design. The first action that starts with the design is the determination of the system architecture, which refers to the hierarchical structure of the program modules and, in addition, is focused on the way its components interact and the structure of the data used by them (Ford et al., 2021).

The system, based on AR, proposed in this work is oriented to the functioning of the human heart and its main objective is to show and obtain an application (software) that helps students of medicine or related areas to identify the parts that make up its functioning in a virtual model through various sensory senses. With the approach shown in (Kleftodimos et al. (2023), the software presented in this work is built to make available to students an application easy to obtain and with the lowest possible cost, since the system can run on a desktop computer or mobile device (usually on a smartphone) where the main requirement is that a video camera is available for the detection of the images that will be processed through AR. This technology makes it possible first, for medical students to learn in a 3D environment and, subsequently, to simulate the physical constitution of a model as well as the interaction of the parts involved in the siological process related to the functioning of the human heart (Tang et al., 2022). Therefore, the creation of a new learning platform, through AR, will allow students in the area of medicine, particularly anatomy and physiology, to obtain quality knowledge, as well as a correct approach to new technologies for the timely execution of their activities in an operating room. As previously mentioned, to acquire know-how competencies, medical students must learn to perform medical procedures with living or dead people, these processes can be simulated with AR (Cofano et al., 2021; Barcali et al., 2022).

RESULTS AND DISCUSSION

System Architecture

After analyzing and understanding the system, with the sole purpose of determining how it works, the requirements to create it are obtained and, based on these requirements, proceed to the elaboration of its design and construction, which will be represented by its general software architecture, interfaces, and algorithms, i.e., the process that translates the requirements into software specifications. The objective of the system design phase is, roughly speaking, to show the behavior of the proposed solution. Likewise, the logical view of the system architecture describes its structure and functionality; for this purpose, a sequence diagram was used where the actions performed by the system entities can be observed, as the AR user focuses the device's camera on the marker that will "detonate" the AR through the learning actions and, finally, the evaluation of the acquired knowledge. The system can be seen in Figure 1, where a diagram shows the actions, starting with the one that gives access to the system, which is stored on a website and contains link buttons that show the functions with the options: video, audio, and learning and where in this last option derives, in turn, an evaluation of the student, which can be stored to later analyze their academic progress.

Figure 1. Sequence diagram of the AR-based system
Source: Author's own elaboration.

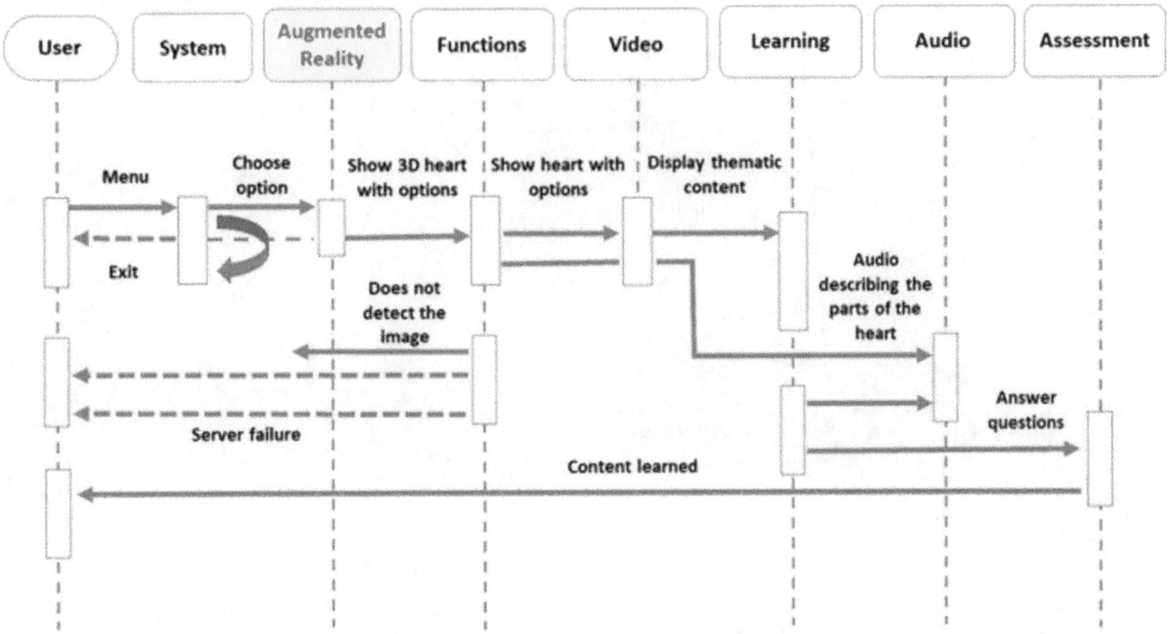

For the development of the system, it was considered that the users already have an academic background and that their disciplinary knowledge is more specific. For this reason, the resources developed, through the AR-based system, include knowledge directed toward professional-level students. Thus, the system proposed in this work starts with a screen showing a MENU (Figure 2).

User interface

When an option is selected from the main MENU, then the AR is displayed with virtual objects that are shown by the association that exists, through a marker (usually with a QR -Quick Response- code), between the initial (2D) image and a final (3D) image (Belin et al., 2018), where the first one is focused to the camera and takes the form of a physiological model of the human heart (it is recalled that the image was created using the SketchUp program and the AR was coded with Javascript and HTML5 in an Aframe platform), same that can be manipulated to be visualized from different positions and angles, giving the appearance of a real physical model (see Figure 3).

In this way, the AR system starts showing a MENU of options (Functions, Audio, Video, Learning), which "trigger/trigger" an event when the user clicks on any of these options (also remember that these actions were programmed with JavaScript code and in a platform called Aframe). Thus, when the user clicks on the Functions option, then a web page will be displayed, which will have the purpose of showing each element involved in the functioning of the human heart, i.e., it will show images and text that describe it more creatively and innovatively (see Figure 3). For example, when the user selects in the MENU the option VIDEO/AUDIO then a multimedia/audio file will be displayed where the main functions of the human heart are presented in a specific way (Figure 4).

Figure 2. Startup of the AR-based system
Source: Author's own elaboration.

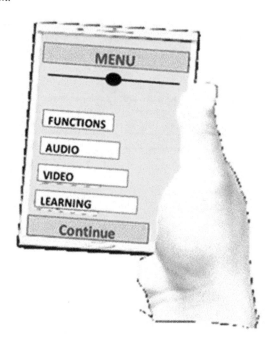

Figure 3. Image of a two-dimensional human heart generated by AR
Source: Author's own elaboration.

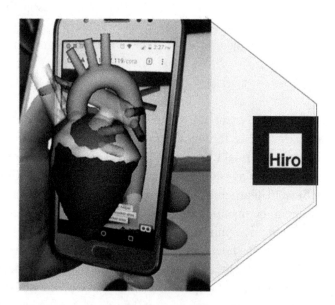

The main MENU of the AR system has an option called FUNCTIONS, where the user can search, using a keyword, for a part of the human heart. When the AR system finds the word, it then displays the image related to that word as well as an audio that explains the most significant part of that part of the human heart. This search option follows the algorithm shown in Figure 5.

Figure 4. Results when selecting some MENU options
Source: Author's own elaboration.

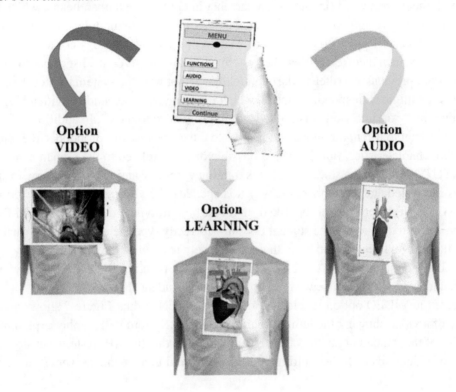

Figure 5. Algorithm for the search of a word in the system with AR
Source: Author's own elaboration.

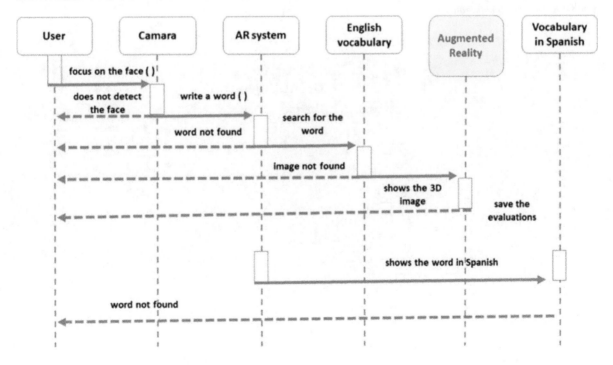

In this module of the AR system, the images used are stored in a database and each one of them is associated with the correct word (in our case a part that integrates the human heart), which the student will consult employing a capture line. This system has two independent modules to motivate the student: MODULE WITH TUTORIAL: When the word written in the capture line is not located in the list of stored words or is written incorrectly, then the system will show the student a list of possible words very similar to the word previously written in the capture line. In that way, the system locates the correct word and associates it with its corresponding image, which is displayed to the student with a message telling the student that the "<desired word> is spelled as follows <word found>". In addition, a button is presented for the student to listen, through an audio file, to the correct way to pronounce the found word as well as its main characteristics, functions, and possible diseases related to the human heart. MODULE WITHOUT TUTORIAL: If the student starts his training without wanting to know how to spell a word (so that he is motivated and remembers the way it is spelled), then he can choose this option from the MENU/FUNCTIONS where he will be asked, in a text box, to type a desired word and thus activate the search process. In this way, if the student does not correctly type the desired word, then the system will display the image, from the database, that most closely resembles the one previously typed on the capture line. If the System with RA does not find any match then it will send the following message "Word not found" and will give a new capture option to the student (Figure 6).

Likewise, if the VIDEO option is selected in the main MENU, then Figure 7 shows an example of the sequence of a video showing the human heart that the AR System will display explaining the main characteristics of that human organ. It is important to mention that the AR System can store a considerable number of videos since all the multimedia files are stored in a backup server. That is, all the files

Figure 6. Response for the search of a word in the system with AR
Source: Author's own elaboration.

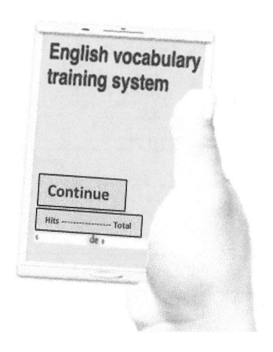

Figure 7. Sequence of a video shown by the AR-based system
Source: Author's own elaboration.

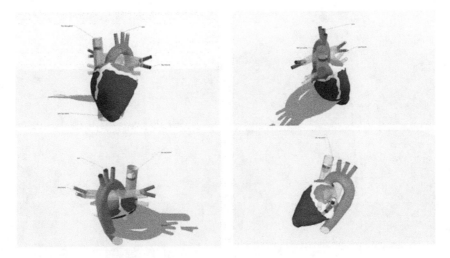

used by this AR System are stored on a server and can be "downloaded" by the user, as long as he/she has started the corresponding session in the AR System.

In the same way, when the user selects the LEARNING option from the main MENU then the system with AR will show a didactic test where the student will have the experience of experimenting and practicing, through AR, the functioning of all the parts of the human heart. In this didactic test it will be possible to accumulate the evolution of their learning (the System shows the option to SAVE the didactic test) and different ascending levels of learning will be shown as if the student were in a video game (see Figure 8).

In this didactic test, a series of several questions are asked to carry out a self-assessment of the student and where, through which, the acquired knowledge can be appreciated. This evaluation contains questions with dichotomous answers (the questions were implemented with JavaScript events and performed on the SDK platform), which serve as input for the system to display the score obtained by the student (see Figure 9).

AR-Based System Evaluation

To evaluate the system presented in this work, a statistically significant sample of 389 students from 4 public universities in the Metropolitan Zone of Mexico City (ZMCM) where undergraduate studies in medicine were being carried out was calculated. This sample was calculated by stratified random sampling with proportional allocation without knowledge of the total population, with 95% confidence, 5% error, and 50% homogeneity (Wu and Thompson, 2020). After the installation of the system, on the functioning of the human heart, on the smartphones of the students who were taking a learning unit specifically related to cardiology, they were shown the system developed in this work. Once the students had the opportunity and the experience of getting to know the system, a survey with 30 questions was applied where each student, previously selected, expressed their experience using an AR App to learn how the human heart works. The purpose of this survey was to determine 4 evaluation parameters, on the objective of this research, i.e., that the students "learn by doing" based on the AR-based system.

Figure 8. Results when selecting the LEARNING option from the MENU
Source: Author's own elaboration.

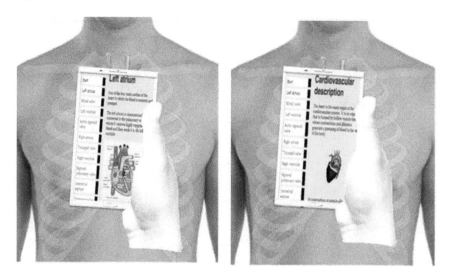

Figure 9. Didactic test (self-evaluation) carried out using an AR-based system
Source: Author's own elaboration.

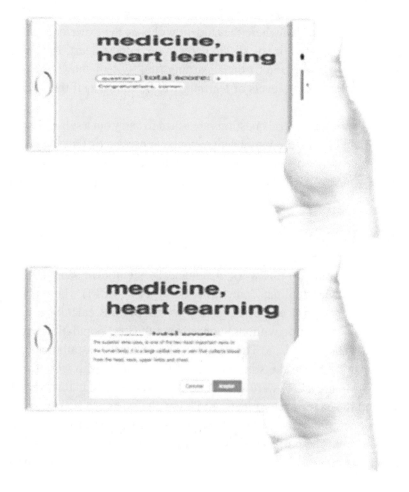

Thus, the first result for this survey was that Cronbach's alpha had a value of 83.1%, which implies that the questionnaire meets the study objective for which it was designed and, therefore, is valid and consistent. Subsequently, for the 4 concepts, the level of knowledge retention was evaluated by comparing the two ways in which the students studied the functioning of the human heart, i.e., with and without the AR. Thus, the first impressions of the students surveyed regarding these 4 items were: 1) Meaningful learning (89.3% with AR and 35.0% without AR); 2) Motivation (94.5% with AR and 35.7% without AR); 3) Ease of use (93.8% with AR and 86.6% without AR) and; 4) Performance (82.0% with AR and 60.0% without AR). Consequently, the implications for each of these 4 criteria evaluated, through an AR-based system, were as follows:

Significant learning. The neural maps made during the activity allowed us to detect significant learning of 89.3%. The second contrast in meaningful learning refers to the fact that the teaching of cognitively complex knowledge, disconnected so many times from the emotional system, is a mistake since nothing is learned if it is not loved or does not mean something. Thus, it was found that the significant learning of 89.3% achieved in the tests, occurred when the students liked and understood what they were doing; the responses of the significant learning category showed that the analysis of the content was easy for them (87.0%); the system showed the learning sequences with an intuitive logic (88.0%); the learning they considered it for their educational level (90.0%) and that it was easy to learn with relatively new technology (92.0%). Consequently, it can be deduced that AR activates the neural networks of the learners to generate thinking based on logical sequences, and, therefore, more complex knowledge is understood and acquired.

Motivation. In this context, it was found that AR motivated medical students in 94.7% with elements that served to use their primary senses. This result was verified through the interviews because the students answered that they liked the images, the audio, and the interaction with AR through the devices and, consequently, they were excited by the use of these superimposed systems in real contexts. In the study, students were cheerful, curious, and encouraged to use these educational tools; the data conjugated with the interviews determined that students liked the AR elements in 95.4%, the structure of the system 93.0%, they would like to learn other subjects with AR in 95.3%, as they felt excited in 95%. These results allow us to argue that AR generates contexts where dopamine overflows with the purpose of including the desire to continue learning, to appropriate this knowledge, and to keep it in their long-term memory.

Easy to use. With the educational resources that were implemented, it was observed that intuitive and easy-to-handle educational elements can be generated; this result was demonstrated with 93.8% since when compared to the percentage obtained with the resources without AR it would seem that it should be equally or less easy than using paper (60% ease), however, the students evaluated it according to what they learned. This result asserted that AR makes it easier for teachers to impart knowledge and for students to obtain it, which was reflected in their learning. Therefore, the implementation of technological resources in the classroom helped to improve the learning process, increased motivation, and considerably facilitated the teacher's work.

Performance. The students obtained a performance of 86.4% because there were many words to learn in a short time. Therefore, this result allows arguing that the learning that is obtained, and that remains in the long-term memory, is easier to obtain when it is understood in a 3D model than when using flat resources (2D). This immediate evaluation of the learner allows decisions to be made at the appropriate time for improvement and also optimizes learner participation and the benefit is reflected in subsequent sessions. The evaluation shown by AR-based systems is carried out at the moment of learning or the end, allowing the student to self-evaluate and, when necessary, continue learning. This result emphasizes that using an AR-based system results in a 26% improvement in student performance. Therefore, it can be affirmed that the evaluation through an AR-based system helps students to generate challenges with themselves, based on the synergy of real and digital contexts, which allows them to increase their performance.

FUTURE RESEARCH DIRECTIONS

The creation of a new learning platform, through AR, will allow students in the area of medicine, particularly in anatomy and physiology, to obtain quality knowledge, as well as a correct approach to new technologies for the timely execution of their activities either in an operating room or in the classroom. It is important to remember that, to acquire the competencies of know-how, medical students must learn to perform medical procedures with living or dead people and, fortunately, through these educational platforms, these processes can be simulated or foreseen through AR. A platform with these qualities is a training medium for each student to evaluate his or her learning before carrying it out with live people.

There are multiple add-ons to make AR a more interesting and engaging experience. For example, we can highlight the use of AR glasses (which can even manage and display certain data when worn), headsets adapted with AR viewers and surround sound, or the latest generation of AR smartphones where video calls can be made using a hologram or Avatar. Concerning holograms, little by little these technological tools are being developed with more complex designs where AI is playing a preponderant role in making these holograms more real but, above all, be an unconditional support for learning in all areas of knowledge. On the other hand, in virtual or mixed environments there is already the possibility of using gloves, screens, or rooms equipped with specific objects to feel and appreciate the virtual extended reality. Undoubtedly, there are multiple options for generating new environments, whether educational or not, where AR is the main tool for their creation or development. These complements and new environments depend on the budget available for their implementation, development, or creation, however, their creation is not too costly. What is clear is that these environments favor and facilitate the learning process of students at any educational level.

CONCLUSION

In addition to verifying the null hypothesis (Ho) proposed in this work, the following results could be obtained: 1) AR is a useful and easy-to-use tool that works to build suitable, innovative and efficient learning environments, which allow students to feel motivated, encouraged and eager to continue learning; 2) With the support of AR it is possible to generate computational systems that help the learning of abstract or difficult to perceive knowledge; 3) Medicine handles models where appearance and shape help to strengthen learning, which can be represented with three-dimensional (3D) entities; 4) The interaction with AR and multimedia materials that are added to the physical reality allow the sensory senses of the human being to be stimulated, thus achieving that students learn in an auditory, visual and kinesthetic way; 5) The cost of the design will depend on how much is willing to invest in accessories or complements to show AR, however, the programming and design of virtual reality (three-dimensional design, simulation and web page) are generally not very expensive. Nevertheless, an advantage of the proposed system is that it could be reusable, i.e., new knowledge and free 3D models on the web can be adapted. Finally, it is worth mentioning that the challenges of AR for educational environments are vast and transcendental so a contribution of this nature allows and will allow to lay the foundations to broaden the current learning horizon and create a new mosaic of knowledge.

REFERENCES

Abad-Segura, E., González-Zamar, M.-D., Luque-de la Rosa, A. L., & Morales Cevallos, M. B. (2020). Sustainability of Educational Technologies: An Approach to Augmented Reality Research. *Sustainability (Basel)*, *12*(10), 4091. doi:10.3390/su12104091

Abuhassna, H., Al-Rahmi, W. M., Yahya, N., Zakaria, M. A. Z. M., Kosnin, A. B. M., & Darwish, M. (2020). Development of a new model for utilizing online learning platforms to improve students' academic achievements and satisfaction. *International Journal of Educational Technology in Higher Education*, *17*(1), 38. doi:10.1186/s41239-020-00216-z

Adebowale, O. J., & Agumba, J. N. (2022). Applications of augmented reality for construction productivity improvement: a systematic review. Smart and Sustainable Built Environment. doi:10.1108/SASBE-06-2022-0128

Andersson, G. (2018). Internet interventions: Past, present and future. *Internet Interventions : the Application of Information Technology in Mental and Behavioural Health*, *12*, 181–188. doi:10.1016/j.invent.2018.03.008 PMID:30135782

Arulanand, N., Ramesh Babu, A., & Rajesh, P. K. (2020). Enriched Learning Experience using Augmented Reality Framework in Engineering Education. *Procedia Computer Science*, *172*, 937–942. doi:10.1016/j.procs.2020.05.135

Barcali, E., Iadanza, E., Manetti, L., Francia, P., Nardi, C., & Bocchi, L. (2022). Augmented Reality in Surgery: A Scoping Review. *Applied Sciences (Basel, Switzerland)*, *12*(14), 6890. doi:10.3390/app12146890

Belin, E., Douarre, C., Gillard, N., Franconi, F., Rojas-Varela, J., Chapeau-Blondeau, F., Demilly, D., Adrien, J., Maire, E., & Rousseau, D. (2018). Evaluation of 3D/2D Imaging and Image Processing Techniques for the Monitoring of Seed Imbibition. *Journal of Imaging*, *4*(7), 83. doi:10.3390/jimaging4070083

Betthäuser, B. A., Bach-Mortensen, A. M., & Engzell, P. (2023). A systematic review and meta-analysis of the evidence on learning during the COVID-19 pandemic. *Nature Human Behaviour*, *7*(3), 375–385. doi:10.1038/s41562-022-01506-4 PMID:36717609

Birdsong, D. (2018). Plasticity, Variability and Age in Second Language Acquisition and Bilingualism. *Frontiers in Psychology*, *9*, 81. doi:10.3389/fpsyg.2018.00081 PMID:29593590

Bloom, D. E., Canning, D., Kotschy, R., Prettner, K., & Schünemann, J. (2024). Health and economic growth: Reconciling the micro and macro evidence. *World Development*, *178*, 106575. doi:10.1016/j.worlddev.2024.106575 PMID:38463754

Bölek, K. A., De Jong, G., & Henssen, D. (2021). The effectiveness of the use of augmented reality in anatomy education: A systematic review and meta-analysis. *Scientific Reports*, *11*(1), 15292. doi:10.1038/s41598-021-94721-4 PMID:34315955

Bozkurt, A., Karakaya, K., Turk, M., Karakaya, Ö., & Castellanos-Reyes, D. (2022). The Impact of COVID-19 on Education: A Meta-Narrative Review. *TechTrends*, *66*(5), 883–896. doi:10.1007/s11528-022-00759-0 PMID:35813033

Bruno, R. R., Wolff, G., Wernly, B., Masyuk, M., Piayda, K., Leaver, S., Erkens, R., Oehler, D., Afzal, S., Heidari, H., Kelm, M., & Jung, C. (2022). Virtual and augmented reality in critical care medicine: The patient's, clinician's, and researcher's perspective. *Critical Care*, *26*(1), 326. doi:10.1186/s13054-022-04202-x PMID:36284350

Bryant, L., & Hemsley, B. (2022). Augmented reality: A view to future visual supports for people with disability. *Disability and Rehabilitation. Assistive Technology*, 1–14. doi:10.1080/17483107.2022.2125090 PMID:36149835

Cao, W., & Yu, Z. (2023). The impact of augmented reality on student attitudes, motivation, and learning achievements-a meta-analysis (2016–2023). *Humanities & Social Sciences Communications*, *10*(1), 352. doi:10.1057/s41599-023-01852-2

Chemnad, K., Alshakhsi, S., Almourad, M. B., Altuwairiqi, M., Phalp, K., & Ali, R. (2022). Smartphone Usage before and during COVID-19: A Comparative Study Based on Objective Recording of Usage Data. *Informatics (MDPI)*, *9*(4), 98. Advance online publication. doi:10.3390/informatics9040098

Cheng, Y., Lee, M.-H., Yang, C.-S., & Wu, P.-Y. (2022). Hands-on interaction in the augmented reality (AR) chemistry laboratories enhances the learning effects of low-achieving students: a pilot study. Interactive Technology and Smart Education. doi:10.1108/ITSE-04-2022-0045

Chien-Huan, C., Chien-Hsu, C., & Tay-Sheng, J. (2010). *An interactive augmented reality system for learning anatomy structure*. Proceedings of the International Multi-Conference of Engineers and Computer Scientists, Hong Kong, China. https://www.iaeng.org/publication/IMECS2010/IMECS2010_pp370-375.pdf

Chien-Yu, L., & Yu-Ming, C. (2015). Interactive augmented reality using Scratch 2.0 to improve physical activities for children with developmental disabilities. *Research in Developmental Disabilities*, *37*, 1–8. doi:10.1016/j.ridd.2014.10.016 PMID:25460214

Cipresso, P., Giglioli, I. A. C., Raya, M. A., & Riva, G. (2018). The Past, Present, and Future of Virtual and Augmented Reality Research: A Network and Cluster Analysis of the Literature. *Frontiers in Psychology*, *9*, 2086. doi:10.3389/fpsyg.2018.02086 PMID:30459681

Cofano, F., Di Perna, G., Bozzaro, M., Longo, A., Marengo, N., Zenga, F., Zullo, N., Cavalieri, M., Damiani, L., Boges, D. J., Agus, M., Garbossa, D., & Calì, C. (2021). Augmented Reality in Medical Practice: From Spine Surgery to Remote Assistance. *Frontiers in Surgery*, *8*, 657901. doi:10.3389/fsurg.2021.657901 PMID:33859995

Dhar, P., Rocks, T., Samarasinghe, R. M., Stephenson, G., & Smith, C. (2021). Augmented reality in medical education: Students' experiences and learning outcomes. *Medical Education Online*, *26*(1), 1953953. doi:10.1080/10872981.2021.1953953 PMID:34259122

Dodds, S., Russell-Bennett, R., Chen, T., Oertzen, A.-S., Salvador-Carulla, L., & Hung, Y.-C. (2022). Blended human-technology service realities in healthcare. *Journal of Service Theory and Practice*, *32*(1), 75–99. doi:10.1108/JSTP-12-2020-0285

Dorloh, H., Li, K.-W., & Khaday, S. (2023). Presenting Job Instructions Using an Augmented Reality Device, a Printed Manual, and a Video Display for Assembly and Disassembly Tasks: What Are the Differences? *Applied Sciences (Basel, Switzerland)*, *13*(4), 2186. doi:10.3390/app13042186

Doshi, R., Hiran, K. K., Gök, M., El-kenawy, E. S. M., Badr, A., & Abotaleb, M. (2023). Artificial Intelligence's Significance in Diseases with Malignant Tumours. *Mesopotamian Journal of Artificial Intelligence in Healthcare*, *2023*, 35–39.

Du, Z., Liu, J., & Wang, T. (2022). Augmented Reality Marketing: A Systematic Literature Review and an Agenda for Future Inquiry. *Frontiers in Psychology*, *13*, 925963. doi:10.3389/fpsyg.2022.925963 PMID:35783783

Dziuban, C., Graham, C. R., Moskal, P. D., Norberg, A., & Sicilia, N. (2018). Blended learning: The new normal and emerging technologies. *International Journal of Educational Technology in Higher Education*, *15*(1), 3. doi:10.1186/s41239-017-0087-5

ECLAC. (2021). *Digital technologies for a new future*. CEPAL. https://www.cepal.org/sites/default/files/publication/files/46817/S2000960_en.pdf

El Filali, Y., & Krit, S. (2020). Augmented Reality Types and Popular Use Cases. In *Proceedings of the 1st International Conference of Computer Science and Renewable Energies-ICCSRE*. ScitePress. ISBN 978-989-758-431-2 10.5220/0009776301070110

El Kassis, R., Ayer, S. K., & El Asmar, M. (2023). Augmented Reality Applications for Synchronized Communication in Construction: A Review of Challenges and Opportunities. *Applied Sciences (Basel, Switzerland)*, *13*(13), 7614. doi:10.3390/app13137614

Eversberg, L., & Lambrecht, J. (2023). Evaluating digital work instructions with augmented reality versus paper-based documents for manual, object-specific repair tasks in a case study with experienced workers. *International Journal of Advanced Manufacturing Technology*, *127*(3-4), 1859–1871. doi:10.1007/s00170-023-11313-4

Ford, N. (2021). *Software Architecture: The Hard Parts: Modern Trade-Off Analyses for Distributed Architectures*. O'Reilly Media.

Fraser, B. J. (2023). The Evolution of the Field of Learning Environments Research. *Education Sciences*, *13*(3), 257. doi:10.3390/educsci13030257

Godber, K. A., & Atkins, D. R. (2021). COVID-19 Impacts on Teaching and Learning: A Collaborative Autoethnography by Two Higher Education Lecturers. *Frontiers in Education*, *6*, 647524. doi:10.3389/feduc.2021.647524

Goo, H. W., Park, S. J., & Yoo, S. J. (2020). Advanced medical use of three-dimensional imaging in congenital heart disease: Augmented reality, mixed reality, virtual reality, and three-dimensional printing. *Korean Journal of Radiology*, *21*(2), 133–145. doi:10.3348/kjr.2019.0625 PMID:31997589

Greengard, S. (2019). *Virtual Reality*. MIT Press Direct., doi:10.7551/mitpress/11836.001.0001

Gruzina, Y., Firsova, I., & Strielkowski, W. (2021). Dynamics of Human Capital Development in Economic Development Cycles. *Economies*, *9*(2), 67. doi:10.3390/economies9020067

Gumbau-Albert, M., & Maudos, J. (2022). The importance of intangible assets in regional economic growth: A growth accounting approach. *The Annals of Regional Science*, *69*(2), 361–390. doi:10.1007/s00168-022-01138-6 PMID:35729957

Guo, L., Wang, D., Gu, F., Li, Y., Wang, Y., & Zhou, R. (2021). Evolution and trends in intelligent tutoring systems research: A multidisciplinary and scientometric view. *Asia Pacific Education Review*, *22*(3), 441–461. doi:10.1007/s12564-021-09697-7

Gupta, A. K., Srinivasulu, A., Hiran, K. K., Sreenivasulu, G., Rajeyyagari, S., & Subramanyam, M. (2022). Prediction of omicron virus using combined extended convolutional and recurrent neural networks technique on CT-scan images. *Interdisciplinary Perspectives on Infectious Diseases*, *2022*, 2022. doi:10.1155/2022/1525615 PMID:36562006

Habil, S. G. M., El-Deeb, S., & El-Bassiouny, N. (2023). The metaverse era: leveraging augmented reality in the creation of novel customer experience. Management & Sustainability: An Arab Review. doi:10.1108/MSAR-10-2022-0051

Haleem, A., Javaid, M., Qadri, M. A., & Suman, R. (2022). Understanding the role of digital technologies in education: A review. *Sustainable Operations and Computers*, *3*, 275–285. doi:10.1016/j.susoc.2022.05.004

Haorongbam, L., Nagpal, R., & Sehgal, R. (2022). *Service Oriented Architecture (SOA): A Literature Review on the Maintainability, Approaches and Design Process. 12th International Conference on Cloud Computing, Data Science & Engineering (Confluence)*, Noida, India. 10.1109/Confluence52989.2022.9734153

Harris, B., Regan, T., Schueler, J., & Fields, S. A. (2020). Problematic Mobile Phone and Smartphone Use Scales: A Systematic Review. *Frontiers in Psychology*, *11*, 672. doi:10.3389/fpsyg.2020.00672 PMID:32431636

Hemanth, J. D., Kose, U., Deperlioglu, O., & de Albuquerque, V. H. C. (2020). An augmented reality-supported mobile application for diagnosis of heart diseases. *The Journal of Supercomputing*, *76*(2), 1242–1267. doi:10.1007/s11227-018-2483-6

Hitzler, P. (2021). A review of the semantic web field. *Communications of the ACM*, *64*(2), 76–83. https://cacm.acm.org/magazines/2021/2/250085-a-review-of-the-semantic-web-field/abstract. doi:10.1145/3397512

Ifanov, Jessica, P., Salim, S., Syahputra, M. E., & Suri, P. A. (2023). A Systematic literature review on implementation of virtual reality for learning. *Procedia Computer Science*, *216*, 260–265. doi:10.1016/j.procs.2022.12.135

Jain, R. K., Hiran, K. K., & Maheshwari, R. (2023, April). Lung Cancer Detection Using Machine Learning Algorithms. In *2023 International Conference on Computational Intelligence, Communication Technology and Networking (CICTN)* (pp. 516-521). IEEE. 10.1109/CICTN57981.2023.10141467

Kamińska, D., Zwoliński, G., Laska-Leśniewicz, A., Raposo, R., Vairinhos, M., Pereira, E., Urem, F., Ljubić Hinić, M., Haamer, R. E., & Anbarjafari, G. (2023). Augmented Reality: Current and New Trends in Education. *Electronics (Basel)*, *12*(16), 3531. doi:10.3390/electronics12163531

Katsumata, S., Ichikohji, T., Nakano, S., Yamaguchi, S., & Ikuine, F. (2022). Changes in the use of mobile devices during the crisis: Immediate response to the COVID-19 pandemic. *Computers in Human Behavior Reports*, *5*, 100168. doi:10.1016/j.chbr.2022.100168 PMID:35079660

Kayapinar, U. (2021). *Teacher Education. New Perspectives*. IntechOpen Book Series. doi:10.5772/intechopen.94952

Kendall, K., & Kendall, J. (2023). *Systems Analysis and Design* (11th ed.). Pearson.

Kessler, G. (2018). Technology and the future of language teaching. *Foreign Language Annals*, *51*(1), 205–218. doi:10.1111/flan.12318

Khurram, J., Wandschneider, K., & Phanindra, V. W. (2007). The effect of political regimes and technology on economic growth. *Applied Economics*, *39*(11), 1425–1432. doi:10.1080/00036840500447906

Kleftodimos, A., Evagelou, A., Gkoutzios, S., Matsiola, M., Vrigkas, M., Yannacopoulou, A., Triantafillidou, A., & Lappas, G. (2023). Creating Location-Based Augmented Reality Games and Immersive Experiences for Touristic Destination Marketing and Education. *Computers*, *12*(11), 227. doi:10.3390/computers12110227

Korkut, E. H., & Surer, E. (2023). Visualization in virtual reality: A systematic review. *Virtual Reality (Waltham Cross)*, *27*(2), 1447–1480. doi:10.1007/s10055-023-00753-8

Kossiakoff, A. (2020). *Systems Engineering Principles and Practice* (3rd ed.). John Wiley & Sons, Inc. doi:10.1002/9781119516699

Kurniawan, M. H., Suharjito, D., & Witjaksono, G. (2018). Human Anatomy Learning Systems Using Augmented Reality on Mobile Application. *Procedia Computer Science*, *135*, 80–88. doi:10.1016/j.procs.2018.08.152

Li, K. C., & Wong, B. T. M. (2022). Research landscape of smart education: A bibliometric analysis. *Interactive Technology and Smart Education*, *19*(1), 3–19. doi:10.1108/ITSE-05-2021-0083

Li, M., & Liu, L. (2022). Students' perceptions of augmented reality integrated into a mobile learning environment. Library Hi Tech. doi:10.1108/LHT-10-2021-0345

Lin, Y., & Yu, Z. (2023). Extending Technology Acceptance Model to higher-education students' use of digital academic reading tools on computers. *International Journal of Educational Technology in Higher Education*, *20*(1), 34. doi:10.1186/s41239-023-00403-8

Lum, H. C., Elliott, L. J., Aqlan, F., & Zhao, R. (2020). Virtual Reality: History, Applications, and Challenges for Human Factors Research. *Proceedings of the Human Factors and Ergonomics Society Annual Meeting, 64*(1), 1263–1268. doi:10.1177/1071181320641300

Mahr, D., & Huh, J. (2022). Technologies in service communication: Looking forward. *Journal of Service Management, 33*(4/5), 648–656. doi:10.1108/JOSM-03-2022-0075

Mathew, M., Thomas, M. J., Navaneeth, M. G., Sulaiman, S., Amudhan, A. N., & Sudheer, A. P. (2023). A systematic review of technological advancements in signal sensing, actuation, control and training methods in robotic exoskeletons for rehabilitation. *The Industrial Robot, 50*(3), 432–455. doi:10.1108/IR-09-2022-0239

McAnally, K., Wallwork, K., & Wallis, G. (2023). The efficiency of visually guided movement in real and virtual space. *Virtual Reality (Waltham Cross), 27*(2), 1187–1197. doi:10.1007/s10055-022-00724-5

McDiarmid, G. W., & Zhao, Y. (2023). Time to Rethink: Educating for a Technology-Transformed World. *ECNU Review of Education, 6*(2), 189–214. doi:10.1177/20965311221076493

Mikhailova, O. (2018). Adoption and implementation of new technologies in hospitals: A network perspective. *IMP Journal, 12*(2), 368–391. doi:10.1108/IMP-05-2017-0027

Mishra, S. K., & Sarkar, A. (2022). Service-oriented architecture for Internet of Things: A semantic approach. *Journal of King Saud University. Computer and Information Sciences, 34*(10, 10 Part A), 8765–8776. doi:10.1016/j.jksuci.2021.09.024

Navab, N., Martin-Gomez, A., Seibold, M., Sommersperger, M., Song, T., Winkler, A., Yu, K., & Eck, U. (2023). Medical Augmented Reality: Definition, Principle Components, Domain Modeling, and Design-Development-Validation Process. *Journal of Imaging, 9*(1), 4. doi:10.3390/jimaging9010004 PMID:36662102

Niknejad, N., Ismail, W., Ghani, I., Nazari, B., Bahari, M., & Hussin, A. R. B. C. (2020). Understanding Service-Oriented Architecture (SOA): A systematic literature review and directions for further investigation. *Information Systems, 91*, 101491. doi:10.1016/j.is.2020.101491

OASIS. (2023). *Advancing open standards for the information society*. OASIS. http://www.c5.cl/ieinvestiga/actas/ribie98/279.html

Okoye, K., Hussein, H., Arrona-Palacios, A., Quintero, H. N., Ortega, L. O. P., Sanchez, A. L., Ortiz, E. A., Escamilla, J., & Hosseini, S. (2023). Impact of digital technologies upon teaching and learning in higher education in Latin America: An outlook on the reach, barriers, and bottlenecks. *Education and Information Technologies, 28*(2), 2291–2360. doi:10.1007/s10639-022-11214-1 PMID:35992366

Parsons, D., & MacCallum, K. (2021). Current Perspectives on Augmented Reality in Medical Education: Applications, Affordances and Limitations. *Advances in Medical Education and Practice, 12*, 77–91. doi:10.2147/AMEP.S249891 PMID:33500677

Passavanti, R., Pantano, E., Priporas, C. V., & Verteramo, S. (2020). The use of new technologies for corporate marketing communication in luxury retailing: Preliminary findings. *Qualitative Market Research, 23*(3), 503–521. doi:10.1108/QMR-11-2017-0144

Piekarski, W., & Thomas, B. (2002). ARQuake: The outdoor augmented reality gaming system. *Communications of the ACM, 45*(1), 36–38. https://dl.acm.org/doi/10.1145/502269.502291. doi:10.1145/502269.502291

Pingxuan, R. (2020). AR 3D Magic Book: A Healthy Interactive Reading Device Based on AR and Portable Projection. *CIPAE 2020: Proceedings of the 2020 International Conference on Computers, Information Processing and Advanced Education*. ACM. 10.1145/3419635.3419714

Pliatsikas, C. (2020). Understanding structural plasticity in the bilingual brain: The Dynamic Restructuring Model. *Bilingualism: Language and Cognition, 23*(2), 459–471. doi:10.1017/S1366728919000130

Qazi, A., Hardaker, G., Ahmad, I. S., Darwich, M., Maitama, J. Z., & Dayani, A. (2021). The Role of Information & Communication Technology in Elearning Environments: A Systematic Review. *IEEE Access : Practical Innovations, Open Solutions, 9*, 45539–45551. doi:10.1109/ACCESS.2021.3067042

Ramasamy, J., Doshi, R., & Hiran, K. K. (2021, August). Segmentation of brain tumor using deep learning methods: a review. In *Proceedings of the International Conference on Data Science, Machine Learning and Artificial Intelligence* (pp. 209-215). ACM. 10.1145/3484824.3484876

Ramasamy, J., Doshi, R., & Hiran, K. K. (2022, October). Detection of Brain Tumor in Medical Images Based on Feature Extraction by HOG and Machine Learning Algorithms. In *2022 International Conference on Trends in Quantum Computing and Emerging Business Technologies (TQCEBT)* (pp. 1-5). IEEE. 10.1109/TQCEBT54229.2022.10041564

Rasa, T., & Laherto, A. (2022). Young people's technological images of the future: Implications for science and technology education. *European Journal of Futures Research, 10*(1), 4. doi:10.1186/s40309-022-00190-x

Rathi, S., Hiran, K. K., & Sakhare, S. (2023). Affective state prediction of E-learner using SS-ROA based deep LSTM. *Array (New York, N.Y.), 19*, 100315. doi:10.1016/j.array.2023.100315

Richards, M., & Ford, N. (2020). *Fundamentals of Software Architecture: An Engineering Approach*. O'Reilly Media.

Roopa, D., Prabha, R., & Senthil, G. A. (2021). Revolutionizing education system with interactive augmented reality for quality education. *Materials Today: Proceedings, 46*(9), 3860–3863. doi:10.1016/j.matpr.2021.02.294

Sailer, M., Murböck, J., & Fischer, F. (2021). Digital learning in schools: What does it take beyond digital technology? *Teaching and Teacher Education, 103*, 103346. doi:10.1016/j.tate.2021.103346

Salina, T. (2023). A Review of Augmented Reality for Informal Science Learning: Supporting Design of Intergenerational Group Learning. *Visitor Studies, 26*(1), 1–23. doi:10.1080/10645578.2022.2075205

Shammar, E. A., & Zahary, A. T. (2020). The Internet of Things (IoT): A survey of techniques, operating systems, and trends. *Library Hi Tech, 38*(1), 5–66. doi:10.1108/LHT-12-2018-0200

Sharma, P., & Harkishan, M. (2022). Designing an intelligent tutoring system for computer programing in the Pacific. *Education and Information Technologies, 27*(5), 6197–6209. doi:10.1007/s10639-021-10882-9 PMID:35002465

Sommerauer, P., & Müller, O. (2014). Augmented Reality in Informal Learning Environments: A Field Experiment in a Mathematics Exhibition. *Computers & Education*, *79*, 59–68. doi:10.1016/j.compedu.2014.07.013

Stocchi, L., Pourazad, N., Michaelidou, N., Tanusondjaja, A., & Harrigan, P. (2022). Marketing research on Mobile apps: Past, present and future. *Journal of the Academy of Marketing Science*, *50*(2), 195–225. doi:10.1007/s11747-021-00815-w PMID:34776554

Szymkowiak, A., Melović, B., Dabić, M., Jeganathan, K., & Kundi, G. S. (2021). Information technology and Gen Z: The role of teachers, the internet, and technology in the education of young people. *Technology in Society*, *65*, 101565. doi:10.1016/j.techsoc.2021.101565

Tang, Y. M., Chau, K. Y., Kwok, A. P. K., Zhu, T., & Ma, X. (2022). A systematic review of immersive technology applications for medical practice and education-Trends, application areas, recipients, teaching contents, evaluation methods, and performance. *Educational Research Review*, *35*, 100429. doi:10.1016/j.edurev.2021.100429

Tezer, M., Yıldız, E. P., Masalimova, A. R. R., Fatkhutdinova, A. M., Zheltukhina, M. R. R., & Khairullina, E. R. (2019). Trends of Augmented Reality Applications and Research throughout the World: Meta-Analysis of Theses, Articles and Papers between 2001-2019 Years. *International Journal of Emerging Technologies in Learning*, *14*(22), 154–174. doi:10.3991/ijet.v14i22.11768

Tilley, S. (2019). *Systems Analysis and Design*. Cengage Learning.

tom Dieck, M. C., Cranmer, E., Prim, A., & Bamford, D. (2023a). Can augmented reality (AR) applications enhance students' experiences? Gratifications, engagement and learning styles. Information Technology & People. doi:10.1108/ITP-10-2021-0823

tom Dieck, M. C., Cranmer, E., Prim, A. L., & Bamford, D. (2023b). The effects of augmented reality shopping experiences: immersion, presence and satisfaction. *Journal of Research in Interactive Marketing*. doi:10.1108/JRIM-09-2022-0268

Ulrich, E., & Sandor, C. (2013). HARP: A framework for visuo-haptic augmented reality. 2013 IEEE Virtual Reality (VR), (pp. 145-146). IEEE. doi:10.1109/VR.2013.6549404

Valverde-Berrocoso, J., Fernández-Sánchez, M. R., Revuelta Dominguez, F. I., & Sosa-Díaz, M. J. (2021). The educational integration of digital technologies preCovid-19: Lessons for teacher education. *PLoS One*, *16*(8), e0256283. doi:10.1371/journal.pone.0256283 PMID:34411161

Vicsek, L. (2021). Artificial intelligence and the future of work–lessons from the sociology of expectations. *The International Journal of Sociology and Social Policy*, *41*(7/8), 842–861. doi:10.1108/IJSSP-05-2020-0174

Villagran-Vizcarra, D. C., Luviano-Cruz, D., Pérez-Domínguez, L. A., Méndez-González, L. C., & Garcia-Luna, F. (2023). Applications Analyses, Challenges and Development of Augmented Reality in Education, Industry, Marketing, Medicine, and Entertainment. *Applied Sciences (Basel, Switzerland)*, *13*(5), 2766. doi:10.3390/app13052766

Wang, H., Tlili, A., Huang, R., Cai, Z., Li, M., Cheng, Z., Yang, D., Li, M., Zhu, X., & Fei, C. (2023). Examining the applications of intelligent tutoring systems in real educational contexts: A systematic literature review from the social experiment perspective. *Education and Information Technologies*, *28*(7), 9113–9148. doi:10.1007/s10639-022-11555-x PMID:36643383

Wang, J., & Qi, Y. (2022). A Multi-User Collaborative AR System for Industrial *Applications. Sensors (Basel)*, *22*(4), 1319. doi:10.3390/s22041319 PMID:35214221

Wang, K., Guo, F., Zhou, R., & Qian, L. (2023). Implementation of augmented reality in BIM-enabled construction projects: a bibliometric literature review and a case study from China. Construction Innovation. ACM. doi:10.1108/CI-08-2022-0196

Wu, Ch., & Thompson, M. E. (2020). *Sampling Theory and Practice*. Springer Nature. doi:10.1007/978-3-030-44246-0

Xiong, J., Hsiang, E.-L., He, Z., Zhan, T., & Wu, S.-T. (2021). Augmented reality and virtual reality displays: Emerging technologies and future perspectives. *Light, Science & Applications*, *10*(1), 216. doi:10.1038/s41377-021-00658-8 PMID:34697292

Yan, J., Ali, I., Ali, R., & Chang, Y. (2022). The Power of Affection: Exploring the Key Drivers of Customer Loyalty in Virtual Reality-Enabled Services. *Frontiers in Psychology*, *13*, 850896. doi:10.3389/fpsyg.2022.850896 PMID:35548514

Yao, Y., Wang, L., & Shen, J. (2022). Features and Applications of QR Codes. *International Journal for Innovation Education and Research*, *10*(5), 166–169. doi:10.31686/ijier.vol10.iss5.3762

Yawised, K., Apasrawirote, D., Chatrangsan, M., & Muneesawang, P. (2022). Turning digital technology to immersive marketing strategy: a strategic perspective on flexibility, agility and adaptability for businesses. *Journal of Entrepreneurship in Emerging Economies*. IEEE.. https://doi.org/ doi:10.1108/JEEE-06-2022-0169

Zarantonello, L., & Schmitt, B. H. (2023). Experiential AR/VR: A consumer and service framework and research agenda. *Journal of Service Management*, *34*(1), 34–55. doi:10.1108/JOSM-12-2021-0479

Žilak, M., Car, Ž., & Culjak, I. A. (2022). Systematic Literature Review of Handheld Augmented Reality Solutions for People with Disabilities. *Sensors (Basel)*, *22*(20), 7719. doi:10.3390/s22207719 PMID:36298070

Chapter 11

A Systematic Review of the Role of Gerontechnology and AI in Revolutionizing the Wellbeing Landscape for Aging Adults

Suyesha Singh

Department of Psychology, Manipal University Jaipur, India

Vaishnavi Nambiar

Department of Psychology, Manipal University Jaipur, India

ABSTRACT

The application of AI in geriatric healthcare has become a revolutionary and essential solution to tackling the problems faced by older people. An important step toward providing patient-centered and cost-effective treatment, the integration of AI in geriatric healthcare will ultimately enhance the standard of life for older people. This chapter is a systematic review of the rapidly developing field of AI applications in geriatric healthcare. It provides a thorough analysis of the impact and potential of AI technologies in addressing the healthcare needs of the aging population. The review was conducted using PRISMA framework. Thirty-three articles were considered for final review from which five themes were deduced. The study will facilitate the development of relevant and inclusive solutions for healthcare of older individuals and hasten the possibility of greater wellbeing and inclusion of older adults in the technological innovativeness of the healthcare facilities.

INTRODUCTION

The need for geriatric healthcare services is growing as the global population ages. The aging population presents particular healthcare issues, such as the requirement for comprehensive care management, various persistent diseases, and memory impairment. In the realm of geriatric healthcare, artificial intelligence (AI) has demonstrated to be an innovative force through delivering novel approaches to boost

DOI: 10.4018/979-8-3693-1123-3.ch011

diagnosis and treatment, enhance patient care, and streamline the distribution of resources. The chapter aims to systematically analyze the recent trends in utilization of AI in the treatment of diverse range of problems faced by geriatric adults and reflect on its benefits and limitations, respectively.

The chapter begins by providing an overview of the relevance and significance of AI in geriatric healthcare, followed by the formulation of research question and strategy for conducting systematic literature review. Based on the selected studies, an elaborative and categorical understanding of the use of AI is provided. Lastly, authors provide the implications of the findings at the organizational and policy levels.

Relevance of Artificial Intelligence in Geriatric Healthcare

Plans for Individualized Treatment

Based on their distinct medical histories, genetic profiles, and preferences, geriatric patients can receive tailored treatment programs from AI-driven systems (Radenkovic et al., 2021; Alowais et al., 2023). These plans take into account an individual's drug schedule, restrictions on food, difficulties with movement, and other aspects to make sure the care is customized to meet their unique needs.

Virtual Surveillance and Telemedicine

Mobility issues or living in rural places can make frequent medical visits difficult for many older persons. Healthcare practitioners may now remotely monitor patients' vital signs, medication compliance, and general well-being thanks to AI-powered remote monitoring and telehealth systems. Additionally, telephone consultations provide older people with a convenient option to get healthcare services (Dantas et al., 2023; Sheikh et al., 2023; Meena et al., 2021), eliminating the need for in-person visits and dispensing prompt medical advice.

Prevention of Falls and Detection

The senior population is particularly vulnerable to falls, which frequently result in severe injuries and hospitalizations. AI-based fall detection systems watch a person's motions and look for odd patterns that might be signs of a fall using cameras, sensors, or wearable technology (Seng et al., 2023; Monge et al., 2023; Ahmed et al., 2024).

Administration of Medications

Elderly individuals may have complicated treatment regimens comprising many medications. AI can help with medication management by reminding patients to take their medications on time (Kolben et al., 2023; Bays et al., 2023), keeping track of drug interactions, and warning medical professionals and caregivers about potential problems.

Analytics for Predicting Medical Re-Admission

For senior patients, readmissions to the hospital are a typical cause for concern because they frequently arise from complications or poor post-discharge care. AI algorithms can examine patient data to forecast the likelihood of readmission and give healthcare professionals useful information to stop such occurrences (Zeinalnezhad & Shishehchi, 2023). The delivery of geriatric healthcare can be more economical and patient-focused by proactively addressing these concerns.

Significance of Using AI in Geriatric Healthcare

Artificial intelligence (AI) has a profound effect on the geriatric healthcare system because it caters to the special issues and requirements of older people.

Screening and Timely Detection

Prediction analytics powered by AI can spot the early warning signals of diseases associated with age including Alzheimer's disease and heart failure (Modi et al., 2023; Sun et al., 2023), enabling prompt treatment.

Individualized Services

By taking into account a patient's genetics, lifestyle, and health status, AI systems can develop tailored care plans, enhancing the efficacy of treatment while reducing negative effects (Alowais et al., 2023, King, 2023; Doshi et al., 2023). Drug administration that is individualized makes sure senior citizens are given the necessary prescriptions on time and in the right amount.

Virtual Observation and Telemedicine

AI-powered remote monitoring enables healthcare professionals to track vital signs and take appropriate action for elderly patients who have mobility challenges or live in remote locations (Ullah et al., 2023).

Caretaker Assistance

AI-powered chatbots and digital assistants can help carers with daily activities, provide information, and remind them to take their medications (Al Kuwaiti et al., 2023). These systems can also keep tabs on the health of senior citizens and notify caretakers or medical personnel of any concerns.

Resource Management and Effectiveness

By anticipating patient demands and streamlining administrative procedures, AI can enhance resource allocation in geriatric healthcare facilities, freeing up staff time for patient care (Haluza & Jungwirth, 2023). In order to enable targeted treatments and lower healthcare expenditures, predictive analytics can identify those who are more likely to require readmission to the hospital.

The value of AI in the elderly healthcare system rests in its capacity to improve resource allocation, diagnostics, early detection, individualized treatment, remote monitoring, caregiver assistance, prescription management, and research.

Formulation of Research Questions

Earlier studies have investigated the emerging prevalence of artificial intelligence in providing effective health treatment for elderly patients. To analyze present status of AI in geriatric healthcare management, a systematic study of related literature is conducted. The research questions that would be answered through this study are:

a)   What is the present status of AI in geriatric healthcare?
b)   What are the challenges faced while implementing AI in geriatric healthcare?
c)   What are the future trends of AI in geriatric healthcare?

METHODOLOGY

A thorough systematic analysis of the literature was done to determine the state of AI in geriatric healthcare. Databases like Science Direct, Emerald, and MDPI were used to retrieve the data. The study was limited to research articles that were released between the years of 2013 and 2023 because it examined current trends in use of AI-based interventions in promoting wellbeing of older adults. Table 1 lists the inclusion and exclusion standards for choosing studies.

The inclusion and exclusion criteria for the systematic review was decided using the SPIDER framework. This framework was selected because of its great compatibility with non-empirical research techniques (Wakida et al., 2018). SPIDER tool was used to frame the study topic, as shown in Table 2.

The selection of the sample marked the beginning of the search for pertinent literature. Curiosity arose over the use of AI interventions to enhance the wellbeing of older adults. The expected outcome of the study—namely, the current models or approaches of AI in addressing the wellbeing and satisfactions of

Table 1. Inclusion and exclusion criteria

Inclusion Criteria	Exclusion Criteria
1. Published Journal Articles	Only Abstracts
2. Articles written in English	Grey literature
3. Articles published between 2013 and 2023.	Book chapters, conference proceedings, and review papers
4. Only empirical research papers	
5. Full and/or open access to the manuscripts	

Table 2. SPIDER framework for research question

Sample	Geriatric or older adults
Phenomenon of interest	Use of technology for wellbeing of older adults
Design	Survey, Interview, Case Studies
Evaluation	Treatment techniques
Research type	Quantitative research design

older adults, their limitations, and future trends—was prioritized when creating the search strategy and selecting the pertinent literature to assist in answering the formulated research question. Search strings used in the paper is given in Table 3.

Preferred Reporting Items for Systematic Reviews and Meta-analysis (PRISMA) guidelines were used to conduct the systematic review. It is equipped to undertake a rigorous systematic review and to take in the wide range of data related to the themes under examination (Moher et al., 2009). PRISMA assesses the research that fits within a specified timeframe, streamlining the search procedure to yield the desired result.

The authors of the study thoroughly examined each article. Regarding the selection criteria for inclusion and exclusion in the study, the two authors had come to an understanding. The articles were downloaded from the databases and manually coded and categorized. The articles that offered insightful information on the subject were sorted. The title, abstract, and keywords of the various articles were examined in the second step. The publications in other languages were omitted since only articles in English were chosen. Manual data screening was done in order to thoroughly synthesize the material that was already available. Later, duplicates were removed from the data by uploading it to Mendeley Reference Manager Software. Then, abstracts were dropped because they didn't include enough information. The remaining complete papers were carefully reviewed to identify themes. The third phase involved repeatedly checking the final collection of data to guard against errors and data repair. The information for the data was manually entered for thematic analysis. The generated PRISMA flowchart is shown in **Figure 1**.

Search Strategy

It entails 3 steps as given below:

a)   Identification

To get the right set of results, the relevant keywords and their synonyms must be searched for. These keywords were chosen after consulting with several experts and reviewing earlier publications (Khan et al., 2023; Hiran et al., 2013). To find previously published publications in databases and journals pertinent to the subject of the study, utilize keyword searches. Science Direct, Emerald, and MDPI databases were used to find the information for this investigation. Science Direct, Emerald, and MDPI were used to retrieve a total of 511650 studies.

b)   Screening

Three factors made up the eligibility criteria during the literature search: the language (English), the time frame (2013-2023), and the study style (empirical, conceptual, review). For review, only journal-published articles with full access were taken into account. There were 486360 articles after the re-

Table 3. Search strings

Search Strings	*"Geriatric adults" OR "healthy ageing" AND "intervention" OR "Internet of Medical Things" OR "digital solution" OR "Artificial Intelligence"*

Figure 1. PRISMA flowchart

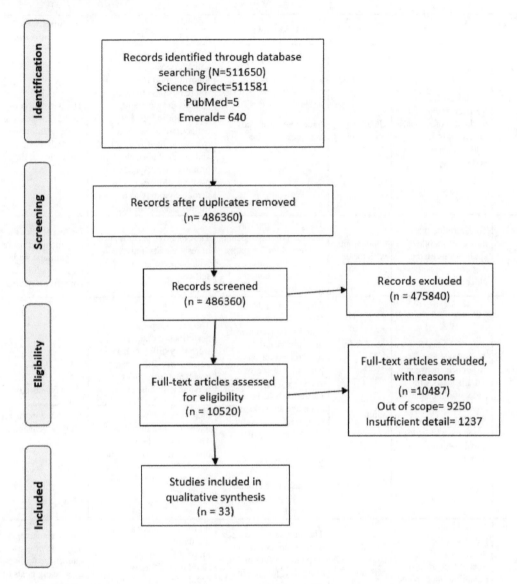

moval of 25290 entries for duplication. In order to completely understand the problem at hand, 475840 articles—389750 from Science Direct and 86090 from Emerald—that only had abstracts were ignored. There were so only 10520 articles left for the review.

c)   Eligibility

After evaluating the first selected articles, recovered articles were used in the SLR's last stage to make sure the final selection of articles satisfied the necessary criteria. The quality of the theoretical underpinning of each work was then closely scrutinized. 33 items were processed for final evaluation, including 12 publications from Science Direct, 16 articles from Emerald, and 5 article from MDPI, due to insufficient elaboration. A list of the papers that were chosen is shown in Table 4.

Table 4. Summary of selected articles

Author and year	Objective	Sample	Methodology	Findings	Limitations/Future Recommendation
Delbreil & Zvobgo (2013)	To understand the perspective of medical professionals towards wireless sensor technology in gerontology	Health professionals	Interview, case study and questionnaire	Considering potential value propositions and innovations at the core of future business models, channel development, and multidisciplinary collaboration that could overcome significant social and political obstacles was prompted by respondents' positive attitudes toward gerontechnology as a way to improve quality of life.	The perception of older adults may be studied. More quantitative research may be conducted in the area
Merilampi et al., (2014)	To determine the impact of mobile applications on the cognitive capacities of older adults	Older adults with mean age of 90	The gaming app was provided to respondents and tested for 3 months. The feedback of the game was obtained through interview.	The cognitive performance of respondents improved with respect to memory and self-care.	Further studies may be conducted using longitudinal studies on older adults having cognitive impairments
Haesner et al., (2015)	To evaluate the differences between older persons with and without cognitive impairment and to assess the potential influence of cognitive impairment on web usability.	50 older adults	On a PC and tablet, 50 senior citizens examined a web-based user interface that was created for this particular user group using a style guide. Participants had to complete six tasks in two sessions. In a third session, senior citizens were left unattended in the lab, where they encountered unforeseen circumstances brought on by the primary investigator.	The two groups' performance outcomes were very different from one another. When using a web platform, older persons with mild cognitive impairment (MCI) required more time and were more likely to make mistakes. The analysis of error data revealed that older persons with MCI made mistakes because websites lacked direction.	More quantitative research can be conducted in the area using larger sample
van den Berg et al., (2015)	To evaluate the efficacy of internet based interactive games on rehabilitation of older adults	58 older adult patients	The interactive exercises were prescribed to respondents for one hour every day, for weight lifting and walking	It promises safety and feasibility to older individuals, but may vary in suitability. This can only be supplemented to the usual routine of exercises	Future researchers may study the use of interactive web-sessions in devising goals of activities.
Vaportzis et al., (2017)	To evaluate the effectiveness of a tablet computer training program for enhancing older individuals' cognitive capacities.	48 elderly adults aged 65-76	Randomized controlled design for intervention on healthy ageing	Improvements in processing speed were linked to participation in a novel, intellectually taxing activity (tablet training).	Future research should look at whether our findings might be replicated beyond the age of 76 as they may not be applicable to older persons older than that. Future research should include people with less technology experience so that the benefits that might be obtained in more naive users versus less naive users can be compared.

continued on following page

Table 4. Continued

Author and year	Objective	Sample	Methodology	Findings	Limitations/Future Recommendation
Khaksar et al., (2017)	To increase knowledge of the significance of social assistive technologies play in helping caregiving organizations use the tenets of the care strategy targeted at the consumers and lessen the perception of consumer vulnerability.	335 caregivers of older adults	Cross-sectional survey was conducted	Social assistive technology help care providers improve the welfare of vulnerable older persons based on their socioeconomic situation and to support the care directed at consumers across care-giving organizations. When using social assistive technologies in their service contexts, older persons may be less vulnerable as a result of care strategies for consumers.	More quantitative research may be applied in the area
Stahl et al., (2017)	To explain the plan and reasoning behind an intervention development study that focuses on the prevention of mental health issues in individuals sixty years and more who are mourning the recent absence of a spousal companion.	Older adults aged above 60 years	Authors designed and standard self-supervision of everyday living preferences through an electronic diary (BSM) in Phase I. We also integrated BSM with motivational interviewing-based lifestyle coaching (BSM + MI) to be given to individuals who were mourning the absence of a loved one.	The best way to enhance health and wellbeing is to involve widows in tech-based lifestyle changes that may both improve their mental health and give them self-confidence.	More quantitative research may be conducted in the area
Couto et al., (2019)	To outline the creation of a multi-domain virtual space for elder persons who are experiencing cognitive deterioration.	Seven medical professionals and 4 elderly patients	Post-Study System Usability Questionnaire System was administered	Medical specialists believed that the system, the data, and the user interface were of high standards. Despite their little digital expertise, older persons believed the smartphone application to be suitable, useful, and simple to use.	Similar studies may be conducted using larger sample
Tang et al., (2019)	To develop a solution for demands of elderly in nursing homes using Internet of Medical things (IoMT)- based Geriatric Care Management	Older adults in Taiwan	Case study	IoMT helps improve the efficacy of monitoring elderly individuals in nursing homes.	The findings cannot be generalized as the sample size is small and specific.
Park & Kim (2020)	To evaluate whether various profiles of elderly diabetic persons could be created based on their Internet usage.	1919 older adults aged above 65 years	The digital activities of the respondents regarding information related to diabetes was classified	In comparison to other groups, consumers of technology were well-informed, rich, and active within the social circle, as well as to have good physiological and psychological functioning.	More quantitative research may be employed for in-depth information in the area

continued on following page

Table 4. Continued

Author and year	Objective	Sample	Methodology	Findings	Limitations/Future Recommendation
Trymbulak et al., (2020)	To test the viability of a unique smartphone app used to remotely monitor overall wellbeing of older persons with atrial fibrillation (AF) for a period of six months.	40 patients of atrial fibrillation	Using a smartphone app and a Fitbit, a 6-minute walk test was performed as part of a 6-component geriatric evaluation that included verified indicators of weakness, mental agility, social interaction, symptoms of depression, eyesight, and auditory.	It is practical for smartphone users to perform periodic assessments on elderly individuals with AF for six months using a wearable activity monitor and a mobile health app.	Future studies can evaluate the acceptance rate of older adults of the mobile applications. Results need to be looked at in a bigger, more varied sample, including those not using mobile phones
Portz et al., (2020)	To study the provision of healthcare through digital platform for older adult using caregivers' perspectives	81 elderly patients and caregivers	Semi-structured interview	The chance to broaden the scope of medical solutions for older adults is provided by digital health. In the COVID-19 pandemic, robust digital solutions might help convoys and patients to more effectively manage oneself and identify individual palliative treatment needs, saving more complex and severe cases for synchronous palliative telehealth.	First, while having a wide age range across patients and convoys, our sample lacks the desired racial and ethnic variety. results are probably skewed toward a marginally fitter sample. The suggestions and observations provided may not include the perspectives of convoys that were less involved. did not discuss the results with those receiving treatment or convoy participants.
Conroy et al., (2020)	To study the viability of employing new technologies to combat senior loneliness, as well as its consequences and responses to the 2019 corona virus illness outbreak	Past studies and elderly adults	Literature review and observations of elderly adults	In spite of the requirement to be physically distant, enhancement in technology have provided opportunities to build associations.	More quantitative research may be conducted in the area
Lund (2021)	To investigate the possible impact of 11 factors on older adults' use of digital technology for family and friend communication, including stress, belongingness to community, mental capacity, control of life events, satisfaction in life, physiological wellbeing.	Health and Retirement survey data of 2018	Correlation and regression were calculated of the obtained data	The usage of digital technology for communication is found to directly affect three traits— mental capacity, self-esteem, and sociability—in statistically meaningful ways. The influences of the remaining eight elements on these three factors itself serve to mitigate their effects.	More quantitative research needs to be conducted in the area to understand the present status in the area

continued on following page

Table 4. Continued

Author and year	Objective	Sample	Methodology	Findings	Limitations/Future Recommendation
Khaksar et al., (2021)	To assess the use of wearable technology in a setting in organizations that provide care-giving can provide better care by working with caregivers.	1031 older individuals from four countries in Asia	Survey was conducted to obtain information	Adoption of Technology among elderly adults lead to positive results in their overall wellbeing	Different results were procured from participants of selected countries. Hence, the study may be replicated for reliable findings
Bianchi (2021)	Examine the key obstacles that older people face while utilizing Internet services and how they might work together with their families to co-create benefits that will enhance their service inclusion and general wellbeing.	24 elderly adults over 75 years	In-depth interview of respondent was conducted	The findings highlight the value co-creation habits of older Internet users, including formal education, following directions, and asking for assistance when they run into technical difficulties. In addition, family members who help and support senior relatives with technology and show patience and tolerance when they require assistance also contribute to the wellbeing of the elderly.	The study may be replicated using larger sample
Murciano-Hueso et al., (2022)	To examine the use of gerontechnology among older population of Spain	497 older adults aged 60-94 years of Spain	Survey design was adopted	Even while the majority of participants believe that technology is valuable in everyday life, there remains less knowledge of its usage, particularly in elderly people. This emphasizes the need of encouraging cocreation of tech-based projects like elder living labs.	It is urged that future studies by other researchers include the perspectives of senior citizens who use gerontechnology.
Qiu et al., (2022)	To ascertain the level of tolerance and acceptance among Chinese older individuals for a focused VR cognitive training program.	14 older individuals	A VR-based curriculum with five games for improving cognitive function was devised. After training, the participants' tolerance and acceptance of the video-based training were evaluated.	Chinese older individuals accepted VR-based cognitive training well, with no serious side events.	To encourage healthy aging, expanding the community's access to focused cognitive training using VR technology may be studied.
Lorusso et al., (2022)	To study the reliability and useability of technology by elderly adults	Elderly adults living in a residential-homes in Italy and Apulia	The research took place in 2 phases. In phase 1, the respondents were involved in an individual interaction about their perception of technology in healthcare. In phase 2, the respondents were trained to use digital devices. Their life quality was measured using questionnaire.	Geriatric adults showed an acceptable level of usage with respect to technology, that is applications for socialization and telepresence robots. Moreover, respondents who had lesser technological skills showed higher anxiety related to health.	Stress experience by respondents may not be compared with their anxiety levels, as not all participants were tested for the same. Hence, the relationship between technology, stress and anxiety may be measured in future research

continued on following page

Table 4. Continued

Author and year	Objective	Sample	Methodology	Findings	Limitations/Future Recommendation
Spargo et al., (2022)	To examine the usage characteristics and operationality of technology by older adults at their home as part of the SHAPES project	30 older adults	A pilot test was conducted wherein a smart device was handed over to respondents to assist their healthcare at their home. The changes in their health will be monitored and observed continuously.	Technology can help improve self-care among older adults, and enhance independence of the elderly	The sample size is small. The study can be replicated to a larger population for effective comprehension of the impact of technology on the wellbeing of elderly
Giannouli et al., (2022)	To evaluate the accuracy and relevance of the speed of walking and space of life measurements provided by the MOBITEC-GP app	57 older individuals	In two testing sessions spaced nine days apart, participants performed a number of speeds of walking tests.	The MOBITEC-GP application is a trustworthy and accurate instrument for evaluating older individuals' life-space parameters and real-world speed of walking.	In order to prevent using inaccurate measures, technical difficulties should be investigated more thoroughly in future investigations.
Villa-Garcia (2022)	To outline structure and growth of the virtual spaces for the creation and supervision of senior citizens who utilize home care services and have complicated care needs.	Geriatric adults, caregivers	Case study, focus group and interview method was used	The strategy used produced digital technology that helps a home care business sustain a person-centered care paradigm.	The findings may not be generalizable to larger population
Kuerbis et al., (2022)	To assess the efficacy of text-based intervention on the use of alcohol by older adults	49 older adults aged between 50 and 65 years	The respondents in the experimental group were provided text messages to monitor their health-related wellbeing	The experimental group reported to have been satisfied with the intervention and is willing to continue the treatment. There was decreased level of alcohol use.	More quantitative research about adoption of messaging individuals personally as an intervention for use of alcohol may be conducted
Cangelosi et al., (2022)	To answer important questions about the role of social media in preventive health-care information collection, social media and networking choices for personalized health care interventions collection, and the kinds of modification in behavior generated in response to PHCI.	936 baby boomers and Generation X individuals	Questionnaire was administered to collect data	The features of the Baby Boomer and Generation X cohorts differ significantly. Consumers of health care from Generation X place more value on social media and networking locations as personalized health care intervention delivery systems. As a result of exposure to PHCI, Generation X customers of medical facilities show more significant modification in behavior.	More quantitative research may be conducted in the area
Ma et al., (2022)	To study about nursing to take an active role in closing the digital gap by examining older individuals' readiness to use cellphones and advance their digital abilities.	23 elderly individuals of China	In-depth interview	Peer learning may be a useful strategy to help older persons in China who are prepared to embrace and utilize cellphones for basic tasks.	Further studies may be conducted in the area for more empirical evidence

continued on following page

Table 4. Continued

Author and year	Objective	Sample	Methodology	Findings	Limitations/Future Recommendation
Hong et al., (2022)	To create and assess a mobile health solution led by nurses focusing on depression in elderly individuals living alone in South Korea	64 elder adults with depression	Quasi-experimental design. The intervention comprised of three parts: a nurse-led mHealth program, a standardized mHealth device training session, and art-related activities.	Particularly when adopting high-tech intervention, nurses must contribute to producing personalized tech-based wellbeing tasks taking into account the elderly individual's independence and supporting decision-making.	The methodological and medical benefits of an ecological momentary evaluation of elderly depression should be maximized in future studies.
Gazit et al., (2022)	To evaluate the effect of older adults' participation in online group of family	427 older adults	Three WhatsApp groups comprising family members were created for older adults	Membership in online intergenerational group of family showed lesser level of loneliness and increased wellbeing and enhance their perspective regarding their age	Future research may examine the impact of participation in other online community platforms and its impact on their wellbeing
Talukder et al., (2022)	To assess the older adults' intention to use wearable health technologies	295 older adults from China	Questionnaire was administered to collect data	The largest factor supporting prolonged WHT use is social value, which is also supported by emotional and epistemic values as well as quality of device. Significant impediments included inertia and technology anxiety.	Study may be replicated in other countries for better generalization of findings
Velciu et al., (2023)	To develop a sustainable technological device to maximize the experience and adoption of users	30 older adults and 32 caregivers of Italy, Romania and Australia	Questionnaire was administered to the respondents to obtain data	Geriatric adults believe that use of technology can increase wellbeing and healthcare experience. Regardless of their health status, seniors prefer using wearable technology to self-monitor their vital signs.	The findings may not be generalized. Future research can use mixed-method to obtain wider understanding in the area
Paimre et al., (2023)	To present the findings of a study examining the associations between older adults aged 50 or older living in Estonia's intention to utilize tech-based resources for health-related information, behavior and openness for vaccination for COVID-19.	501 individuals aged 50 years	Cross-sectional study was conducted	Higher need for health-related data prompted respondents to use higher level of internet, and led to higher level of motivation for vaccination.	The study may be replicated in other regions for better generalization of findings

continued on following page

Table 4. Continued

Author and year	Objective	Sample	Methodology	Findings	Limitations/Future Recommendation
Cook et al., (2023)	An automated, self-reported geriatric assessment tool was developed to expand older persons with cancer's (>65 years old) access to GA and enhance treatment choice making. A thorough evaluation of My Plan was created.	17 Older adults over the age 65	The layout and content of the tool were developed through user-centered design workshops with older persons with cancer. They then took part in usability testing to evaluate the tool's usability (ease of use, acceptability, etc.). To create the tool's clinician interface, design meetings involving cancer clinicians (oncologists and nurses) were also held.	The tool's usability was praised by both older persons and medical professionals. Functional status, falls risk, cognitive impairment, nutrition, medication review, social supports, depression, substance use disorder, and other topics were included in the final CHAMP tool's domains (along with questions and suggestions).	The study may be replicated using larger sample
Zhao et al., (2023)	To investigate how Chinese older individuals and their families feel about smart nursing homes in terms of expectations and acceptance	28 elderly patients aged between 60 and 75, and 6 children	Semi-structured interview and focus groups	Governments and societies demand smart nursing homes to provide high-quality care, as well as smart technology applications, access to basic medical services, a team of qualified healthcare professionals, integration of medical services, and smart technology itself.	Small sample, mainly from rural regions were selected. It's possible that older persons from less affluent backgrounds were either unavailable or unable to participate, which could have resulted in an insufficient grasp of attitudes about modern nursing facilities.
Alam & Khanam (2023)	To investigate the perception of older adults about mHealth	271 older women users of mHealth in Bangladesh	Survey method was adopted to collect data	The study found that factors such as perceived reliability, perceived utility, pricing value, and technological fear significantly influenced the adoption of mHealth. The uptake of mHealth services was not influenced by their simplicity of use.	The study may be replicated in other countries for widened understanding in the area
Papachristou et al., (2023)	To evaluate the Life Champs, a virtual platform in implementation's viability, usability, acceptability, fidelity, adherence, and safety aspects.	Older adults (above 65) with cancer in Greece, Spain, Sweden and UK	Mixed methods design	Future geriatric oncology practices will begin implementing AI digital technologies like LifeChamps to aid in gathering, storing, integrating, and disseminate large amount of information from diverse sources to enable excessive in-depth and extensive supervising of patients and promoted making decisions for clinical problems.	More quantitative research may be applied in the area

continued on following page

Table 4. Continued

Author and year	Objective	Sample	Methodology	Findings	Limitations/Future Recommendation
Edna Mayela et al., (2023)	To evaluate the impact on older persons' physical performance (PP) of a multi-component online physical exercise intervention (MPE).	110 older individuals	In a controlled experiment, participants were randomly distributed to the MPE groups or the control group.	Online MPE intervention is successful in improving community-dwelling older persons' PP, which may help this demographic have less functional reliance.	To determine whether a treatment can enhance the quality of life of the aged population, it is important to conduct more clinical studies with a variety of geriatric populations in the long run, which can be covered in further research

The authors then carefully read the selected pieces to gain a thematic understanding of the problem at hand. Thematic analysis is the best method for synthesis of the articles, according to Vaismoradi et al. (2013), as it provides for reasonably flexible result interpretation. The thematic analysis begins with the development of topics. To do this, important common themes were found and linked studies were merged for a comprehensive study. Five themes were identified in relation to the use of AI interventions to support wellbeing of geriatric adults.

First, a publication timeline for the selected papers is shown. Second, a graphic representation of the nations where the chosen studies were carried out was included.

Timeline of Selected Articles

The 33 articles that were published between 2013 and 2023 were given final review consideration. The year 2022 had the most articles (12), followed by 2023 (7), as illustrated in **Figure 2**.

Thematic Discussion of Findings

The thematic understanding of the results from the systematic literature review is presented in the section. The review included 33 papers. The findings are categorized into 5 groups based on the thematic analysis as shown in **Figure 3**.

Emerging Trends in the Use of AI in Gerontology

Upon conducting the systematic literature review, it was found that there was a commendable number of studies examining the significance of AI in improving cognitive performance of older adults. For example, Merilampi et al., (2014) studied the impact of mobile applications in *accelerating the rate of memory* in older adults. Through detailed interview of the participants, it was understood that mobile applications were useful in improving the memory of geriatric adults. Similarly, Qiu et al., (2022) suggests through the study's findings that an effective VR curriculum program targeted at geriatric adults help *improve their cognitive performance.*

On familiar grounds, AI was also used to understand its relevance in *expanding the mental wellness* or mHealth of older adults. For instance, Trymbulak et al., (2020) assessed the general wellbeing of

Figure 2. Timeline of selected articles

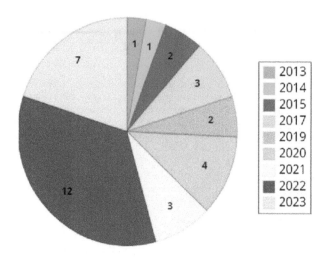

Figure 3. Theme-based segregation of papers

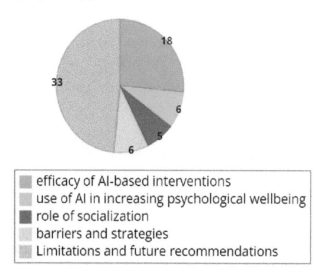

older adults undergoing atrial fibrillation. The study made use of mobile applications in measuring the overall functioning of geriatric adults, including speed of walking, sleep cycle, mental agility, social interactions and signs of depression.

AI was also found to be relevant in observing and treating older adults with *physical ailments* such as diabetes. Park and Kim (2020) through the use of digital applications found that those older adults who used mobile applications had higher level of awareness about diabetes and the ways to improve their quality of life through beneficial activities such as walking and maintaining a quiet diet.

Efficacy of Technological Interventions in Improving Physical Wellness

van den Berg et al., (2015) evaluated the impact of *tech-based interactional game* on the physical performance of 58 older adults. Results declared that the older adults were convinced of the safety and reliability the digital intervention offered them in order to improve their physiological health. Similarly, Khaksar (2017) studied the application of *social assistive technology* in promoting the ability of healthcare organizations in adopting consumer-directed care. Through a cross-sectional study of 355 caregivers and older adults technology can help enhance the wellbeing of those older adults that feel vulnerable due to their socio-economical standing.

Tang et al., (2019) developed an intervention using the *Internet of Medical Things (IoMT)* to satisfy the demands of geriatric population of Taiwan with respect to medical interventions. A case study design was employed. Findings show that IoMT helps efficiency of monitoring facilities for older adults in nursing homes in Taiwan. Identical results were procured by Park and Kim (2020), Portz et al., (2020), Trymbulan et al., (2020), Conroy et al., (2020), Khaksar (2021), and Lorusso et al., (2022). Older adults reveal a higher affinity for technology for obtaining health-related information. Moreover, tech-based medical assistance improves scope for self-care and autonomy of older adults with everyday functioning and decision-making with respect to availing medical treatment (Spargo et al., 2022).

Giannouli et al., (2022) through an app called *MOBITEC-GP*, found that the older adults perceive the sense of trust in older adults with respect to the efficacy of the app. The app shared accurate data on older adults' life quality and speed of walking. Nevertheless, the popularity of home-based treatment for older adults has only increased, especially after the global pandemic that hit the world in 2020. This is particularly evident in the findings provided by Villa-Garcias (2022), that virtual platforms aid home-based medical assistance services in providing individualized treatments.

In an experimental study of 49 older adults aged between 50 and 65 years by Kuerbis et al., (2022), it was observed that the group of respondents that were exposed to technology expressed a persistent willingness to pursue intervention, and depicted lower risk for alcohol use. Additionally, personalized messages for respondents increased the efficacy of their efforts in increasing overall wellbeing. Velciu et al., (2023) obtained data on 30 geriatric adults and 32 caregivers belonging to Italy, Romania, and Australia. The respondents believed that technology has the capability to increase wellbeing among older adults and their general experience in healthcare organizations. The *Wearable Health Technology (WHT)* is preferred among older adults to monitor self-care. The results resemble with that of Paimre et al., (2023), wherein older adults showed a higher reliance on technology to obtain health-related data. Similarly Geriatric Adults Tool was perceived to be useful in receiving information regarding fall risks, diet and medication (Cook et al., 2023).

Additionally, perceived reliability, utility, pricing and fear for technological innovations influence adoption of *mHealth interventions* (Alam & Khanam, 2023). An identical tool, named LifeChamps designed by Papachristou et al., (2023), helps in gathering and organizing data on healthcare and enable monitoring of patients and clinical decision making. Similarly, Edna & Mayela (2023) suggest through their study results that *online Multicomponent Physical Exercise Intervention* is found successful in elderly individuals dwelling in communities for increasing physical fitness and reduces functional reliance.

Use of Artificial Intelligence on Psychological Performance of Older Adults

Merilampi et al., (2014) that assessed the efficiency of *mobile applications* in enhancing the cognitive capacities of older adults with an average age of 90 years for 3 months, found that the mobile applications improved the cognitive performance of older adults, particularly, the memory skills and autonomy functioning. Similarly, AI based facilities increase speed of functioning of older adults and also postpones cognitive decline of performance of older adults, thereby influencing the perspective of older adults on ageing process. This was further evidenced in the study by Couto et al., (2019), Park and Kim (2020), Lund (2021) and Qiu et al., (2022).

Stahl et al., (2017) developed an intervention plan for older adults over age 60 years for treating depression and anxiety due to loss of their spousal companion. The respondents were observed daily through their electronic dairy and motivational interviews. It was shown that introducing *tech-based lifestyle* improves the wellbeing of widows and their mental health and self-confidence as they are regularly guided by personalized interventions (Lakhwani et al., 2020; Ramasamy et al., 2022; Patel et al., 2022).

Role of Socialization in Enhancing Efficacy of AI Interventions in Geriatric Healthcare

Delbreil & Zvobgo (2013) suggest that there is scope for technology to be integrated in future geriatric treatment as it helps surpass certain socio-political concerns and help improve the quality of treatment, thereby attracting more geriatric patients, and influencing their attitude towards gerontechnology. Bianchi (2021) asserts through his findings that older users of technology often rely on assistance from others, especially family members. When receiving proper guidance from family and communal members, the overall wellbeing of older adults elevates to a higher platform and therefore increases their sense of enjoyment, personal discovery, and autonomy. The findings closely resonate to that in Gazit et al., (2022) and Park and Kim (2020), which suggested that *virtual socialization* decreased the feeling of loneliness and depression and in turn improved their wellbeing. It was nonetheless, observed that Gen X consumers of technology value social media and networking in obtaining information related to physical fitness and healthcare. It is interesting to notice that *Wearable Health Technologies (WHT)* are usually preferred by older adults as it increases emotional satisfaction due to its ease of use and availability at times of emergency (Talukder et al., 2022).

Barriers and Strategies While Implementing AI in Geriatric Healthcare

Haesner et al., (2015), who studied the differences between functioning of elderly that have and do not have deteriorations in mental capacity, and the relevance of technology in improving mental ability of the older adults, depicted that those virtual facilities that do not provide right guidance and enable independent functioning of older adults can have negative effect on significance of technology in healthcare. Similarly, Lund (2021) asserts that those older adults who have *less technical proficiency* shows higher rate of technological anxiety with respect to obtaining right information about health.

Muciano-Hueso et al., (2022) and Ma et al., (2022) recommends the *need for further training* in gerontechnology so as to provide conducive and effective treatment to older adults and the need to close the digital divide that exists against the older adults so as to promote their use of technology. Hong et al., (2022) on the other hand through their study found that nurses are required to be cautious while implementing interventions using mHealth, in a way that it positively impacts the autonomy and decision-making skills of older adults.

Government and community members demand the introduction of *smart nursing homes*, wherein there is inclusive access to digital medical solutions and proficient healthcare providers (Zhao et al., 2023).

Limitations and Recommendations for Future Research Deduced From Selected Articles

The most common limitation observed across the selected articles were the *incapability to produce generalizable findings* (Vaportzis et al., 2017; Couto et al., 2019; Tang et al., 2019; Trymbulak et al., 2020; Portz et al., 2020; Bianchi, 2020; Spargo et al., 2022; Villa-Garcias, 2022; Talukder et al., 2022; Velciu et al., 2023; Paimre, 2023; Cook et al., 2023; Zhao et al., 2023; Alam & Khanam, 2023).

This highlights the *need for more quantitative research* in the area (Delbreil & Zvobgo, 2013; Merilampi et al., 2014; Haesner et al., 2015; Khaksar et al., 2017; Stahl et al., 2017; Park & Kim, 2020; Conroy et al., 2020; Lund, 2021; Khaksar et al., 2021; Ginnouli et al., 2022; Kuerbis et al., 2022; Cangelosi et al., 2022; Ma et al., 2022; Hong et al., 2022; Velciu et al., 2023; Papachristou et al., 2023; Edna Mayela et al., 2023).

Other notable recommendations for future research included use of interactive web sessions for sharing healthcare information (van den Berg, 2015), studying older adults with reduced technological proficiency for conducting a comparative study (Vaportzis et al., 2017); acceptance rate of technology among older adults with respect to receiving medical treatment (Trymbulak et al., 2020), perspective of older adults regarding gerontechnology (Murciano-Heuso et al., 2022), training professionals for cognitive functioning using VR at community level (Qiu et al., 2022), assessing the relationship between technology, anxiety, and stress (Lorusso et al., 2022), and participation in online community platforms and its impact on wellbeing of older adults (Gazit et al., 2022).

LIMITATIONS AND FUTURE DIRECTIONS FOR RESEARCH

This section describes the limitation and potential future directions for this area of research. This study set out to conduct a thorough literature evaluation on the application of AI in geriatric healthcare system. Priority was given to comprehending how interventions have been written to foster possibility for the same.

The major limitation of the study was that the number of reviewed studies were few. This was due to the narrowed availability of research in the area due to the gradual emergence of gerontechnology.

Future research recommendations are made after carefully reviewing the research gaps, as shown in Table 5. These recommendations clear the way for an improved medical assistance to both healthcare professionals and older adults.

The mentioned future recommendations may be integrated in the future to advance research in the area.

Implication of the Study

The results of a thorough literature analysis on the use of AI to geriatric care will have a big impact on organizational and policy issues. Such a review influences health approaches, informs decision-making, and directs the distribution of funds.

Table 5. Recommendations for future scope of research

Future scope of directions	Key areas for future research
Theoretical constructs	*1. Creating conceptual frameworks that assist in educating healthcare professionals and older adults about the significance of integrating technology in medical treatments* *2.* *3. Use the Human-Robotic interaction theory to understand the perception of healthcare professionals and older adults with respect to engaging with AI in healthcare environment*
Methodology	• *Better strategies may be implemented by conducting more empirical research on interventions focused on improving wellbeing of older adults using technology.* • *Carrying out longitudinal research using a pre-post intervention to increase wellness of older adults in order to comprehend their long-term implications.* • *Doing research in developing and disadvantaged nations to comprehend cultural variations in perception and acceptance of technology by health professionals and geriatric population.*
Context	• *Research must be conducted in all countries, especially where the technological advancements are ow, so as to improve the quality of medical interventions* *The perception of youth and older generations regarding technology along with the differences in effect of mHealth on both populations may be studied.*

At Organizational Level

- The results of the literature review can be used by organizations to create well-informed strategies for applying AI in geriatric healthcare, including hospitals and long-term care facilities. This entails deciding on the best artificial intelligence (AI) methods, comprehending their advantages and disadvantages, and creating deployment strategies that are based on the unique requirements and financial capabilities of the firm.

- Effective resource allocation is made possible by the review. It can assist them in identifying the areas wherein investing in AI infrastructure as well as technology is predicted to result in improved patient care, lower costs, and better efficiency in operations.

- The knowledge and abilities needed for healthcare practitioners to properly use AI technologies can be identified by organizations. This information may guide training activities and workforce development plans, assuring that workers can make the best use of AI tools.

- The evaluation can assist companies in comprehending how AI can be incorporated into healthcare designs, placing an emphasis on customized therapies, higher patient engagement, and greater interaction for elderly patients.

- The review's insights, which highlight effective AI treatments and standards of excellence in elderly medical care, may assist in guide efforts to improve quality. Organizations can improve the standard of care they offer to senior citizens by implementing evidence-based strategies.

At Policy Level

- The research findings can be used by policymakers to create and revise regulatory frameworks that control the use of AI in geriatric healthcare. To promote safe and moral AI deployment, this includes creating standards for data protection, security, informed consent, and algorithm assessment.

- When creating reimbursement and financing policies, policymakers might take the cost-effectiveness and outcomes of artificial intelligence projects into consideration. The incorporation of AI technologies that enhance treatment quality and lower healthcare costs can align incentives and reimbursement mechanisms.
- Certain populations comprising elderly individuals may have varying levels of exposure to powered by AI health measures, which can be solved through policy considerations. For marginalized communities in particular, strategies might be developed to guarantee egalitarian availability of AI-enhanced elderly treatment.
- To make it easier for AI systems to integrate with the current healthcare infrastructure, policymakers might seek to establish interoperability standards. This encourages communication and cooperation between artificial intelligence researchers and medical providers.

CONCLUSION

To answer the specific research questions for the study, a thorough evaluation of the literature from databases like Science Direct, Emerald, and MDPI was conducted. This endeavor was performed in an effort to analyze the current developments in the industry. Moreover, challenges/restrictions, as well as potential long-term repercussions of the examined wellbeing programs and regulations.

Overall, use of technology in treatment of geriatric patients resulted in positive outcomes, particularly, reflected in increased physical and cognitive fitness. The main challenge while implementing AI in geriatric healthcare was the lack of technical training of both health professionals and older adults, which in turn affected the efficiency of the treatment.

By enhancing detection early on, customizing treatment approaches, permitting surveillance from afar, promoting safety, and optimizing care delivery, artificial intelligence is changing elderly treatment. The inclusion of AI in geriatric healthcare systems is crucial for assuring older persons receive high-quality, easily accessible, and reasonably priced treatment in light of the aging population's continued growth. We may anticipate even more improvements in the field as technology evolves, which will ultimately improve senior people's well-being and standard of life.

REFERENCES

Ahmed, S. F., Alam, M. S. B., Afrin, S., Rafa, S. J., Rafa, N., & Gandomi, A. H. (2024). Insights into Internet of Medical Things (IoMT): Data fusion, security issues and potential solutions. *Information Fusion, 102*, 102060. doi:10.1016/j.inffus.2023.102060

Al Kuwaiti, A., Nazer, K., Al-Reedy, A., Al-Shehri, S., Al-Muhanna, A., Subbarayalu, A. V., Al Muhanna, D., & Al-Muhanna, F. A. (2023). A Review of the Role of Artificial Intelligence in Healthcare. *Journal of Personalized Medicine, 13*(6), 951. doi:10.3390/jpm13060951 PMID:37373940

Alam, M. Z., & Khanam, L. (2023). Understanding the determinants of adoption of mHealth services among older women's perspective in Bangladesh. *International Journal of Pharmaceutical and Healthcare Marketing, 17*(1), 132–152. doi:10.1108/IJPHM-05-2021-0055

Alowais, S. A., Alghamdi, S. S., Alsuhebany, N., Alqahtani, T., Alshaya, A. I., Almohareb, S. N., Al-dairem, A., Alrashed, M., Bin Saleh, K., Badreldin, H. A., Al Yami, M. S., Al Harbi, S., & Albekairy, A. M. (2023). Revolutionizing healthcare: The role of artificial intelligence in clinical practice. *BMC Medical Education*, *23*(1), 689. doi:10.1186/s12909-023-04698-z PMID:37740191

Bays, H. E., Fitch, A., Cuda, S., Gonsahn-Bollie, S., Rickey, E., Hablutzel, J., Coy, R., & Censani, M. (2023). Artificial intelligence and obesity management: An Obesity Medicine Association (OMA) Clinical Practice Statement (CPS) 2023. *Obesity Pillars*, *6*, 100065. doi:10.1016/j.obpill.2023.100065 PMID:37990659

Bianchi, C. (2021). Exploring how internet services can enhance elderly well-being. *Journal of Services Marketing*, *35*(5), 585–603. doi:10.1108/JSM-05-2020-0177

Cangelosi, J., Damron, T. S., & Kim, D. (2022). Preventive health care information and social media: A comparison of Baby Boomer and Generation X health care consumers. *International Journal of Pharmaceutical and Healthcare Marketing*, *16*(2), 282–296. doi:10.1108/IJPHM-04-2021-0042

Cook, S., Munteanu, C., Papadopoulos, E., Abrams, H., Stinson, J. N., Pitters, E., & Puts, M. (2023). The development of an electronic geriatric assessment tool: Comprehensive health assessment for my plan (CHAMP). *Journal of Geriatric Oncology*, *14*(1), 101384. doi:10.1016/j.jgo.2022.09.013 PMID:36216760

Couto, F., de Lurdes Almeida, M., dos Anjos Dixe, M., Ribeiro, J., Braúna, M., Gomes, N., Caroço, J., Monteiro, L., Martinho, R., Rijo, R., & Apóstolo, J. (2019). Digi&Mind: Development and validation of a multi-domain digital cognitive stimulation program for older adults with cognitive decline. *Procedia Computer Science*, *164*, 732–740. doi:10.1016/j.procs.2019.12.242

Dantas, M. A., Da Silva, J. D., Tkachenko, N., & Paneque, M. (2023). Telehealth in genetic counselling consultations: The impact of COVID-19 in a Portuguese genetic healthcare service. *Journal of Community Genetics*, *14*(1), 91–100. doi:10.1007/s12687-022-00618-8 PMID:36414926

Delbreil, E., & Zvobgo, G. (2013). Wireless sensor technology in dementia care: Caregiver perceptions, technology take-up and business model innovation. *EuroMed Journal of Business*, *8*(1), 79–97. doi:10.1108/EMJB-05-2013-0019

Doshi, R., Hiran, K. K., Gök, M., El-kenawy, E. S. M., Badr, A., & Abotaleb, M. (2023). Artificial Intelligence's Significance in Diseases with Malignant Tumours. *Mesopotamian Journal of Artificial Intelligence in Healthcare*, *2023*, 35–39.

Edna Mayela, V. C., Miriam, L. T., Ana Isabel, G. G., Oscar, R. C., & Alejandra, C. A. (2023). Effectiveness of an online multicomponent physical exercise intervention on the physical performance of community-dwelling older adults: A randomized controlled trial. *Geriatric Nursing*, *14*(54), 83–93. doi:10.1016/j.gerinurse.2023.08.018 PMID:37716123

Gazit, T., Nisim, S., & Ayalon, L. (2023). Intergenerational family online community and older adults' overall well-being. *Online Information Review*, *47*(2), 221–237. doi:10.1108/OIR-06-2021-0332

Giannouli, E., Kim, E. K., Fu, C., Weibel, R., Sofios, A., Infanger, D., Portegijs, E., Rantanen, T., Huang, H., Schmidt-Trucksäss, A., Zeller, A., Rössler, R., & Hinrichs, T. (2022). Psychometric properties of the MOBITEC-GP mobile application for real-life mobility assessment in older adults. *Geriatric Nursing*, *48*, 273–279. doi:10.1016/j.gerinurse.2022.10.017 PMID:36334468

Haddaway, N. R., Macura, B., Whaley, P., & Pullin, A. S. (2018). ROSES Reporting standards for Systematic Evidence Syntheses: Pro forma, flow-diagram and descriptive summary of the plan and conduct of environmental systematic reviews and systematic maps. *Environmental Evidence*, *7*(1), 1–8. doi:10.1186/s13750-018-0121-7

Haesner, M., Steinert, A., O'Sullivan, J. L., & Steinhagen-Thiessen, E. (2015). Evaluating an accessible web interface for older adults–the impact of mild cognitive impairment (MCI). *Journal of Assistive Technologies*, *9*(4), 219–232. doi:10.1108/JAT-11-2014-0032

Haluza, D., & Jungwirth, D. (2023). Artificial Intelligence and Ten Societal Megatrends: An Exploratory Study Using GPT-3. *Systems*, *11*(3), 120. doi:10.3390/systems11030120

Hiran, K. K., & Doshi, R. (2013). An artificial neural network approach for brain tumor detection using digital image segmentation. *Brain*, *2*(5), 227–231.

Hong, S., Lee, S., Song, K., Kim, M., Kim, Y., Kim, H., & Kim, H. (2023). A nurse-led mHealth intervention to alleviate depressive symptoms in older adults living alone in the community: A quasi-experimental study. *International Journal of Nursing Studies*, *138*, 104431. doi:10.1016/j.ijnurstu.2022.104431 PMID:36630872

Khaksar, S. M. S., Jahanshahi, A. A., Slade, B., & Asian, S. (2021). A dual-factor theory of WTs adoption in aged care service operations–a cross-country analysis. *Information Technology & People*, *34*(7), 1768–1799. doi:10.1108/ITP-10-2018-0449

Khaksar, S. M. S., Shahmehr, F. S., Khosla, R., & Chu, M. T. (2017). Dynamic capabilities in aged care service innovation: The role of social assistive technologies and consumer-directed care strategy. *Journal of Services Marketing*, *31*(7), 745–759. doi:10.1108/JSM-06-2016-0243

Khan, N., Okoli, C. N., Ekpin, V., Attai, K., Chukwudi, N., Sabi, H., & Uzoka, F. M. (2023). Adoption and utilization of medical decision support systems in the diagnosis of febrile Diseases: A systematic literature review. *Expert Systems with Applications*, *220*, 119638. doi:10.1016/j.eswa.2023.119638

King, M. R. (2023). The future of AI in medicine: A perspective from a Chatbot. *Annals of Biomedical Engineering*, *51*(2), 291–295. doi:10.1007/s10439-022-03121-w PMID:36572824

Kolben, Y., Azmanov, H., Gelman, R., Dror, D., & Ilan, Y. (2023). Using chronobiology-based second-generation artificial intelligence digital system for overcoming antimicrobial drug resistance in chronic infections. *Annals of Medicine*, *55*(1), 311–318. doi:10.1080/07853890.2022.2163053 PMID:36594558

Kuerbis, A., Behrendt, S., Arora, V., & Muench, F. J. (2022). Acceptability and preliminary effectiveness of a text messaging intervention to reduce high-risk alcohol use among adults 50 and older: An exploratory study. *Advances in Dual Diagnosis*, *15*(2), 100–118. doi:10.1108/ADD-11-2021-0012

Lakhwani, K., Bhargava, S., Hiran, K. K., Bundele, M. M., & Somwanshi, D. (2020, December). Prediction of the onset of diabetes using artificial neural network and Pima Indians diabetes dataset. In *2020 5th IEEE International Conference on Recent Advances and Innovations in Engineering (ICRAIE)* (pp. 1-6). IEEE. 10.1109/ICRAIE51050.2020.9358308

Lorusso, L., Mosmondor, M., Grguric, A., Toccafondi, L., D'Onofrio, G., Russo, S., Lampe, J., Pihl, T., Mayer, N., Vignani, G., Lesterpt, I., Vaamonde, L., Giuliani, F., Bonaccorsi, M., La Viola, C., Rovini, E., Cavallo, F., & Fiorini, L. (2023). Design and Evaluation of Personalized Services to Foster Active Aging: The Experience of Technology Pre-Validation in Italian Pilots. *Sensors (Basel)*, *23*(2), 797. doi:10.3390/s23020797 PMID:36679590

Lund, B. (2021). Predictors of use of digital technology for communication among older adults: Analysis of data from the health and retirement study. *Working with Older People (Brighton, England)*, *25*(4), 294–303. doi:10.1108/WWOP-01-2021-0002

Ma, T., Zhang, S., Zhu, S., Ni, J., Wu, Q., & Liu, M. (2022). The new role of nursing in digital inclusion: Reflections on smartphone use and willingness to increase digital skills among Chinese older adults. *Geriatric Nursing*, *48*, 114–122. doi:10.1016/j.gerinurse.2022.09.004 PMID:36155310

Meena, G., Dhanwal, B., Mahrishi, M., & Hiran, K. K. (2021, August). Performance comparison of network intrusion detection system based on different pre-processing methods and deep neural network. In *Proceedings of the International Conference on Data Science, Machine Learning and Artificial Intelligence* (pp. 110-115). ACM. 10.1145/3484824.3484878

Merilampi, S., Sirkka, A., Leino, M., Koivisto, A., & Finn, E. (2014). Cognitive mobile games for memory impaired older adults. *Journal of Assistive Technologies*, *8*(4), 207–223. doi:10.1108/JAT-12-2013-0033

Modi, K., Singh, I., & Kumar, Y. (2023). A Comprehensive Analysis of Artificial Intelligence Techniques for the Prediction and Prognosis of Lifestyle Diseases. *Archives of Computational Methods in Engineering*, *30*(8), 1–24. doi:10.1007/s11831-023-09957-2

Moher, D., Liberati, A., Tetzlaff, J., & Altman, D. G.The PRISMA Group. (2009). *Preferred Reporting Items for Systematic Reviews and Meta-Analyses: The PRISMA Statement. PLoS Medicine*, *6*(6), e1000097. doi:10.1371/journal.pmed.1000097 PMID:19621072

Monge, J., Ribeiro, G., Raimundo, A., Postolache, O., & Santos, J. (2023). AI-Based Smart Sensing and AR for Gait Rehabilitation Assessment. *Information (Basel)*, *14*(7), 355. doi:10.3390/info14070355

Murciano-Hueso, A., Martín-Lucas, J., Serrate González, S., & Torrijos Fincias, P. (2022). Use and perception of gerontechnology: Differences in a group of Spanish older adults. *Quality in Ageing : Policy, Practice and Research*, *23*(3), 114–128. doi:10.1108/QAOA-02-2022-0010

Paimre, M., Virkus, S., & Osula, K. (2023). Health information behavior and related factors among Estonians aged≥ 50 years during the COVID-19 pandemic. *The Journal of Documentation*, *79*(5), 1164–1181. doi:10.1108/JD-10-2022-0217

Papachristou, N., Kartsidis, P., Anagnostopoulou, A., Marshall-McKenna, R., Kotronoulas, G., Collantes, G., & Bamidis, P. D. (2023, May). A Smart Digital Health Platform to Enable Monitoring of Quality of Life and Frailty in Older Patients with Cancer: A Mixed-Methods, Feasibility Study Protocol. In *Seminars in Oncology Nursing* (p. 151437). WB Saunders. doi:10.1016/j.soncn.2023.151437

Park, S., & Kim, B. (2020). Readiness for utilizing digital intervention: Patterns of internet use among older adults with diabetes. *Primary Care Diabetes*, *14*(6), 692–697. doi:10.1016/j.pcd.2020.08.005 PMID:32839128

Patel, S., Vyas, A. K., & Hiran, K. K. (2022). Infrastructure health monitoring using signal processing based on an industry 4.0 System. *Cyber-Physical Systems and Industry*, *4*, 249–260.

Portz, J. D., Ford, K. L., Doyon, K., Bekelman, D. B., Boxer, R. S., Kutner, J. S., Czaja, S., & Bull, S. (2020). Using grounded theory to inform the human-centered design of digital health in geriatric palliative care. *Journal of Pain and Symptom Management*, *60*(6), 1181–1192. doi:10.1016/j.jpainsymman.2020.06.027 PMID:32615298

Qiu, R., Gu, Y., Xie, C., Wang, Y., Sheng, Y., Zhu, J., Yue, Y., & Cao, J. (2022). Virtual reality-based targeted cognitive training program for Chinese older adults: A feasibility study. *Geriatric Nursing*, *47*, 35–41. doi:10.1016/j.gerinurse.2022.06.007 PMID:35839753

Radenkovic, D., Zhavoronkov, A., & Bischof, E. (2021). AI in Longevity Medicine. In *Artificial Intelligence in Medicine* (pp. 1–13). Springer International Publishing. doi:10.1007/978-3-030-58080-3_248-1

Ramasamy, J., & Doshi, R. (2022). Machine learning in cyber physical systems for healthcare: brain tumor classification from MRI using transfer learning framework. In *Real-Time Applications of Machine Learning in Cyber-Physical Systems* (pp. 65–76). IGI global. doi:10.4018/978-1-7998-9308-0.ch005

Seng, K. P., Ang, L. M., Peter, E., & Mmonyi, A. (2023). Machine Learning and AI Technologies for Smart Wearables. *Electronics (Basel)*, *12*(7), 1509. doi:10.3390/electronics12071509

Sheikh, Y., Ali, A., Khasati, A., Hasanic, A., Bihani, U., Ohri, R., Muthukumar, K., & Barlow, J. (2023). Benefits and Challenges of Video Consulting for Mental Health Diagnosis and Follow-Up: A Qualitative Study in Community Care. *International Journal of Environmental Research and Public Health*, *20*(3), 2595. doi:10.3390/ijerph20032595 PMID:36767957

Spargo, M., Goodfellow, N., Scullin, C., Grigoleit, S., Andreou, A., Mavromoustakis, C. X., Guerra, B., Manso, M., Larburu, N., Villacañas, Ó., Fleming, G., & Scott, M. (2021). Shaping the future of digitally enabled health and care. *Pharmacy (Basel, Switzerland)*, *9*(1), 17. doi:10.3390/pharmacy9010017 PMID:33445509

Stahl, S. T., Emanuel, J., Albert, S. M., Dew, M. A., Schulz, R., Robbins-Welty, G., & Reynolds, C. F. III. (2017). Design and rationale for a technology-based healthy lifestyle intervention in older adults grieving the loss of a spouse. *Contemporary Clinical Trials Communications*, *8*, 99–105. doi:10.1016/j.conctc.2017.09.002 PMID:29170758

Sun, J., Dong, Q. X., Wang, S. W., Zheng, Y. B., Liu, X. X., Lu, T. S., Yuan, K., Shi, J., Hu, B., Lu, L., & Han, Y. (2023). Artificial intelligence in psychiatry research, diagnosis, and therapy. *Asian Journal of Psychiatry*, *87*, 103705. doi:10.1016/j.ajp.2023.103705 PMID:37506575

Talukder, M. S., Laato, S., Islam, A. N., & Bao, Y. (2021). Continued use intention of wearable health technologies among the elderly: An enablers and inhibitors perspective. *Internet Research*, *31*(5), 1611–1640. doi:10.1108/INTR-10-2020-0586

Tang, V., Choy, K. L., Ho, G. T., Lam, H. Y., & Tsang, Y. P. (2019). An IoMT-based geriatric care management system for achieving smart health in nursing homes. *Industrial Management & Data Systems*, *119*(8), 1819–1840. doi:10.1108/IMDS-01-2019-0024

Trymbulak, K., Ding, E., Marino, F., Wang, Z., & Saczynski, J. S. (2020). Mobile health assessments of geriatric elements in older patients with atrial fibrillation: The Mobile SAGE-AF Study (M-SAGE). *Cardiovascular Digital Health Journal*, *1*(3), 123–129. doi:10.1016/j.cvdhj.2020.11.002 PMID:35265884

Ullah, M., Hamayun, S., Wahab, A., Khan, S. U., Rehman, M. U., Haq, Z. U., Rehman, K. U., Ullah, A., Mehreen, A., Awan, U. A., Qayum, M., & Naeem, M. (2023). Smart technologies used as smart tools in the management of cardiovascular disease and their future perspective. *Current Problems in Cardiology*, *48*(11), 101922. doi:10.1016/j.cpcardiol.2023.101922 PMID:37437703

Vaismoradi, M., Turunen, H., & Bondas, T. (2013). Content analysis and thematic analysis: Implications for conducting a qualitative descriptive study. *Nursing & Health Sciences*, *15*(3), 398–405. doi:10.1111/nhs.12048 PMID:23480423

van den Berg, M., Sherrington, C., Killington, M., Smith, S., Bongers, B., Hassett, L., & Crotty, M. (2016). Video and computer-based interactive exercises are safe and improve task-specific balance in geriatric and neurological rehabilitation: A randomised trial. *Journal of Physiotherapy*, *62*(1), 20–28. doi:10.1016/j.jphys.2015.11.005 PMID:26701163

Vaportzis, E., Martin, M., & Gow, A. J. (2017). A tablet for healthy ageing: The effect of a tablet computer training intervention on cognitive abilities in older adults. *The American Journal of Geriatric Psychiatry*, *25*(8), 841–851. doi:10.1016/j.jagp.2016.11.015 PMID:28082016

Velciu, M., Spiru, L., Dan Marzan, M., Reithner, E., Geli, S., Borgogni, B., Cramariuc, O., Mocanu, I. G., Kołakowski, J., Ayadi, J., Rampioni, M., & Stara, V. (2023). How Technology-Based Interventions Can Sustain Ageing Well in the New Decade through the User-Driven Approach. *Sustainability (Basel)*, *15*(13), 10330. doi:10.3390/su151310330

Villa-García, L., Puig, A., Puigpelat, P., Solé-Casals, M., & Fuertes, O. (2022). The development of a platform to ensure an integrated care plan for older adults with complex care needs living at home. *Journal of Integrated Care*, *30*(4), 310–323. doi:10.1108/JICA-01-2022-0010

Wakida, E. K., Talib, Z. M., Akena, D., Okello, E. S., Kinengyere, A., Mindra, A., & Obua, C. (2018). Barriers and facilitators to the integration of mental health services into primary health care: A systematic review. *Systematic Reviews*, *7*(1), 1–13. doi:10.1186/s13643-018-0882-7 PMID:30486900

Zeinalnezhad, M., & Shishehchi, S. (2023). An integrated data mining algorithms and meta-heuristic technique to predict the readmission risk of diabetic patients. *Healthcare Analytics*, 100292.

Zhao, Y., Sazlina, S. G., Rokhani, F. Z., Su, J., & Chew, B. H. (2023). The expectations and acceptability of a smart nursing home model among Chinese older adults and family members: A qualitative study. *Asian Nursing Research*, *17*(4), 208–218. doi:10.1016/j.anr.2023.08.002 PMID:37661084

Chapter 12
Robotics Rx:
A Prescription for the Future of Healthcare

Jaspreet Kaur
Chandigarh University, India

ABSTRACT

"Robotics Rx: A Prescription for the Future of Healthcare" provides a forward-thinking road plan for the implementation of robotics in the medical field. The purpose of this study is to investigate the revolutionary potential of robots in terms of boosting diagnostic accuracy, enhancing patient care, and revolutionising surgical procedures. This prescription illustrates a future in which artificial intelligence, machine learning, and precision robotics work together in a seamless manner with medical professionals, thereby enhancing their ability to perform and ultimately redefining the standards of medical practise. This is accomplished by delving into the advancements that have been made in these areas.

INTRODUCTION

The field of healthcare has witnessed the emergence of robotics as a transnational force, which has revolutionized the delivery of medical services, the administration of therapies, and the provision of patient care. Over the course of the last few decades, there has been a significant increase in the utilization of robots in the healthcare industry. This has resulted in the development of novel solutions, increases in precision, and improvements in the results for patients (Valles-Peris & Domènech, 2023).

Within the realm of healthcare, the utilization of robotics spans a broad spectrum of applications, spanning from diagnostics and patient care to surgical operations and rehabilitation. The purpose of designing and programming robots is to provide assistance to medical professionals in a variety of capacities. These robots offer an unprecedented level of accuracy, efficiency, and consistency in the execution of tasks that were previously completely dependent on the intervention of humans. It is impossible to exaggerate the relevance of incorporating robotics into the healthcare infrastructure. Within the field of surgical operations, one of the most significant advantages can be obtained. It is becoming increasingly common for surgeons to execute complex procedures with the assistance of robotic-assisted surgery, which enables them to achieve higher precision while minimizing the amount of pervasiveness involved.

DOI: 10.4018/979-8-3693-1123-3.ch012

Surgeons are provided with cutting-edge equipment that improve their dexterity, control, and visualization capabilities. As a result, the number of complications that occur during surgical procedures is reduced, recuperation times are shortened, and patient outcomes are improved (Deo & Anjankar 2023).

In addition, robotics is increasingly being utilized in the field of rehabilitation therapy. Robots designed for rehabilitation assist patients in regaining their motor functions following injuries or surgical procedures. In order to provide patients with the opportunity to participate in individualized therapy sessions that are adapted to their specific requirements, these assistive devices support repetitive and targeted motions. By utilizing robots in the field of rehabilitation, medical professionals are able to improve the efficiency of the recovery process and speed up the process of patients returning to their functional independence.

The field of diagnostic robots is another one that is experiencing substantial forward movement. Robots that are outfitted with advanced sensors and the ability to perform artificial intelligence are able to perform tasks such as analyzing medical images, carrying out tests, and interpreting data with an incredible level of precision. Not only does this speed up the diagnosis process, but it also helps medical practitioners make decisions about patient treatment that are better informed and based on accurate information (Ragno et al., 2023).

In addition, the incorporation of robots into patient care services is becoming increasingly common. These technologies are reducing the load that is placed on healthcare personnel while simultaneously improving the quality of life for patients. Examples of these technologies include robotic companions for the elderly, automated medication dispensers, and support systems and assistance systems for people with impairments (Kumar et al., 2023; Minopoulos et al., 2023).

Numerous advantages are brought about as a result of the use of robotics into the healthcare industry. It is possible for medical experts to carry out difficult treatments with an accuracy that is unmatched and a margin of error that is significantly decreased because to the emphasis placed on efficiency and precision. Because robotics reduces the dangers that are connected with invasive procedures and treatments, patient safety is also considerably improved as a result of this technology. In addition, the utilization of these technology results in shorter hospital stays, faster healing times, and ultimately, a more cost-effective healthcare system (Minopoulos et al., 2023).

As we get further into this chapter, we will investigate a variety of aspects of robotics in the medical field using robotics. Within the context of the medical industry, we will investigate the development of robotics by analyzing its historical trajectory as well as the significant technological developments that have been the driving force behind its growing popularity. In addition, we will conduct an analysis of the current state of robotics in the healthcare industry, focusing on the various uses of these technologies as well as the impact they have on patient care and medical practise. In addition, the chapter will look into the difficulties and ethical problems that are linked with the incorporation of robotics into the healthcare industry. It is essential to navigate the ethical landscape of robotic intervention in healthcare in order to ensure its responsible and effective implementation. Concerns over the possible displacement of jobs, as well as ethical difficulties surrounding autonomy and decision-making, are examples of the factors that constitute this landscape (Khaddad at al., 2023).

The final part of this discussion will focus on the prospects for the future and the developing patterns in the arena of healthcare robotics. We will investigate the current state of robotics in the healthcare business and how it has the ability to revolutionize the industry in generations to come. This will include the development of increasingly advanced robotic systems as well as the incorporation of machine learning, AI, and other algorithms. The field of healthcare has witnessed the emergence of robotics as a transformation force, which has revolutionized the delivery of medical services, the administration of therapies, and the provision of patient care. Over the course of the last few decades, there has been a significant increase in the utilization of robots in the healthcare industry. This has resulted in the development of novel solutions, increases in precision, and improvements in the results for patients (Kim et al.,2023; Srinivasulu et al., 2022). Within the realm of healthcare, the utilization of robotics spans a broad spectrum of applications, spanning from diagnostics and patient care to surgical operations and rehabilitation. The purpose of designing and programming robots is to provide assistance to medical professionals in a variety of capacities. These robots offer an unprecedented level of accuracy, efficiency, and consistency in the execution of tasks that were previously completely dependent on the intervention of humans. It is impossible to exaggerate the relevance of incorporating robotics into the healthcare infrastructure. Within the field of surgical operations, one of the most significant advantages can be obtained. It is becoming increasingly common for surgeons to execute complex procedures with the assistance of robotic-assisted surgery, which enables them to achieve higher precision while minimizing the amount of pervasiveness involved. Surgeons are provided with cutting-edge equipment that improve their dexterity, control, and visualization capabilities. As a result, the number of complications that occur during surgical procedures is reduced, recuperation times are shortened, and patient outcomes are improved (Rivero-Moreno et al., 2023; Ramasamy et al., 2022).

In addition, robotics is increasingly being utilized in the field of rehabilitation therapy. Robots designed for rehabilitation assist patients in regaining their motor functions following injuries or surgical procedures. In order to provide patients with the opportunity to participate in individualized therapy sessions that are adapted to their specific requirements, these assistive devices support repetitive and targeted motions. By utilizing robots in the field of rehabilitation, medical professionals are able to improve the efficiency of the recovery process and speed up the process of patients returning to their functional independence. The field of diagnostic robots is another one that is experiencing substantial forward movement. Robots that are outfitted with advanced sensors and the ability to perform artificial intelligence are able to perform tasks such as analyzing medical images, carrying out tests, and interpreting data with an incredible level of precision. Not only does this speed up the diagnosis process, but it also helps medical practitioners make decisions about patient treatment that are better informed and based on accurate information (Yeisson et al., 2023).

In addition, the incorporation of robots into patient care services is becoming increasingly common. These technologies are reducing the load that is placed on healthcare personnel while simultaneously improving the quality of life for patients. Examples of these technologies include robotic companions for the elderly, automated medication dispensers, and support systems and assistance systems for people with impairments. Numerous advantages are brought about as a result of the use of robotics into the healthcare industry. It is possible for medical experts to carry out difficult treatments with an accuracy that is unmatched and a margin of error that is significantly decreased because to the emphasis placed on efficiency and precision. Because robotics reduces the dangers that are connected with invasive procedures and treatments, patient safety is also considerably improved as a result of this technology. In addition, the utilization of these technology results in shorter hospital stays, faster healing times, and ultimately, a more cost-effective healthcare system.

As we get further into this chapter, we will investigate a variety of aspects of robotics in the medical field using robotics. Within the context of the medical industry, we will investigate the development of robotics by analyzing its historical trajectory as well as the significant technological developments that have been the driving force behind its growing popularity. In addition, we will conduct an analysis of the current state of robotics in the healthcare industry, focusing on the various uses of these technologies as well as the impact they have on patient care and medical practices. In addition, the chapter will look into the difficulties and ethical problems that are linked with the incorporation of robotics into the healthcare industry. It is essential to navigate the ethical terrain of robotic involvement in medical care in order to ensure its accountable and successful implementation. Concerns over the possible displacement of jobs, as well as ethical difficulties concerning liberty and making choices, are examples of the factors that constitute this landscape (Lochan et al., 2023; Ramasamy et al., 2021). The final part of this discussion will focus on the prospects for the future and recent developments in the field of healthcare automation. We will investigate the trajectory of robotics in the healthcare business and its potential to revolutionize the industry in the years to come. This will include the development of increasingly advanced robotic systems as well as the incorporation of machine learning, AI, and other algorithms.

Medical Robotic Applications

Surgical Robotics: The field of surgical robotics has brought about a considerable transformation in the landscape of modern medicine, thereby revolutionizing the way in which complex surgeries are carried out. In this particular field, the da Vinci Surgical System is one of the most notable developments that has taken place. This robotic platform gives surgeons the ability to do minimally invasive surgery with a level of precision and control that is virtually unmatched. With the da Vinci Surgical System, surgeons are able to move robotic arms that have been fitted with surgical instruments with the use of a terminal console. These devices have a greater range of motion in comparison to the human's hand, which enables surgeons to conduct delicate man-oeuvres with a higher degree of precision with these instruments. A magnified, high-definition, three-dimensional view of the surgical site is provided by the device, which can be of great assistance to surgeons in terms of enhanced visualization (Schönmann et al., 2023).

There are many different uses for surgical robotics, and they can be found in a wide range of medical disciplines. The da Vinci system is utilized in the field of urology for the purpose of performing protectorates and hysterectomies. This results in decreased hemorrhaging, fewer nights in the hospital, as well as quicker recovery times for patients recovering from these procedures. During gynecological treatments, such as hysterectomies. Additionally, the da Vinci system is not the only example of advancements in surgical robots. New technologies are always being investigated by researchers and developers. Some examples of these technologies are bendable robotics for endoscopic treatments, micro bots for targeted administration of medication within the body, and independent robotic surgeons that are capable of performing predetermined tasks with minimal assistance from humans (Matsuzaki et al., 2023; Lakhwani et al., 2020; Jain et al., 2023).

Rehabilitation Robotics: Rehabilitating robotics has established itself as a game-changer in the field of physical therapy. It provides patients with unique solutions to assist them in regaining their motor capabilities and improving their quality of life. People who have movement difficulties as a result of injuries, cerebrovascular accidents, or neurological disorders can receive assistance from these robots to help them overcome those symptoms. One of the most prominent examples of rehabilitation robotics is the use of exoskeletons. The motions of a patient are supported and enhanced by these wearable devices, which also contribute to the improvement of muscular strength and gait development. Their ability to enable persons to stand and walk with the assistance of an external support system is especially advantageous for those individuals who are undergoing rehabilitation following spinal cord injuries (Kato et al., 2023).

The usage of robotic-assisted therapeutic equipment is yet another key application of this technology. To aid in the process of motor recovery, these devices make use of movements that are both repeated and targeted. As an example, robotic arms encourage patients who have suffered a stroke to participate in individualized therapy sessions that are suited to their particular rehabilitation requirements. This helps these patients restore functionality in their upper limbs. Robotics in rehabilitation have an impact that extends beyond the realm of physical therapy. These technologies not only hasten the process of recuperation, but they also stimulate neurolinguistics, which helps in the rebuilding of cerebral connections and fosters functional improvements in patients who are suffering from neurological diseases. Robotic Prostheses and Assistance Gadgets: Recent developments in robotics have resulted in extraordinary advancements in prostheses and assistive devices, which have considerably improved the quality of life for people who have lost limbs or who have disabilities. It is possible to achieve enhanced functionality and natural mobility with prosthetic limbs that are fitted with robotic components. These prosthetic limbs closely resemble the abilities of human appendages (Ohneberg et al., 2023).

One primary example is the use of muscle impulses to regulate movement in prosthetic limbs, which is accomplished through the use of myoelectric prostheses. These technologies make it possible for users to carry out complex activities with a greater degree of both ease and precision. Furthermore, developments in sensor technology have led to the creation of prosthetic limbs that are equipped with sensory feedback. These prosthetic limbs enable users to experience sensations such as touch and pressure more accurately. In addition to prosthetics, assistive robots are an essential component in the process of assisting people with disabilities in their day-to-day activities responsibilities. These gadgets enable individuals and promote independence. An example of one such item is a robotic wheelchair that is integrated with intelligent navigation systems. Another example is a robotic companion that provides social contact and help. The incorporation of robotics into prostheses and assistive devices is continuously evolving, with the primary focal points being the enhancement of user comfort, the improvement of durability, and the refinement of control mechanisms. The ultimate objective is to provide consumers with seamless connectivity and natural functionality, thereby bridging the gap among human capability and technical enhancement (Alowais et al., 2023).

In a nutshell the applications of robots in healthcare, which include surgical procedures and rehabilitation as well as prostheses and assistive technology, represent a trans-formative age in the field of modern medicine. Not only do these improvements raise the bar for patient care, but they also prepare the path for a future in which technology will complement and enhance human talents, therefore radically altering the face of healthcare as depicted in figure 1 below:

Robotics in Diagnostics and Imaging

Diagnostic technologies that are powered by artificial intelligence (AI) and robotics: The combination of artificial intelligence (AI) and robots has brought about on an entirely novel phase of diagnostic precision within the healthcare industry. Artificial intelligence-driven diagnostic tools utilize the power of artificially intelligent algorithms to process vast amounts of medical data, which ultimately results in diagnoses that are more accurate and time-efficient (Kaur, 2023).

The analysis of complex datasets, in particular medical pictures such as a series of magnetic resonance imaging (MRI), computed tomography (CT), and histopathology images, is one of the most significant contributions that artificial intelligence makes to the field of diagnosis. Deep learning algorithms, which are a subset of artificial intelligence, are very good at pattern recognition. This gives them the ability

Figure 1. Medical robotic applications

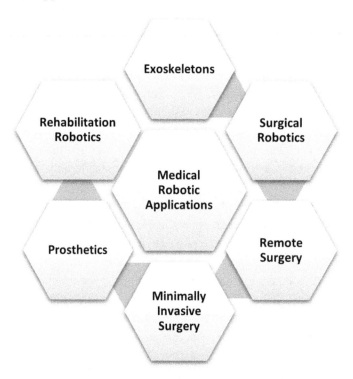

to identify minor irregularities that may be missed by human observers. Systems that are powered by artificial intelligence, for instance, are able to quickly identify early indicators of diseases such as cancer by analyzing radio-logical pictures with greater precision and speed than traditional approaches. Incorporating artificial intelligence algorithms into robotic systems results in an increase in diagnostic capabilities. Image analysis, pattern recognition, and initial diagnosis are just some of the jobs that can be performed by robots that are equipped with artificial intelligence to provide assistance to medical personnel. This integration not only lessens the amount of labour that medical professionals have to do, but it also improves diagnosis accuracy by reducing the number of mistakes that are made by humans. In addition, diagnostic robots that are powered by artificial intelligence speed up the process of generating diagnostic reports, which ensures that interventions and therapies are administered in a timely manner. These systems are always learning and improving from the data that they analyse, which allows them to refine their diagnostic abilities over time and potentially reduce diagnostic errors, which in turn improves patient care dramatically (Kaur, 2023).

Innovative Integration of Imaging Technologies: There are a multitude of applications that have been made possible as a result of the convergence of robotics and imaging technologies. These applications offer significant benefits across a variety of medical fields. Medical imaging methods have been completely transformed as a result of the integration of robotics with imaging technologies. The use of robotic systems in conjunction with imaging technologies enables precise and controlled motions to be made during imaging, hence reducing the number of errors that occur and enhancing the overall quality of the images that are captured. Robots that are integrated into magnetic resonance imaging (MRI) scanners, for example, ensure that patients are positioned in a consistent and exact manner, thereby eliminating motion artifacts and improving imaging quality. The combination of robots and imaging modalities has made it possible to perform minimally invasive operations with an unprecedented level of precision in the field of intervention radiology. It is now possible for medical professionals to navigate through complex anatomical structures with greater precision thanks to robotic devices that are guided by real-time imaging techniques like fluoroscope or ultrasound. When performing procedures such as biopsies or catheter placements, this improves accuracy, which in turn reduces risks and leads to better outcomes for patients (Harry, 2023).

In addition, robotics has been instrumental in the creation of capsule endoscopy, which is a minimally invasive imaging technique in which patients are required to swallow a small capsule that contains a little camera. During their journey through the digestive tract, these capsules take pictures and then send them to devices that are located outside of the body. The utilization of robotics is of critical importance in the process of strengthening the maneuverability and control of these capsules, which in turn guarantees complete imaging coverage and accurate diagnostics. Beyond the benefits of accuracy and precision, the combination of imaging techniques and robots offers another set of advantages. Because of these integration's, the duration of the treatment is shortened, the patient experiences less discomfort, and the recovery period is shortened accordingly. In addition, the real-time input that is supplied by imaging technology is used to direct robotic systems, which makes surgeries safer and more efficient while simultaneously reducing the hazards which patients face (Ali, 2023).

In nutshell, the combination of artificial intelligence (AI)-driven diagnostic tools and robots, in conjunction with the incorporation of imaging technologies, constitutes a revolutionary step forward in the field of healthcare diagnostics. Not only do these developments improve diagnosis accuracy, but they also revolutionize imaging techniques, which promises to make patient care more effective and personalized. The persistent development of these technologies carries with it a tremendous potential for more innovations and enhancements in diagnostic capacities within the healthcare sector (Ahmad et al., 2023).

Remote Surgery and Teleoperation

Satellite imagery Surgery and Teleoperation: The development of telemedicine, in conjunction with the progress made in robotics, has made it possible for surgeons to do surgeries on patients who are located in a different geographical area. This is a revolutionary notion that has been made possible by the advent of teleoperative technology. The utilization of robotic equipment to carry out surgical procedures under the direction of a skilled surgeon who is operating from a remote location is an essential component of remote surgery. Teleoperation is a major component of remote surgery. The use of high-speed internet connections and cutting-edge robotic equipment that are able to relay real-time video feedback between the operating room and the person doing the surgery is essential to the viability of remote surgery. The implementation of this technology has the potential to overcome geographical constraints, making it possible for patients living in under-served or rural places to gain access to specialized surgical knowledge (Ali, 2023; Gupta et al., 2022; Goel et al., 2023).

On the other hand, remote surgery involves a number of significant problems. To ensure that the surgeon's directions and the movements of the robotic system are in perfect sync with one another and that there is no interruption in communication, this is one of the key issues. As a result of the fact that delays or disruptions in data transmission could put the success of the surgery in jeopardy, it is essential to have networks that are both dependable and have an extremely low latency (Abbasimoshaei et al., 2023).

In addition, it is of the utmost importance to guarantee the safety of patients and to ensure compliance with ethical and regulatory standards. The presence of reliable systems and robust security measures is essential for robotic systems, since they are designed to avoid counterattacks or breakdowns in operation that might potentially threaten the health of patients.

Remote patient monitoring and virtual consultations: Through the utilization of telemedicine and robotics, online counselling and remote patient monitoring are able to facilitate medical procedures that do not require the patient's physical presence. A multitude of benefits can be gained from utilizing these practices, particularly in circumstances whereby visitation in person are either difficult or unnecessary. It is possible for patients to communicate with medical professionals remotely through the use of virtual consultations. This allows patients to receive medical advice, prescriptions, and assistance without having to physically visit a clinic. The use of telepresence robots that are equipped with audiovisual capabilities is an example of how robotics can be utilized in this context. These robots enable medical professionals to remotely inspect patients and deliver consultations in real (Mahmoud et al., 2023; Doshi et al., 2023).

The process of remotely monitoring patients comprises the utilization of detectors and wearable devices that are combined with robotic systems in order to monitor the health parameters of patients from a different location. By transmitting data to healthcare providers, including blood pressure or blood glucose levels, these devices make it possible for them to take preventative measures in the event that anomalies occur.

There are several drawbacks associated with these approaches, despite the fact that they improve accessibility and ease. Among the difficulties that arise are the inability to perform hands-on examinations and the constraints that come with evaluating particular medical issues without the need for direct physical contact. In addition, significant gaps exist between patients in terms of their access to technology and their level of digital literacy, which may impede the widespread use of remote monitoring and virtual consultations. Furthermore, the transmission of sensitive medical information over networks raises concerns regarding data privacy and security, highlighting the importance of implementing effective encryption and adhering to legislation governing the protection of healthcare data (Stasevych & Zvarych, 2023).

In nutshell, the incorporation of videoconferencing and robotics into surgical procedures performed remotely, virtual visits, and monitoring patients remotely has the potential to bring about a revolutionary change in the delivery of healthcare. It is essential to address technologically regulatory, and ethical problems in order to guarantee the safe and successful application of these technologies, which will ultimately result in improved patient care and connectivity to healthcare services as represented in figure 2 below:

Despite the fact that these advancements offer unparalleled access and convenience, it is essential to address these challenges (Murakami et al., 2023).

Ethical and Regulatory Considerations

Concerns Regarding Ethical Issues in Healthcare Robotics The use of robotics into healthcare presents significant ethical concerns that need to be thoroughly investigated. The degree to which robotic systems are able to function independently is a fundamental concern. As these technologies continue to advance in their level of sophistication, problems arise concerning the degree of autonomy in decision-making that is provided to technology. To ensure the safety of patients and to maintain ethical standards in practise, it is essential to strike a balance between the autonomy of robots and human oversight and accountability. Confidentiality is also another essential ethical consideration. The huge volumes of sensitive patient data

Figure 2. Remote surgery and teleoperation

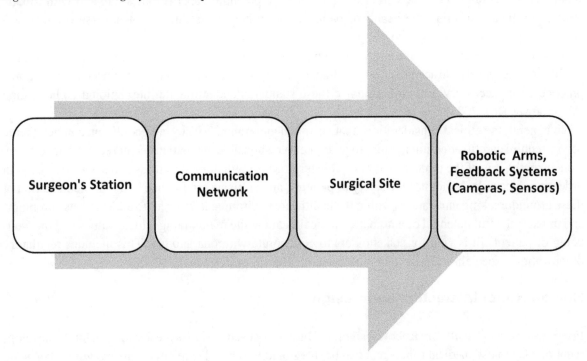

that are collected by healthcare robots raise problems regarding the ownership, privacy, and confidentiality of the data. It is absolutely necessary to protect sensitive information from being accessed or used inappropriately by unauthorized parties in order to maintain the trust of patients and adhere to ethical standards. In addition, it is essential to create and continue to sustain confidence between individuals, medical professionals, and robotic systems inside the healthcare system. It is imperative that patients receive reassurance that the technologies in question are dependable, risk-free, and supportive of their well-being. For the purpose of fostering trust, it is vital to have open dialogue regarding the roles that robotic systems play in patient care, as well as transparency regarding the strengths and weaknesses of robotic systems (Stasevych & Zvarych, 2023).

The Frameworks for Regulatory Compliance and Safety Standards: The legal structures and safety standards that are in place in the healthcare industry have a considerable impact on the acceptance as well as implementation of robotic technologies. The development, implementation, and use of these innovations are all subject to the oversight of regulatory authorities, which play a crucial role in ensuring that these technologies comply with moral and safety norms (Al Kuwaiti et al., 2023).

Regulatory agencies, such as the FDA, or Food and Drug Administration, in the United States and the European Medicines Agency (EMA) in Europe, need severe reviews and permissions for healthcare robots. These agencies are responsible for their respective regions. The purpose of these studies is to determine whether or not robotic systems are safe, effective, and reliable before they are implemented in clinical settings. It is not only the compliance with these standards that guarantees the safety of patients, but it also instills confidence in both the healthcare professionals and the affected individuals (Božić, 2023).

There are design requirements, performance measurements, and risk assessments that are included in the safety standards that are specific to robotics in the healthcare industry. The observance of these standards is absolutely necessary in order to reduce the potential hazards that are linked with robotic treatments, hence ensuring the health of patients and reducing the number of adverse occurrences. Nevertheless, negotiating regulatory regimes on a global scale presents problems, such as the possibility that different regions may have different approval procedures and requirements. When it comes to facilitating the worldwide acceptance of healthcare robotics while preserving uniform safety and ethical practices, it is necessary to both harmonize these standards and stimulate international collaboration (Varshney & Dev, 2023).

In general, the ethical considerations that surround autonomy, privacy, and confidence in healthcare robots require careful attention in order to guarantee a responsible and patient-centered implementation. Concurrently, it is of the utmost need to establish rigorous regulatory structures and safety standards in order to reduce risks, guarantee the safety of patients, and cultivate confidence in the implementation of these groundbreaking innovations within the healthcare environment. In order to address these problems and unleash the full potential of automation in healthcare while maintaining ethical values and the well-being of patients, it is vital for stakeholders to collaborate with one another. This includes regulatory organizations, specialists from the industry, and healthcare professionals.

Human-Robot Interaction and Design

Friendly for Users Healthcare Robot Designing: Human-focused design is the foundation for the development of easy to use medical robots that can be integrated into healthcare environments without causing any disruptions. This strategy places an emphasis on gaining an understanding of the requirements, abilities, and individual needs of patients as well as healthcare providers in order to develop robotic systems that contribute to an improved user experience and increased efficiency. For medical robots to be considered user-friendly, it is essential that they have interfaces that are easy to understand and utilize. The creation of user interfaces that are concise, ergonomic, and simple to use is a factor that contributes to interactions between people and robots that are more seamless. Controls and feedback mechanisms that are easy to understand are absolutely necessary in order to guarantee that medical personnel are able to operate these systems effectively (Nwadiokwu, 2023).

Furthermore, it is essential to take into consideration the particular physical environment in which these robots function. It is of the utmost importance to develop robots that are capable of navigating through therapeutic environments without generating any disturbances or risks. For the purpose of successfully integrating medical robots into healthcare facilities, it is essential to take into consideration a number of factors, including their size, mobility, and adaptation to many different contexts (Kaur, 2024).

When it comes to the development of medical robots, continuous input from users and iterative design procedures are absolutely necessary. Iterative enhancements are made possible by the collection of insights from medical personnel and patients. This helps to ensure that these systems continue to adapt to meet the ever-changing demands and preferences of patients. Elements of interactions between humans and robots in Healthcare That Feature Psychological Considerations: As a result of the advent of robots in healthcare settings, psychological factors that influence the interaction between humans and robots have presented themselves. Addressing the worries of patients and ensuring that they are willing to adopt new technologies is essential for the successful integration of these technologies (Wang et al., 2023).

It is possible for patients to develop worry or apprehension when engaging with healthcare robots due to the fact that they are unfamiliar with the technology or they are concerned about its dependability. Therefore, it is essential to have communication techniques that are effective in order to notify patients about the tasks and abilities of robots related to their care. Building trust with patients and easing their anxieties can be accomplished through communication that is both open and compassionate from health-care providers. An additional factor that contributes significantly to the development of acceptance is the professionalization and customization of interactions. Increasing the degree of comfort experienced by patients and making interactions more seamless can be accomplished by tailoring interactions to the preferences of individual patients. It is possible for robots that are built to demonstrate social cues or personalized interactions, such as utilizing patients' names or adjusting to cultural norms, to boost the human-like features of interaction, which in turn promotes patient acceptance (Tigard et al., 2023).

It is equally important to have a solid understanding of the psychological effects that human-robot contact has on medical researchers and practitioners. Concerns can be alleviated and a smoother incor-poration into clinical workflows can be achieved through the implementation of training programme that familiarize healthcare personnel with robotic systems and the capabilities they possess. In addition, it is important to place an emphasis on ethical considerations concerning the outsourcing of work to robots and the preservation of the human-centered aspect of healthcare delivery. It is important to emphasize that robots are not intended to replace human care but rather to supplement it. This will help to encourage acceptability along with cooperation between healthcare personnel and robotic systems (Tang et al., 2023).

In nutshell principles of human-focused design are essential for the development of medical robots that are convenient to use and can be integrated into healthcare environments without any difficulty. It is essential to address the psychological components of human-robot interaction, such as patient wor-ries and acceptance, in order to guarantee a successful integration and to cultivate an environment that encourages collaboration between humans and robots in the delivery of healthcare. When it comes to unlocking the full potential of medical robots while concurrently placing an emphasis on patient-centered care, continuous improvement and considerate consideration of user wants and preferences are essential components (Tukhtakhodjaeva & Khayitova, 2023).

Recent Developments in Healthcare Robotics and the Potential Plans for the Future

When it comes to the use of robotics in the healthcare industry, the problems that you have mentioned—namely, the cost, the technological barriers, and the societal acceptance—are absolutely essential. On the other hand, the prospects for the future of healthcare robotics are encouraging, with a number of untapped frontiers and opportunities. Due to the significant initial investments required for research, implementation, and maintenance, robotics in the healthcare industry frequently incurs high costs. It is possible that expenses will decrease over time as technology continues to progress and become more popular. There is a pressing need to investigate the means by which these technologies might be made more inexpensive without sacrificing their quality (Tang et al., 2023).

The application of robotics in the medical field necessitates the utilization of cutting-edge technolo-gies such as neural networks, machine learning, and smart sensors. One of the most important things that needs to be done is to overcome the technical obstacles that are associated with accuracy, flexibility to different healthcare settings, compatibility with current technologies, and maintaining data security and privacy.

Acceptance by society: It is crucial that patients, healthcare providers, and society as a whole come to terms with the situation. In order to build trust in robotic technology, it is necessary to address issues around job relocation, dependability, moral concerns, and the idea that robots have supplanted human interaction & compassion in the healthcare industry.

The Prospects of the Future and the Uncharted Landscape: By analyzing huge volumes of patient data, robotics can support accurate and personalized treatments, which in turn enables individualized therapies and interventions. Precision medicine and personalized care are two fields that are becoming increasingly important (Firoozi & Firoozi, 2023).

Telehealth and Distant Medical Care: Improved robotics could make it possible to implement more advanced telemedicine practices, which would make it possible to do remote diagnostics, surgeries, and monitoring, particularly in locations that are under-served or more remote.

Robotics for Assistive Assistance and Rehabilitation: The ongoing development of robotics has the potential to revolutionize rehabilitation procedures, thereby assisting patients in regaining their mobility and independence following injuries or surgical procedures (Sahoo & Goswami, 2023).

Nanotechnology and Pharmaceutical Delivery: Miniaturized robots could be built to carry pharmaceuticals to specific places within the body, which could potentially reduce the number of adverse effects and improve the effectiveness of treatment (Fidan et al., 2023).

Surgical Robotics and Minimally Invasive Procedures: Robotics has the potential to continue develop in order to enable more precise and less invasive procedures, hence reducing the amount of time it takes for patients to recuperate and problems that may arise. Support for Mental Health Robots that are equipped with artificial intelligence could give support for mental health by assisting counsellor while offering camaraderie to patients. This would be especially useful in situations when there are few human resources available. When it comes to ethical and regulatory considerations, there is a need for continuous discussion and the establishment of rigorous ethical frameworks and laws. This is necessary in order to guarantee the responsible and ethical utilization of robots in patient care. The foreseeable future of medical robotics holds enormous potential, but in order to overcome hurdles and open these undiscovered frontiers in a responsible and ethical manner, it will take collaboration from technological designers, medical professionals, regulators, and the general public (Ramezani & Mohd, 2023).

Healthcare robotics has made considerable advancements recently, with robots playing important roles in patient care, surgery, and rehabilitation. Surgical robotics, such as the da Vinci Surgical System, have made significant advancements by allowing for precise and minimally invasive surgeries, ultimately decreasing patient trauma and recovery time. Robotic exoskeletons are now being used as effective tools in rehabilitation to help individuals with mobility problems regain movement and independence. In the future, healthcare robotics have great potential. Innovations may involve incorporating artificial intelligence to improve robot autonomy and decision-making skills, enabling the completion of more intricate tasks with increased efficiency and precision. Robots have the potential to take on increased responsibilities in telemedicine by aiding healthcare personnel in monitoring patients remotely and delivering care. Healthcare robots is advancing rapidly and has the potential to transform medical procedures, leading to better patient results and increased healthcare availability (Kaur,2023).

Augmented reality (AR) is growing rapidly into a revolutionary tool in healthcare robotics, transforming patient care, medical training, and surgical procedures. Augmented reality (AR) improves the functionality of robotic systems in many healthcare settings by superimposing digital data onto the real world as presented in figure 3 below:

AR-equipped robots in surgical settings offer surgeons immediate visual guidance by showing important information including patient anatomy, surgical planning, and instrument location immediately in their line of sight. This enhanced visualization enhances surgical accuracy, minimizes mistakes, and

Figure 3. Benefits of augmented reality (AR) in healthcare

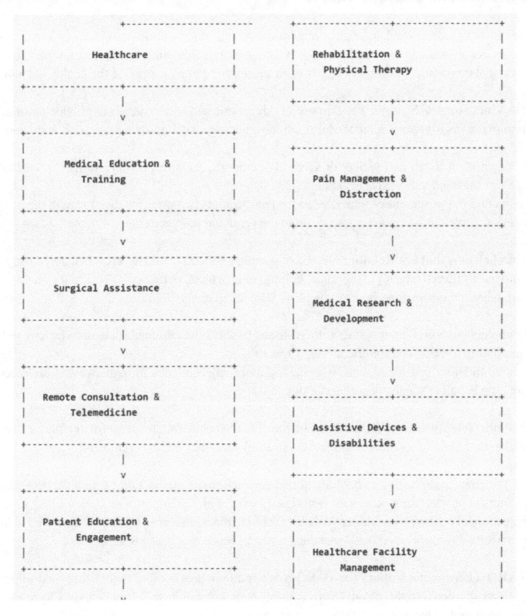

decreases operation duration's, ultimately resulting in improved patient results. AR-enhanced training modules allow medical personnel to practise difficult procedures in a realistic virtual environment, improving their skills and proficiency without endangering patient safety. Advancements in integrating augmented reality with healthcare robotics offer benefits that go beyond the operating room. Telemedicine consultations can utilize augmented reality (AR) to allow specialists in faraway regions to offer immediate guidance and assistance to healthcare providers in different areas. AR-enabled robotic exoskeletons and rehabilitation equipment provide personalized therapy experiences to assist patients in their recovery. Augmented reality shows great potential in improving healthcare robotics, which can lead to better patient care, enhanced medical education, and increased access to new medicines (Khaddad et al., 2023).

Case Studies and Success Stories

Robotics in the medical field has had a revolutionary impact, revolutionizing patient care, surgical procedures, rehabilitation, and other areas of healthcare. The following are some examples from the real world that demonstrate how robotics has been successfully implemented in the healthcare industry:

1. **Da Vinci Surgical System:** The purpose of this robotic surgical system is to provide assistance in minimally invasive surgical procedures while simultaneously improving precision and control.

    Implementation: Used in a variety of surgical operations, including hysterectomies, protectorates, and repair of the heart valve (Shakeel et al., 2023).
    A reduction in the amount of time needed for recuperation, a shorter length of stay in the hospital, and superior surgical outcomes in comparison to conventional procedures.

2. **Exoskeletons that are Robotic:** The use of wearable robotic exoskeletons is beneficial for people who have suffered injuries to the spinal column or neurological diseases because they assist in the rehabilitation process and improve mobility (Dicuonzo et al., 2023).

    The implementation of devices such as ReWalk and EksoGT, which enable patients who have reduced limb immobility to walk, is a significant step forward.
    Restored mobility, greater muscle strength, and more independence for patients who are receiving rehabilitation are all examples of successful outcomes.

3. **Robotic Telepresence Systems:** Through the use of a mobile robotic platform, telepresence robots make it possible to conduct healthcare counselling and track patients remotely.

    The implementation of this technology allows for the remote connection of medical professionals with patients in hospitals and other care facilities (Biswas et al., 2023).
    It is successful because it enables specialists to travel to places that are not adequately served, it makes timely consultations easier, and it reduces the amount of travel that patients need to do.

4. **PARO Therapeutic Robot:** The PARO robot is a therapeutic robot that is supposed to provide patients, particularly the elderly, with comfort and companionship. It is designed to resemble a newborn seal (Khang et al., 2023).

    In order to alleviate feelings of tension and loneliness among patients, this implementation is utilized in residential care facilities and hospitals.
    Patients have shown to experience an improvement in their mood, a reduction in stress, and an increase in social engagement that is successful.

5. **Automated Pharmacy Procedures Assisted by Robots:** In pharmacies, automated robots are responsible for the distribution of medications, the packaging of those medications, and the maintenance of inventory.

Utilization: Employed in healthcare facilities and drugstores to reduce the number of errors caused by human intervention and to streamline the distribution of medications.

Achieved success: increases accuracy, decreases the amount of time patients have to wait, and improves the overall efficiency of the pharmacy (Khang et al., 2023).

6. **Robert for Interactive Body Assistance, or RIBA:** Developed to provide assistance to healthcare professionals in the process of carrying and transporting patients, with the goal of lowering the likelihood of musculoskeletal injuries occurring.

Implementation: A tool that is utilised in healthcare facilities and hospitals to facilitate the transportation of patients (George et al., 2023).

Reduces the amount of physical strain that healthcare personnel are under, hence reducing the number of injuries that occur on the job and improving the safety of patient handling.

7. **The MiroSurge Surgical Robotic System:** A surgical robotic system of the next generation designed for minimally invasive surgical procedures.

Implementation: Used in a variety of surgical operations, including urological interventions and surgeries on the gastrointestinal tract (Hastuti, 2023).

This product is successful because it provides improved dexterity and precision, which ultimately results in improved surgical outcomes and less patient trauma. These examples illustrate the various applications of robotics in the healthcare industry, demonstrating how improvements in patient care, rehabilitation, surgical procedures, and overall medical management have been brought about by the implementation of these technologies. In spite of the fact that technological advancements are still being made, the possibility that robotics will further revolutionize healthcare remains hopeful.

Collaboration and Integration of Robotics

In order to push innovation and address complicated challenges, interdisciplinary collaboration is a cornerstone in the process of integrating robotics into healthcare. This collaboration helps to develop synergy across many fields, which promotes creativity. In order to successfully bridge the gap between robots and healthcare, it is necessary for specialists in engineering, medicine, ethics, and a variety of other fields to collaborate extensively. This collaboration presents its own unique set of problems, but it also offers a wide range of rewards over its whole (Kaur,2023).

The Advantages of Working With People From Different Fields

Combining the knowledge and experience of specialists from a variety of fields results in the generation of a pool of distinct viewpoints, which in turn leads to creativity and the resolution of problems. Within the fields of robotics and healthcare, this collaboration results in a variety of benefits, including the following:

Creative and Diverse ideas: Engineers, doctors, health care ethicists, and designers each contribute their own distinct ideas to the table, which helps to stimulate the development of creative robotic solutions that are specifically designed to meet the requirements of the healthcare industry. For example, the combination of the technical expertise of engineers with the awareness of patient requirements that clinicians possess results in robotic devices that are more effective and focused on the patient when used together (Hastuti, 2023).

Multidisciplinary problem-solving skills: Complex problems in healthcare demand solutions that take into account multiple dimensions. The capacity to work together makes it possible to take a holistic approach, which takes into account not only the technological feasibility but also the ethical ramifications, usability, and therapeutic efficacy of the solution. This results in solutions that are more complete and take into consideration a variety of other areas of patient care (George et al., 2023).

Enhanced Design and Execution: Teams from different disciplines expedite the establishment procedure through incorporating feedback from a wide variety of stakeholders at each stage. This results in accelerated development and implementation. This results in the developing, evaluating, and execution of technological advances in robotics in clinical settings occurring at a faster pace, hence accelerating the transition of these technologies from the laboratory to applications in the real world. Cooperation ensures that the final goods, such as robot medical equipment or structures, are more easy to use and matched with the requirements of both patients and healthcare practitioners. This results in an improved user experience. As a consequence, there is a rise in the acceptance and use of robotic technologies within the healthcare industry.

Problems That Arise While Working With People From Different Fields

Despite the fact that the benefits are enormous, managing interdisciplinary collaboration in the fields of robots and healthcare isn't devoid its difficulties:

Interaction Barriers: Professionals from various fields frequently have their own language and terminology that they use in their working lives. Filling in these interactions gaps is absolutely necessary in order to guarantee successful collaboration. Both misunderstandings and misinterpretations have the potential to impede progress and result in goals that are not aligned (George et al., 2023).

Differences in Priorities and Perspectives: various disciplines may place various parts of a project at the forefront of their priorities. For example, engineers may place a higher priority on the feasibility of the technical aspect, whereas healthcare providers may place a greater emphasis on the clinical effectiveness and patient safety. Creating solutions that are advantageous to both parties needs negotiation and compromise in order to achieve a balance between these interests.

The allocation of resources and the acquisition of funds might be difficult when it comes to projects that include multiple disciplines. It may be challenging for multidisciplinary groups to gain access to the resources they require since funding authorities may have stringent criteria or may favour research that is conducted within a single discipline (Khang et al., 2023).

Leadership and Team Dynamics: Managing diverse teams demands employing strong leadership and creating a work climate that is conducive to productivity. It is of the utmost importance to promote teamwork within the context of recognizing different skills and viewpoints. In order to achieve success, it is necessary to have leadership that encourages candid debate and mutual respect. The takeaway is that interdisciplinary collaboration in the field of robotics and healthcare is certainly beneficial, as it provides novel solutions that are tailored to meet the requirements of a wide range of healthcare requirements. In order to fully exploit the advantages of this joint method, it is essential to overcome obstacles to communication, to align priorities, to get finance, and to cultivate good team dynamics. Collaboration between disciplines will play a growing part in determining the future environment of robotic uses in healthcare as technological continues to evolve at a rapid pace. This framework provides a balanced analysis of this essential component by covering the benefits and limitations of multidisciplinary collaboration in robotics and healthcare within a scope of one thousand words. multidisciplinary collaboration is an important aspect. When necessary, adjustments can be made based on certain areas of attention or additional details that are desired.

Economic Viability of Healthcare Robotics

However, the economic sustainability of healthcare robots is still a complicated interplay of various aspects, despite the fact that it presents a potential route for revolutionizing medical practises. In the beginning, the beginning costs that are involved with the development and implementation of robots technology might be quite high. This encompasses activities such as research and development, as well as the acquisition of advanced machinery. Nevertheless, the potential cost reductions become apparent over time as a result of enhanced efficiency, precision, and a reduction in the amount of human error. Robotics has the potential to simplify repetitive procedures, improve workflows, and improve surgical precision, which will ultimately result in less time in the hospital, fewer problems, and reduced overall healthcare costs in the long run (Khang et al., 2023).

Additionally, as technology continues to progress and become more popular, economics of scale may bring down initial costs, which will make automation cheaper to use for a wider variety of healthcare settings. However, additional factors include the price of continuous maintenance and improvements, as well as professional development. In addition, while determining the financial viability of healthcare robots, it is essential to strike a balance between the initial expense and long-term cost savings. This balance is a significant factor in determining whether or not healthcare robotics will be adopted and integrated into healthcare systems around the world (Kaur,2023).

CONCLUSION

Robotics is entwined with the future health sector in ways that have the potential to revolutionize patient care, expedite processes, and improve medical outcomes. As we come to the end of this investigation into the possibilities that robots could bring to the field of healthcare, it is abundantly clear that these technologies have a great deal of promise. Professionals in the medical field can rely on robots as trusted allies because of their accurateness, efficiency, and capacity to carry out activities that must be performed repeatedly without error. They not only contribute to the enhancement of human abilities but also limit the margin for error, whether they are used to assist in surgical procedures or to handle regular procedures. In addition, the use of artificial intelligence (AI) makes it possible for robots to acquire knowledge, modify their behaviour, and personalize patient care, which results in individualized therapies and enhanced diagnostics. This combination of artificial intelligence and robotics has the potential to democratize healthcare by making specialized therapies more accessible on a global scale.

In spite of the fact that the future appears to be bright, difficulties still exist. There are a number of issues that need to be carefully considered, including the ethical use of artificial intelligence, the protection of data, and the eventual elimination of specific jobs due to automation. The success of this marriage between robots and healthcare is contingent on collaboration between several parties, including scientists, engineers, healthcare professionals and legislators. Managing obstacles and realizing the full capabilities of robotics in the healthcare industry can be accomplished through the promotion of inter-disciplinary collaboration. In summary, the recommendation for the foreseeable future of healthcare is to embrace robotics as a force that can alter the industry. We are able to set out on an adventure towards a healthcare landscape that is more effective, readily available and patient-centered if we harness their capabilities in a responsible and ethical manner.

REFERENCES

Abbasimoshaei, A., Chinnakkonda Ravi, A. K., & Kern, T. A. (2023). Development of a New Control System for a Rehabilitation Robot Using Electrical Impedance Tomography and Artificial Intelligence. *Biomimetics*, 8(5), 420. doi:10.3390/biomimetics8050420 PMID:37754171

Ahmad, A., Tariq, A., Hussain, H. K., & Gill, A. Y. (2023). Revolutionizing Healthcare: How Deep Learning is poised to Change the Landscape of Medical Diagnosis and Treatment. Journal of Computer Networks. *Architecture and High-Performance Computing*, 5(2), 458–471. doi:10.47709/cnahpc.v5i2.2350

Al Kuwaiti, A., Nazer, K., Al-Reedy, A., Al-Shehri, S., Al-Muhanna, A., Subbarayalu, A. V., Al Muhanna, D., & Al-Muhanna, F. A. (2023). A Review of the Role of Artificial Intelligence in Healthcare. *Journal of Personalized Medicine*, 13(6), 951. doi:10.3390/jpm13060951 PMID:37373940

Ali, M. (2023). A Comprehensive Review of AI's Impact on Healthcare: Revolutionizing Diagnostics and Patient Care. *BULLET: Jurnal Multidisiplin Ilmu*, 2(4), 1163–1173.

Alowais, S. A., Alghamdi, S. S., Alsuhebany, N., Alqahtani, T., Alshaya, A. I., Almohareb, S. N., Al-dairem, A., Alrashed, M., Bin Saleh, K., Badreldin, H. A., Al Yami, M. S., Al Harbi, S., & Albekairy, A. M. (2023). Revolutionizing healthcare: The role of artificial intelligence in clinical practice. *BMC Medical Education*, 23(1), 689. doi:10.1186/s12909-023-04698-z PMID:37740191

Biswas, S., Pillai, S., Kadhim, H. M., Salam, Z. A., & Marhoon, H. A. (2023, September). Building business resilience and productivity in the healthcare industry with the integration of robotic process automation technology. In AIP Conference Proceedings (Vol. 2736, No. 1). AIP Publishing. doi:10.1063/5.0171098

Deo, N., & Anjankar, A. (2023). Artificial intelligence with robotics in healthcare: A narrative review of its viability in India. *Cureus*, 15(5). doi:10.7759/cureus.39416 PMID:37362504

Dicuonzo, G., Donofrio, F., Fusco, A., & Shini, M. (2023). Healthcare system: Moving forward with artificial intelligence. *Technovation*, 120, 102510. doi:10.1016/j.technovation.2022.102510

Doshi, R., Hiran, K. K., Gök, M., El-kenawy, E. S. M., Badr, A., & Abotaleb, M. (2023). Artificial Intelligence's Significance in Diseases with Malignant Tumours. *Mesopotamian Journal of Artificial Intelligence in Healthcare*, 2023, 35–39.

Fidan, I., Huseynov, O., Ali, M. A., Alkunte, S., Rajeshirke, M., Gupta, A., Hasanov, S., Tantawi, K., Yasa, E., Yilmaz, O., Loy, J., Popov, V., & Sharma, A. (2023). Recent inventions in additive manufacturing: Holistic review. *Inventions (Basel, Switzerland)*, 8(4), 103. doi:10.3390/inventions8040103

Firoozi, A. A., & Firoozi, A. A. (2023). A systematic review of the role of 4D printing in sustainable civil engineering solutions. *Heliyon*, 9(10), e20982. doi:10.1016/j.heliyon.2023.e20982 PMID:37928382

George, A. S., George, A. H., & Martin, A. G. (2023). ChatGPT and the Future of Work: A Comprehensive Analysis of AI's Impact on Jobs and Employment. *Partners Universal International Innovation Journal, 1*(3), 154–186.

Goel, P., Jhanwar, N., Jain, P., Khatri, S., & Hiran, K. K. (2023, August). Efficient Blood Availability for Targeted Individuals Through Cloud Computing Web Application. In *2023 International Conference on Emerging Trends in Networks and Computer Communications (ETNCC)* (pp. 1-7). IEEE. 10.1109/ETNCC59188.2023.10284940

Gupta, A. K., Srinivasulu, A., Hiran, K. K., Sreenivasulu, G., Rajeyyagari, S., & Subramanyam, M. (2022). Prediction of omicron virus using combined extended convolutional and recurrent neural networks technique on CT-scan images. *Interdisciplinary Perspectives on Infectious Diseases, 2022*, 2022. doi:10.1155/2022/1525615 PMID:36562006

Harry, A. (2023). The Future of Medicine: Harnessing the Power of AI for Revolutionizing Healthcare. *International Journal of Multidisciplinary Sciences and Arts, 2*(1), 36–47. doi:10.47709/ijmdsa.v2i1.2395

Hastuti, R., & Syafruddin. (2023). Ethical Considerations in the Age of Artificial Intelligence: Balancing Innovation and Social Values. *West Science Social and Humanities Studies, 1*(02), 76–87. doi:10.58812/wsshs.v1i02.191

Jain, R. K., Hiran, K. K., & Maheshwari, R. (2023, April). Lung Cancer Detection Using Machine Learning Algorithms. In *2023 International Conference on Computational Intelligence, Communication Technology and Networking (CICTN)* (pp. 516-521). IEEE. 10.1109/CICTN57981.2023.10141467

Kato, K., Yoshimi, T., Aimoto, K., Sato, K., Itoh, N., & Kondo, I. (2023). Reduction of multiple-caregiver assistance through the long-term use of a transfer support robot in a nursing facility. *Assistive Technology, 35*(3), 271–278. doi:10.1080/10400435.2022.2039324 PMID:35320681

Kaur, J. (2023). Robotic Process Automation in Healthcare Sector. In *E3S Web of Conferences* (Vol. 391, p. 01008). EDP Sciences.

Kaur, J. (2023, May). How is Robotic Process Automation Revolutionising the Way Healthcare Sector Works? In International Conference on Information, Communication and Computing Technology (pp. 1037-1055). Singapore: Springer Nature Singapore. 10.1007/978-981-99-5166-6_70

Kaur, J. (2024). Green Finance 2.0: Pioneering Pathways for Sustainable Development and Health Through Future Trends and Innovations. In Sustainable Investments in Green Finance (pp. 294-319). IGI Global.

Khaddad, A., Bernhard, J. C., Margue, G., Michiels, C., Ricard, S., Chandelon, K., Bladou, F., Bourdel, N., & Bartoli, A. (2023). A survey of augmented reality methods to guide minimally invasive partial nephrectomy. *World Journal of Urology, 41*(2), 335–343. doi:10.1007/s00345-022-04078-0 PMID:35776173

Khang, A., Hahanov, V., Litvinova, E., Chumachenko, S., Hajimahmud, A. V., Ali, R. N., & Anh, P. T. N. (2023). The Analytics of Hospitality of Hospitals in a Healthcare Ecosystem. In *Data-Centric AI Solutions and Emerging Technologies in the Healthcare Ecosystem* (pp. 39–61). CRC Press. doi:10.1201/9781003356189-4

Kim, M., Zhang, Y., & Jin, S. (2023). Soft tissue surgical robot for minimally invasive surgery: A review. *Biomedical Engineering Letters*, *13*(4), 1–9. doi:10.1007/s13534-023-00326-3 PMID:37872994

Kumar, P., Chauhan, S., & Awasthi, L. K. (2023). Artificial intelligence in healthcare: Review, ethics, trust challenges & future research directions. *Engineering Applications of Artificial Intelligence*, *120*, 105894. doi:10.1016/j.engappai.2023.105894

Lakhwani, K., Bhargava, S., Hiran, K. K., Bundele, M. M., & Somwanshi, D. (2020, December). Prediction of the onset of diabetes using artificial neural network and Pima Indians diabetes dataset. In *2020 5th IEEE International Conference on Recent Advances and Innovations in Engineering (ICRAIE)* (pp. 1-6). IEEE. 10.1109/ICRAIE51050.2020.9358308

Lochan, K., Suklyabaidya, A., & Roy, B. K. (2023). Medical and healthcare robots in India. In *Medical and Healthcare Robotics* (pp. 221–236). Academic Press. doi:10.1016/B978-0-443-18460-4.00010-X

Mahmoud, H., Aljaldi, F., El-Fiky, A., Battecha, K., Thabet, A., Alayat, M., & Ibrahim, A. (2023). Artificial Intelligence machine learning and conventional physical therapy for upper limb outcome in patients with stroke: A systematic review and meta-analysis. *European Review for Medical and Pharmacological Sciences*, *27*(11). PMID:37318455

Matsuzaki, H., & Gliesche, P. (2023). Robots and Norms of Care: A Comparative Analysis of the Reception of Robotic Assistance in Nursing. In Social Robots in Social Institutions (pp. 90-99). IOS Press. doi:10.3233/FAIA220607

Minopoulos, G. M., Memos, V. A., Stergiou, K. D., Stergiou, C. L., & Psannis, K. E. (2023). A Medical Image Visualization Technique Assisted with AI-Based Haptic Feedback for Robotic Surgery and Healthcare. *Applied Sciences (Basel, Switzerland)*, *13*(6), 3592. doi:10.3390/app13063592

Murakami, Y., Honaga, K., Kono, H., Haruyama, K., Yamaguchi, T., Tani, M., Isayama, R., Takakura, T., Tanuma, A., Hatori, K., Wada, F., & Fujiwara, T. (2023). New Artificial Intelligence-Integrated Electromyography-Driven Robot Hand for Upper Extremity Rehabilitation of Patients With Stroke: A Randomized, Controlled Trial. *Neurorehabilitation and Neural Repair*, *37*(5), 15459683231166939. doi:10.1177/15459683231166939 PMID:37039319

Nwadiokwu, O. T. (2023). Examining the Impact and Challenges of Artificial Intelligence (AI) in Healthcare. *Edward Waters University Undergraduate Research Journal, 1*(1).

Ohneberg, C., Stöbich, N., Warmbein, A., Rathgeber, I., Mehler-Klamt, A. C., Fischer, U., & Eberl, I. (2023). Assistive robotic systems in nursing care: A scoping review. *BMC Nursing*, *22*(1), 1–15. doi:10.1186/s12912-023-01230-y PMID:36934280

Ragno, L., Borboni, A., Vannetti, F., Amici, C., & Cusano, N. (2023). Application of Social Robots in Healthcare: Review on Characteristics, Requirements, Technical Solutions. *Sensors (Basel)*, *23*(15), 6820. doi:10.3390/s23156820 PMID:37571603

Ramasamy, J., & Doshi, R. (2022). Machine learning in cyber physical systems for healthcare: brain tumor classification from MRI using transfer learning framework. In *Real-Time Applications of Machine Learning in Cyber-Physical Systems* (pp. 65–76). IGI global. doi:10.4018/978-1-7998-9308-0.ch005

Ramasamy, J., Doshi, R., & Hiran, K. K. (2021, August). Segmentation of brain tumor using deep learning methods: a review. In *Proceedings of the International Conference on Data Science, Machine Learning and Artificial Intelligence* (pp. 209-215). ACM. 10.1145/3484824.3484876

Ramezani, M., & Mohd Ripin, Z. (2023). 4D printing in biomedical engineering: Advancements, challenges, and future directions. *Journal of Functional Biomaterials*, *14*(7), 347. doi:10.3390/jfb14070347 PMID:37504842

Rivero-Moreno, Y., Echevarria, S., Vidal-Valderrama, C., Stefano-Pianetti, L., Cordova-Guilarte, J., Navarro-Gonzalez, J., & Avila, G. L. D. (2023). Robotic Surgery: A Comprehensive Review of the Literature and Current Trends. *Cureus*, *15*(7). doi:10.7759/cureus.42370 PMID:37621804

Sahoo, S. K., & Goswami, S. S. (2023). A comprehensive review of multiple criteria decision-making (MCDM) Methods: Advancements, applications, and future directions. *Decision Making Advances*, *1*(1), 25–48. doi:10.31181/dma1120237

Schönmann, M., Bodenschatz, A., Uhl, M., & Walkowitz, G. (2023). The Care-Dependent are Less Averse to Care Robots: An Empirical Comparison of Attitudes. *International Journal of Social Robotics*, *15*(6), 1–18. doi:10.1007/s12369-023-01003-2 PMID:37359432

Shakeel, T., Habib, S., Boulila, W., Koubaa, A., Javed, A. R., Rizwan, M., Gadekallu, T. R., & Sufiyan, M. (2023). A survey on COVID-19 impact in the healthcare domain: Worldwide market implementation, applications, security and privacy issues, challenges and future prospects. *Complex & Intelligent Systems*, *9*(1), 1027–1058. doi:10.1007/s40747-022-00767-w PMID:35668731

Srinivasulu, A., Gupta, A., Hiran, K., Barua, and, T., & Sreenivasulu, G. Omi-cron Virus Data Analytics Using Extended RNN Technique. *Int J Cancer Res Ther, 7*(3), 122.

Stasevych, M., & Zvarych, V. (2023). Innovative robotic technologies and artificial intelligence in pharmacy and medicine: Paving the way for the future of health care—a review. *Big Data and Cognitive Computing*, *7*(3), 147. doi:10.3390/bdcc7030147

Tang, L., Li, J., & Fantus, S. (2023). Medical artificial intelligence ethics: A systematic review of empirical studies. *Digital Health*, *9*, 20552076231186064. doi:10.1177/20552076231186064 PMID:37434728

Tigard, D. W., Braun, M., Breuer, S., Ritt, K., Fiske, A., McLennan, S., & Buyx, A. (2023). Toward best practices in embedded ethics: Suggestions for interdisciplinary technology development. *Robotics and Autonomous Systems*, *167*, 104467. doi:10.1016/j.robot.2023.104467

Tukhtakhodjaeva, F. S., & Khayitova, I. I. (2023). APPLICATION AND USE OF AI (ARTIFICIAL INTELLIGENCE) IN MEDICINE. *Educational Research in Universal Sciences*, *2*(9), 302–309.

Vallès-Peris, N., & Domènech, M. (2023). Caring in the in-between: A proposal to introduce responsible AI and robotics to healthcare. *AI & Society*, *38*(4), 1685–1695. doi:10.1007/s00146-021-01330-w

Wang, C., Liu, S., Yang, H., Guo, J., Wu, Y., & Liu, J. (2023). Ethical considerations of using ChatGPT in health care. *Journal of Medical Internet Research*, *25*, e48009. doi:10.2196/48009 PMID:37566454

Yeisson, R. M., Sophia, E., Vidal-Valderrama, C., Luigi, P., Jesus, C. G., Navarro-Gonzalez, J., & Katheryn, A. A. (2023). Robotic Surgery: A Comprehensive Review of the Literature and Current Trends. *Cureus*, *15*(7). PMID:37621804

Chapter 13
Augmented Reality Gamification for Promoting Healthy Lifestyles and Wellbeing in Children

Kali Charan Modak
https://orcid.org/0000-0002-2980-5422
IPS Academy, India

Sanju Mahawar
IPS Academy, India

Pallabi Mukherjee
IPS Academy, India

ABSTRACT

In recent years, the merging of augmented reality (AR) technology and gamification has received substantial attention, providing fresh pathways for engaging youngsters in encouraging healthy lifestyles and general well-being. This book chapter delves into the intersection of augmented reality and gamification as a novel method to addressing the growing concerns about childhood health issues. This chapter investigates how these technologies might effectively grab children's interest and empower them to make healthier choices by synergistically combining the immersive experiences of AR with the motivational features of gamification. This chapter elucidates the psychological underpinnings of gamification through a thorough assessment of relevant literature, emphasising its ability to inspire intrinsic motivation, foster skill development, and increase engagement. Furthermore, it delves into the pedagogical ideas that underpin great AR design, emphasising the significance of developing immersive and interactive experiences that smoothly integrate with real-world environments.

INTRODUCTION

Augmented Reality, Gamification, and Both Combined

Gamification of augmented reality (AR) entails incorporating aspects of game mechanics and design into augmented reality experiences. In numerous situations, this combination improves user experiences,

DOI: 10.4018/979-8-3693-1123-3.ch013

interaction, and engagement. Augmented reality (AR) projects pictures, animations, or information from the digital world onto the physical world. Mobile phones, tablets, augmented reality (AR) glasses, and another wearable tech are frequently used to experience this. By introducing interactive virtual features, augmented reality (AR) enhances the physical environment.

Gamification is the application of game-like components to non-game environments, such as rewards, challenges, and competition. It seeks to engage and inspire people by appealing to their innate urges for success, rivalry, and advancement. When AR and gamification are combined, an engaging and dynamic experience is produced. AR enables the insertion of digital items into the user's actual surroundings. These objects may be used as challenges, characters, or other game components. Users may use their smartphones to engage physically with these items. User engagement is boosted through gamification principles like points, badges, leaderboards, and awards. Higher levels of engagement and sustained interest in the AR experience may result from this.

Users are frequently encouraged by Augmented Reality Gamification (ARG) to explore their environment in order to find buried game features. The experience may be made more immersive and interesting by tying this discovery to incentives or goals. ARG may be applied to education to make learning more engaging and fun. Users can answer questions or perform activities to learn more about an area, for instance, by using AR material to bring historical sites to life (Barua et al., 2020; Skouby et al., 2022).

Businesses employ augmented reality gamification to develop engaging brand experiences. Scavenger hunts, interactive ads, or user-participable promotions can all be used in this way. Users are encouraged to collaborate and engage in friendly rivalry through leaderboards and social sharing tools, which also encourage them to tell others about their experiences. ARG can be used to promote exercise. During outdoor activities, fitness applications may utilize augmented reality to replicate virtual challenges or rewards. By fusing digital and physical aspects, gamification-based AR experiences and games may provide fun on a whole new level (Srinivasulu et al., 2022; Jain et al., 2024).

It should be noted that creating successful ARG experiences necessitates a thorough comprehension of both AR technology and game design fundamentals. Engagement, usability, and meaningful interactions are all balanced in successful implementations. The potential for inventive and imaginative ARG experiences will probably increase as technology progresses across a range of sectors and areas.

Impact and Uses in Augmented Reality in Variety of Disciplines

There are many uses for augmented reality (AR) in a variety of disciplines and sectors. In order to improve our perception and engagement with the environment, it includes superimposing digital information, objects, or experiences over the actual world. Here are some essential augmented reality uses:

Gaming and entertainment: By fusing virtual aspects with the actual environment, augmented reality has revolutionized gaming. Players are drawn into actual spaces by immersive experiences created by games like Pokémon GO and augmented reality escape rooms.

Retail and e-commerce: Before making a purchase, shoppers may see things in their actual surroundings thanks to augmented reality (AR). AR may improve the shopping experience with virtual try-ons for apparel, furniture layout, and cosmetics simulations, for instance.

Education and Training: AR provides visual and interactive learning opportunities. Through interactive textbooks, historical reenactments, and 3D models, students may investigate challenging ideas. Additionally, it is utilized to simulate real-world situations for technical training (Rathi et al., 2023; Patel et al., 2022).

Healthcare: During surgical training, augmented reality (AR) can help surgeons visualize anatomical features or facilitate procedure practice. By superimposing medical data on patient bodies, AR also helps doctors plan operations and diagnose illnesses (Doshi et al., 2023).

Architecture and design: Using augmented reality, architects and designers may see their creations in actual environments. Before construction even starts, clients may view how a structure or interior design will appear.

Travel & tourism: By offering interactive guides, historical details, and virtual tours of places, AR improves travel and tourist experiences. More interesting ways for visitors to learn about their surroundings are available (Hiran et al., 2023).

Advertising and marketing: Companies employ augmented reality to make interactive commercials that draw in customers. Interactive material from AR campaigns may bring traditional media, like as posters and billboards, to life.

Automotive Industry: AR head-up displays (HUDs) project information onto a vehicle's windscreen, such as speed, navigation, and warnings. This technology minimizes distractions while keeping drivers informed (Mishra et al., 2021).

Real estate: Home and flat purchasers may digitally tour properties using augmented reality. This saves time and enables prospective buyers to see a room equipped.

Manufacturing and maintenance: AR may direct employees through challenging maintenance and assembly procedures. It immediately overlays information and directions onto the machinery.

Social media and Communication: On apps like Snapchat and Instagram, augmented reality (AR) filters and effects have gained popularity, enabling users to include virtual components in their images and videos.

Sports and fitness: By offering real-time data overlays during broadcasts, augmented reality improves sports experiences. Athletes to train by visualizing motions and evaluating performance may use AR.

Museums and cultural landmarks: AR brings historical artifacts and settings to life in these settings. Visitors may engage in interactive virtual displays while learning about history.

Emergency Services: AR helps first responders by giving them up-to-the-second knowledge of their surroundings. While exploring new places, firefighters are able to examine floor layouts and other important information.

Navigation and way finding: AR navigation applications direct users by superimposing virtual arrows and markers over the actual world, making it simpler to get around inconvenient places.

These are only a handful of the numerous uses for augmented reality. As technology develops, new applications for augmented reality (AR) are opening up in a variety of sectors, providing creative ways to improve user experiences, education, productivity, and more.

Augmented Reality in Health

By utilizing its interactive and immersive features, augmented reality (AR) has the potential to benefit health in a number of ways. Here are some ways that AR may support the advancement of health and wellbeing:

Fitness and physical activity: By making physical activity into a game, AR may promote fitness and physical activity. Users of fitness applications may create interactive challenges that encourage them to run, walk, or carry out particular activities by superimposing virtual components on the actual environment. With the help of gamification, exercise becomes more interesting and enjoyable.

Healthy Eating Patterns: AR can offer visual signals to assist consumers in selecting healthier foods. Through a smartphone camera, apps might superimpose nutritional data, serving sizes, and advice for healthy meals on actual goods.

Medical Education and Training: AR may be used to improve training and education for medical practitioners. Surgeons may practice treatments on virtual patients before conducting them on real ones, and medical students can visualize intricate anatomical features in 3D.

Physical Rehabilitation: By guiding patients through exercises and movements, AR can help with physical therapy and rehabilitation. Virtual coaching and real-time feedback can assist guarantee optimal technique and advancement.

Stress management and mindfulness: AR apps may lead users through meditation and relaxation techniques, fostering a virtual environment that promotes stress management and mental health.

Disease Awareness and Prevention: AR may offer engaging learning opportunities to spread knowledge about illnesses, their causes, and effective preventative methods. Users can discover health dangers and management techniques (Gupta et al., 2022).

Patient Education: Using AR, patients' comprehension of medical issues and treatment regimens can be improved. It can help people better understand their medical conditions by visualizing difficult medical ideas.

Remote Consultations: By enabling healthcare professionals to conduct patient assessments remotely, augmented reality technology can support telemedicine. During virtual consultations, doctors can overlay medical information on a patient's body to provide visual explanations.

Pharmacy and medication management: By scanning prescription labels, augmented reality (AR) apps may assist users identify drugs and give dose guidelines, reminders, and potential interactions.

Social Support and Connection: AR-based online forums and support groups can link people with related health objectives or issues. Users can exchange stories, suggestions, and words of support.

Injury Prevention: Using augmented reality (AR), users may learn how to avoid injuries by simulating risky circumstances.

Healthy Workplace Procedures: In order to decrease strain and advance employee wellbeing, ergonomic procedures, appropriate posture, and frequent breaks may all be promoted in the workplace via AR.

Visualizing Health Data: AR makes it simpler to track progress and make wise health decisions by superimposing current health information, such heart rate and step count, into the user's field of view.

Medication Adherence: Using AR reminders and visual cues, users may be reminded to take their prescriptions on schedule and in the proper dosage.

Recreation and mental health: AR may provide immersive spaces for stress-relief, meditation, and relaxation, which supports general mental health.

These apps might enable people to take a more active part in their health and well-being by using AR's capacity to increase engagement and interaction. However, it's crucial to make sure that accuracy, security, and user privacy are all taken into consideration while developing AR health apps.

Augmented Reality in Education

A potent tool in teaching is augmented reality (AR), a technology that projects digital material over the physical world. Augmented reality in learning offers a wide range of advantages that change how students interact with educational information by fusing virtual and real-world aspects. The potential of augmented reality to improve interactive learning, increase student engagement, and increase information retention are highlighted in this article's discussion of the nine advantages of augmented reality in education.

By providing improved interactive learning experiences, augmented reality revolutionizes traditional education. Through immersive and interactive components, augmented reality (AR) allows students to actively engage with the subject matter, in contrast to passive learning approaches. For instance, by enabling students to see three-dimensional models of molecules or explore virtual settings replicating scientific events, augmented reality (AR) in science lectures may bring complicated scientific concepts to life. With this hands-on method, kids may engage with the material in a concrete and meaningful way while also fostering their curiosity and encouraging discovery. As students may participate in group activities where they collaborate to complete virtual simulations or solve issues, AR also encourages collaborative learning. The interactive element of augmented reality in education improves student engagement while also deepening their comprehension and memory of material.

Improved interaction while learning: Students typically want for more engaging and dynamic learning experiences because traditional classroom environments sometimes depend on passive learning techniques. However, augmented reality transforms the educational scene by providing improved interactive learning options. AR helps students to actively connect with the material by integrating virtual components, making theoretical notions into concrete experiences. For instance, by enabling students to see three-dimensional models or carry out virtual experiments, augmented reality (AR) may bring complicated scientific phenomena to life in science lectures.

Increased involvement of students: The capacity of augmented reality to greatly raise student involvement is one of the major advantages of the technology in education. Sometimes traditional lectures and texts fail to hold students' interest and provide inert learning experiences. However, using augmented reality for learning modifies the procedure by generating an engaging environment that captures the attention of pupils. AR makes subjects come to life by superimposing digital material on the actual world, which makes studying more enjoyable and engaging.

Enhanced memory for information: A potential answer to the problem of information retention in education is augmented reality. Since students may find it difficult to relate abstract ideas to practical applications, traditional teaching approaches sometimes struggle to ensure long-term retention of information. But augmented reality (AR) offers a holistic learning environment that improves memory retention and recall.

Personalized education: For each learner, a unique learning experience may be created using augmented reality. AR may offer individualized help and challenges by changing the material and interactions based on a student's development and skills. Virtual reality (AR) can accommodate various learning methods, paces, and preferences through adaptive feedback and specialized virtual settings. This tailored approach improves student understanding and engagement, which results in more successful learning outcomes.

Application in the real world: The capacity of augmented reality (AR) in education to close the gap between classroom learning and practical application is one of its great advantages. By superimposing virtual features over actual settings, augmented reality (AR) helps pupils relate their academic knowledge to real-world situations. The use of augmented reality (AR) immerses students in actual experiences, preparing them for future occupations and real-life issues. Examples include understanding architecture through the construction of virtual buildings or practicing medical procedures on fictitious patients.

Cultural and global viewpoints: Through the use of augmented reality, students may access viewpoints from around the world and from various cultural backgrounds. Students may experience foreign cultures, customs, and languages without leaving the classroom thanks to augmented reality (AR) through virtual travel experiences, language translations, or interactive cultural displays. Students are better prepared to succeed in a globalized environment because to this exposure to many cultures, which also promotes empathy, cultural awareness, and global citizenship.

Motivation and game development: Augmented reality has the ability to make use of gamification components, turning the educational process into a fun and inspiring adventure. With the use of game-like elements like challenges, prizes, and progress monitoring, augmented reality (AR) may make learning fun and promote healthy competition among students. Since students are motivated by their desire to complete tasks, gain badges, or advance to higher levels, gamification in education using augmented reality (AR) encourages intrinsic motivation. The motivation, perseverance, and general enjoyment of the learning process among students are all increased by this gamified method.

By delivering improved interactive learning experiences, raising student engagement, and enhancing information retention, augmented reality is reshaping the educational environment. It is clear from real-world applications of augmented reality in education that this technology has the ability to transform conventional learning by making it more engaging, interactive, and efficient. Teachers have the chance to develop engaging learning environments that educate students for the possibilities and challenges of the future as they embrace modern technology and take use of its advantages. We can usher in a new era of education that promotes creativity, critical thinking, and lifelong learning by using the potential of augmented reality in the classroom.

How ARG Can Be Used for Promoting Health and Wellbeing in Children

Gamification of augmented reality can be an effective strategy for encouraging kids to lead healthy lives and to take care of themselves. You can inspire kids to be more active, make healthier choices, and form good habits by fusing interactive technology with fun games.

Here are some suggestions about how to use ARG towards this goal:

- **Outdoor Adventure Quests:**

Make an augmented reality game that takes kids on outdoor adventures to collect virtual prizes, solve puzzles, or accomplish tasks. Kids could be inspired by these adventures to explore their neighborhoods, parks, or nature trails, developing a passion for the great outdoors.

- **Virtual Fitness Challenges:**

Create an augmented reality program that monitors physical activity like running, leaping, and walking. By completing tasks, kids may receive points and prizes, which would motivate them to keep active while having fun.

- **Healthy Eating Choices:**

Use augmented reality to superimpose virtual healthy food products on actual things. These virtual delicacies were available for kids to "collect" and receive points for throughout the day when they made healthier dietary choices.

- **Interactive Learning:**

Create augmented reality (AR) experiences that teach children about nutrition, portion control, and the advantages of various foods. Children may learn the value of a balanced diet by making learning interactive and aesthetically appealing.

- **Mindfulness and Relaxation:**

Create augmented reality (AR) experiences that lead kids through simple yoga positions, breathing exercises, or mindfulness activities. These pursuits can support mental health and stress reduction.

- **Gardening and Nature Connection:**

Create an augmented reality (AR) software that educates children about gardening and links them to nature. As kids study various plants and their life cycles, virtual garden plots might be maintained and grown.

- **Hydration Reminder Games:**

Make augmented reality games that motivate youngsters to frequently drink water. Children could see fictitious water droplets or figures, encouraging them to drink water throughout the day.

- **Virtual Pet and Avatar:**

Create an augmented reality game where youngsters look after an avatar or virtual pet. The health of the pet may be related to actual behaviors, such going for walks or consuming nutritious foods.

- **Community Challenges:**

Create online contests where kids may work together or compete to accomplish health-related objectives. These tests might be based on the number of steps taken, the number of fruits and vegetables ingested, or the number of hours spent exercising.

- **Reward System:**

Create a system of rewards whereby kids may collect virtual money or stuff to use in customizing their avatars or unlocked new augmented reality activities. This encourages continuing use of the software.

- **Educational Workshops:**

Workshops on subjects like physical fitness, healthy eating, and mental wellbeing should be combined with AR. Children might take part in online activities that teach and encourage good behaviors.

- **Family Engagement:**

Create AR games that parents and kids may play together to promote family interaction. This encourages the family unit to take a comprehensive approach to health and wellbeing.

Age-appropriate content, safety precautions, and user experience are all important factors to take into account when building AR gamification experiences for children to promote a healthy lifestyle and well-being. Your AR gamification efforts can benefit children's lives if you collaborate with specialists in child development, health, and education.

REVIEW OF LITERATURE

In this article, Raja, M., & Priya, G. L. (2023, p. 311) explore AR and VR for sustainable education using a relative framework. This study's purpose is to understand AR and VR applications to encourage students' desire to study. This article describes why the extensive acceptance of AR and VR in education and the reason behind this may be the technology revolution which helps the many constraints and glitches that face the implementation of AR and VR in education. AR and VR applications enhance educational experiences by providing elements of diverse sensory with multimodal atmosphere. The study concludes the unique strategies that encourage students' desire to study using AR and VR application.

Bakır et al (2023, p.1) explains that Augmented reality, or AR, is a relatively new technology that enhances one's experience of reality by combining virtual and physical environments. With the use of computer-generated atmosphere, augmented reality (AR) creates a unique view of reality that is interactive and real-time, connecting virtual and real-world objects. Recently, the use of augmented reality (AR) technology in medicine has grown significantly along with other aided technologies, ranging from clinical practice to teaching. AR immersions have been made possible by the capacity to widely deploy the real atmosphere, which offers advantages over conventional techniques. The study's goal is to perform a systematic evaluation of AR usage in order to gain a better understanding of how gamification and AR use may impact patients in mental health-related scenarios.

Singh, G. et al (2023, p. 93) stated that the development of immersive technologies, fusing the real world with virtual reality has made it feasible to produce immersive experiences. Digital technologies and affordances that duplicate reality in different ways comprise augmented reality (AR), virtual reality (VR), and mixed reality (MR). By offering extended reality views, immersive technology in clinical research, psychology, and medical science can benefit physicians, surgeons, and patients. Creating an environment that is stimulating is greatly aided by immersive technologies like virtual reality and augmented reality.

Blanco, D. et al (2023, p. 1) Virtual reality environments (VREs) are becoming more and more popular in psychological assessment and treatment. Fewer studies have examined the use of VREs with children and adolescents; the majority of research has been on its application in adult psychological illnesses. In order to give an overview of the current status of the literature and suggest future research paths, a comprehensive scoping review of the literature was conducted to determine how VREs have been employed in the assessment and treatment of mental health issues in children. Additionally, there is growing evidence in favour of VRE deep breathing exercises for anxiety, VRE-assisted treatment for internet gaming problems and anorexia nervosa, and VRE body image assessment in anorexia nervosa patients. The study comes to the conclusion that there is some potential for using VRE assessments and therapies for childhood mental health issues in the current literature, especially for anxiety-related illnesses including social anxiety and specific phobias.

Chamberland, C. et al (2024, p. 153) in this research it is demonstrated that the use of virtual reality as a non-pharmacological intervention can effectively reduce anxiety in pediatric patients. In addition to having certain useful advantages over virtual reality, augmented reality is a more recent immersive technology that also appears to have positive effects on anxiety. This study's primary goal was to ascertain whether augmented reality could help pediatric patients having elective day operations feel less anxious before surgery.

AR and gamification are emerging as potent tools for encouraging healthy lifestyles and general well-being in youngsters. (Bacca et al., 2014) highlight the potential of AR in education, paving the way for its use in health awareness and habit formation in youngsters. (Brown and Cairns 2016) investigate the immersive aspect of gamification, showing how including game components might magnify health interventions via AR, making the experience interesting for youngsters. By building on prior research, (Chapman and Chapman 2018) focus on AR's involvement in health behavior interventions, emphasizing its ability to inspire healthy living among children. The meta-analysis conducted by (Gong and Tarasewich 2019) explores the influence of gamification-based mobile apps on health outcomes, indicating the effectiveness of gamification in AR applications for children's health. Hussain et al., 2016) investigate educational AR applications on mobile devices, claiming that AR gamification can make health learning interesting and beneficial for youngsters. These studies highlight the potential of AR gamification in promoting healthy behaviors in children, such as nutrition education, physical activity, and overall wellness.

Augmented reality (AR) and gamification have developed as creative and promising techniques to address health concerns in children, with the goal of promoting healthy lifestyles and overall wellness. (Bacca et al., 2014) conducted a foundational study that highlights the pedagogical potential of AR as a stepping stone for using this technology to health awareness and habit formation in young people. Their systematic research demonstrates how the interactive and immersive characteristics of AR may produce engaging teaching experiences, paving the way for its use in health promotion. Brown and Cairns (2016) expand on this by delving into the complex area of gamification, illustrating how the strategic integration of game components can significantly improve health interventions using AR. Their investigation on the immersive features of gamification offers insight on the ability of AR-enhanced experiences to fascinate youngsters, making health-focused activities more entertaining, memorable, and likely to result in good behavior changes.

Chapman and Chapman (2018) make a substantial contribution by investigating the unique role of AR in health behavior interventions, emphasizing its potential to enhance healthy living among children by leveraging previous research. Their analysis broadens our understanding of AR's use in promoting healthy habits, providing insights into effective tactics for building health-focused AR experiences. Simultaneously, Gong and Tarasewich's (2019) meta-analysis gives a comprehensive evaluation of gamification-based mobile apps, revealing empirical data supporting the incorporation of gamification features into AR applications intended at improving children's health. Their findings validate the promise of AR as a medium for such therapies, revealing light on the concrete influence of gamification on health outcomes.

(Hussain et al., 2016) give a comprehensive analysis of educational AR applications for mobile devices as we investigate the educational aspects of AR gamification. This comprehensive analysis not only highlights the potential for AR gamification in health-related education, but it also emphasizes the importance of engaging, dynamic, and entertaining experiences when teaching youngsters about health and wellness. Their work emphasizes the importance of a user-centric approach in ensuring that AR gamification connects with youngsters and effectively transmits essential health messages by drawing parallels between educational and health-focused applications.

(Lu et al., 2018) focus on kid obesity, a significant topic that necessitates novel solutions. Their study focuses on the effectiveness of health video games as a forerunner to the incorporation of similar ideas into AR gamification, demonstrating the promise of this method in combating childhood obesity. Their work provides a template for building interesting, interactive, and health-promoting AR experiences for children by identifying the areas where AR can boost the impact of such activities. This is especially important in today's digital age, when technology plays such an important role in children's lives that it is critical to use these platforms for beneficial health outcomes.

Ma and Jain's (2014) extensive resource on serious games and edutainment delves deeper into the nexus of education and health. This work is a great reference, showcasing the possible application of serious games in children's education and health promotion. Their findings lay a solid foundation for comprehending the concepts underlying engaging and educational games, a paradigm that can be extended to AR gamification. (Marschollek et al., 2012) work focuses our attention to the collaborative and AR-based features of telemedicine, suggesting possible applications in encouraging healthy lifestyles among youngsters as we explore deeper into the possibilities of AR.

Effective design principles serve as the foundation for effective treatments, and (Miller et al., 2014) investigation of gamification design principles in mHealth applications has a direct impact on the design of AR gamification experiences for enhancing children's health. Their research gives important suggestions, emphasizing the need of motivation, engagement, and user-centered design, all of which are critical for the success of any health-focused AR application aimed at children. Understanding the aspects that contribute to gamification's effectiveness in promoting health allows us to personalize AR experiences to maximize their impact on children's habits and behaviors.

(Neri et al., 2016) change the focus to health professions education, looking into the effect of serious games in improving children's health-related knowledge. Their thorough review not only confirms the effectiveness of serious games in education, but it also underlines the possibility of adapting these results to health promotion activities. Their work provides vital insights into how AR gamification might be developed to educate youngsters about health while keeping them engaged and motivated by finding common themes and outcomes.

(O'Leary et al., 2016) investigate the potential influence of AR gamification on healthcare staff by discussing the novel usage of web-based games in training healthcare personnel about pediatric respiratory disorders. This viewpoint broadens the scope of AR gamification, implying that it can play a critical role in training healthcare professionals, raising health awareness, and ensuring that healthcare providers are well-equipped to address the health requirements of children. This is consistent with the overarching goal of developing a holistic approach to health promotion in which AR gamification not only reaches children directly but also empowers others responsible for their care.

Papastergiou's (2009) research investigates the effect of digital game-based learning on educational efficacy and student motivation. This study is important because it highlights the broader implications of gamification, implying that the concepts that make educational games entertaining may be used to benefit children's health. We get a better knowledge of how to design AR gamification experiences that not only inform but also encourage positive health-related behaviors in children by investigating how game aspects promote motivation and learning.

(Peng et al., 2012) extend this approach by looking into the motivational determinants of exergames. This investigation gives critical insights into the factors that motivate people to engage in physical activity in a game-like setting. When we evaluate the relevance of physical activity in promoting children's health, we can easily translate these findings into building AR gamification experiences that encourage exercise, combat sedentary behaviors, and improve overall wellness.

(Randel et al., 1992) provide historical context for the usefulness of games for educational purposes, reminding us that the integration of technology into education and health promotion is not a new concept. It demonstrates how these approaches have evolved through time, culminating in the revolutionary possibilities of AR gamification. We can grasp the revolutionary influence that AR has the potential to bring to children's health and wellbeing by knowing the roots of educational games.

The development of skills is an important factor, particularly in the context of good behaviors and welfare. (Rosenbaum et al., 2001) dive into this topic, providing important insights into how augmented reality gamification might be intentionally constructed to promote the development of beneficial health behaviors in children. We can design AR experiences that not only engage but also aid the acquisition and reinforcement of healthy habits by matching game mechanics with learning objectives.

The authors (Sailer et al., 2017) return our attention to the motivating benefits of gamification features. Their research provides useful guidance for combining these components within

AR experiences focused on encouraging youngsters to live healthy lifestyles. We can develop AR gamification tactics that effectively attract children's attention, keep their interest, and ultimately lead to the adoption of healthy habits provided we understand what inspires and drives their engagement.

(Santos et al., 2016) present additional insights into serious games in health professions education, validating the approach's potential for developing health-related knowledge among youngsters. We acquire a better understanding of how AR gamification might bridge the gap between learning and healthy behavior adoption in children by drawing parallels between educational and health-focused uses of serious games.

(Schneider et al., 2004) investigated the impact of virtual reality patient simulation on medical education. It demonstrates the potential of augmented reality gamification in engaging children in health-related issues. AR can provide children with vital insights into health by mimicking medical settings, helping them to understand and take care of their own well-being.

(Thompson et al., 2007) describe the design and methods of a serious video game aimed at increasing fruit and vegetable consumption in youth, highlighting the feasibility of similar approaches for promoting healthy eating in children using augmented reality gamification. This study emphasizes the significance of nutrition education, which may be smoothly integrated into AR gamification to make learning about healthy eating fun and impactful for youngsters.

(White et al., 2015) describe a game-based rehabilitation platform for children with cerebral palsy, which provides insights into the potential of augmented reality gamification for increasing physical activity and general wellness in children with diverse health conditions. This application broadens the area of AR gamification, implying that it has the potential to significantly improve the quality of life for youngsters experiencing health issues.

By concentrating on an augmented reality-based mobile learning system for science education, (Yang et al., 2016) provide a valuable perspective. Their findings show that similar techniques to promoting health education and healthy behaviors in youngsters can be used. We can design AR experiences that not only enlighten children about health but also empower them to make informed decisions about their well-being by integrating the educational components of AR with health-related material.

(Yen et al., 2015) investigated the impact of an augmented reality-based mobile learning environment on student learning successes and motivations, which provides useful insights into the potential of comparable approaches for health education in children. This study supports the notion that augmented reality has the ability to make learning more entertaining and motivating, which is critical for teaching youngsters about health and wellness.

The overview of augmented reality in education by Yuen and Yaoyuneyong (2012) provides intriguing avenues for its application in enhancing health education and general welfare in children. Their work demonstrates the adaptability of AR as a medium, demonstrating how it can be used to create engaging and interactive experiences that resonate with youngsters while effectively communicating important health messages.

The assessment of the literature on education and augmented reality by (Zammitto et al., 2017) provides vital insights into the potential of augmented reality in health education and supporting healthy lifestyles in children. This review gives a complete grasp of the field's existing expertise, opening the path for novel applications of AR in children's health promotion.

The practical guidance on creating game mechanics published by Zichermann and Cunningham (2011) is a helpful resource. It lays the groundwork for creating effective AR gamification experiences intended at enhancing children's health and overall well-being. We can construct AR experiences that fascinate and motivate youngsters, leading to the adoption of better habits, by understanding game design principles.

Zuckerman and Gal-Oz (2012) conducted a fascinating study on boosting physical activity in youngsters using a wearable activity tracker and an augmented reality incentive system. This study shows how augmented reality gamification can be used to encourage healthy behaviours. We can build personalised and interactive experiences that reward physical activity by using wearable technology and augmented reality, ensuring that children remain active and engaged in their pursuit of health.

Cairns, Cox, and Day's (2014) evaluation of smartphone apps for smoking cessation are must-read. While the emphasis is on adult smoking cessation, the implications for fostering healthy behaviours in children are clear. This evaluation highlights the potential of similar apps, such as augmented reality gamification, for teaching positive health habits in children, whether it's through physical activity, healthy eating, or other health-related behaviours.

Healthymagination, a mobile phone application aimed to help healthcare in underdeveloped countries, is introduced by (Chen et al., 2011). While the immediate focus is on healthcare in impoverished areas, the principle of using technology to promote health is global. This application demonstrates that similar approaches, regardless of geographic location, can be adjusted to boost health and general wellbeing in children.

The seminal work by (Deterding et al., 2011) in defining "gamification" is crucial. It presents a conceptual framework for understanding how game design aspects might be used to build interesting and inspiring augmented reality experiences for children to promote healthy lifestyles. We can ensure that AR experiences are not only informative but also pleasant by understanding the core concepts of gamification, encouraging youngsters to embrace healthy behaviours with excitement.

(Deterding et al., 2013) investigate the intrinsically motivating features of games, providing useful insights into the design principles that generate participation. Their investigation into what makes games intrinsically engaging lays the groundwork for developing effective augmented reality gamification tactics to promote children's health and overall well-being.

Finally, the combination of these research reviews highlights the enormous potential of augmented reality gamification in promoting healthy lifestyles and general well-being in children. The evidence is clear: AR gamification has the power to engage, motivate, and empower children to make healthier choices, from educational applications to health behavior interventions, from nutrition education to physical activity encouragement, and from serious games to wearable technology integration. We can build novel solutions that resonate with children by adding gaming aspects, leveraging educational ideas, and harnessing the fascinating nature of AR experiences, making the pursuit of health a worthwhile and pleasant journey. To guarantee that AR gamification becomes a cornerstone in molding healthier, happier futures for children globally, we must prioritize user-centered design, evidence-based techniques, and interdisciplinary collaboration as we continue to explore this dynamic sector.

CONCEPTUAL MODEL

Interpretation of Conceptual Model

The first category of the conceptual model, "Application," which involves identifying specific areas where virtual reality (VR) can be advantageous for children's health and lifestyle. For illustration, in the category of "fitness," VR applications can simulate engaging exercise routines or sports activities that encourage physical activity. In the category of "learning," educational VR experiences can transport children to historical events, outer space, or underwater ecosystems, promoting curiosity and knowledge acquisition. Furthermore, VR can improve "well-being" by offering relaxation and mindfulness exercises, immersive nature experiences, or therapeutic interventions for dealing stress or anxiety. Moving on to the next "Category," this point categorizes the identified applications into different thematic areas, such as fun, fitness, well-being, entertainment, happiness, joy, and learning, to ensure a comprehensive coverage of potential benefits. Next, the third stage, "Hardware and Software Requirements," includes the requirement of physical devices and software components for implementing virtual reality (VR)

Figure 1. Conceptual model

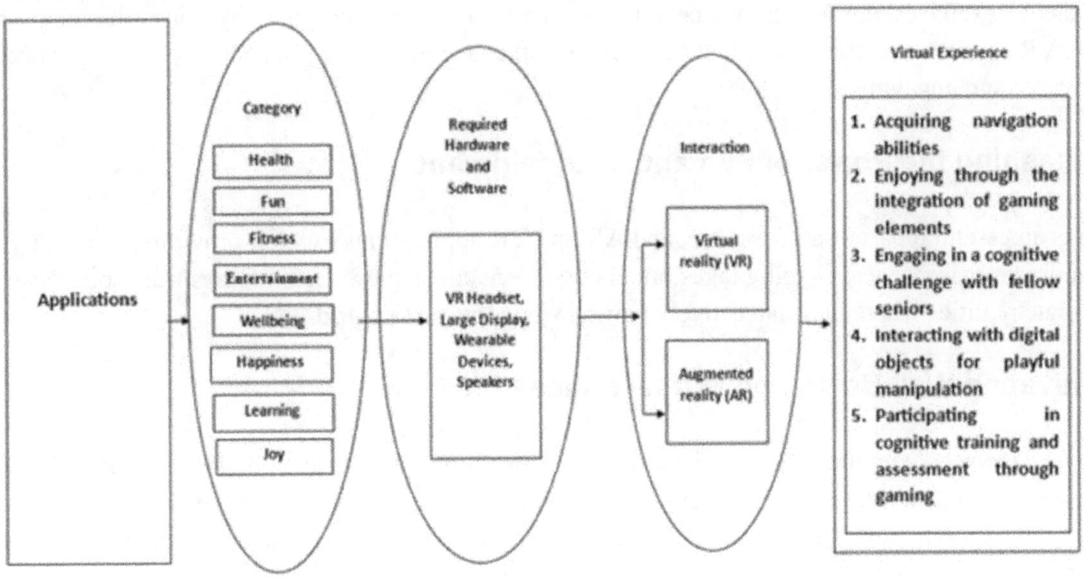

experiences. This may include VR headsets like Oculus Quest or HTC Vive, wearing devices such as haptic feedback vests or gloves, speakers for audio immersion, and display devices like high-resolution monitors or projection screens. In the fourth stage, "Interaction," the model outlines between virtual reality and augmented reality interaction modes. For example, a VR application may fully immerse children in a digital environment, while an augmented reality experience overlays digital content onto the real world, providing interactive learning opportunities. Finally, the fifth category, "Virtual Experience," emphasizes the creation of compelling and tailored VR experiences that align with the identified application areas and cater to children's interests and developmental needs. These experiences may range from interactive storytelling adventures to gamified fitness challenges, each designed to enrich children's lives and promote healthy habits in an engaging and immersive manner.

The world of technology is constantly evolving, and with it comes the rise of innovative tools that have the potential to revolutionize the way we live, learn, and interact. Among these tools, Augmented Reality (AR) and Virtual Reality (VR) have emerged as captivating platforms with a vast array of applications. In recent years, adolescents have eagerly embraced AR and VR, harnessing their power to cater to their diverse needs, ranging from health and fitness to well-being and mental peace.

The model proposes utilizing AR and VR applications tailored for adolescents. These applications can be conveniently accessed through various devices like mobile phones, tablets, desktop computers, and handheld devices. The needs of adolescent users can be categorized into two main groups: physical fitness and emotional well-being. There are instances where users might fall into both of these categories simultaneously.

The applications can be primarily grouped into seven distinct categories: Health, Physical Fitness, Fun, Entertainment, Learning, Wellbeing, Happiness and Joy.

A Multifaceted Approach to Health and Physical Fitness

Adolescents are known for their vibrant energy and eagerness to explore. AR and VR applications offer an engaging way for them to pursue their health and fitness goals. Imagine a scenario where a teenager uses AR to project a virtual personal trainer right into their living room. With real-time guidance and interactive exercises, this technology becomes a dynamic tool for improving physical well-being. Similarly, VR can immerse users in virtual environments that encourage physical activity, making workouts enjoyable and engaging.

Unleashing the Power of Fun and Entertainment

Fun is an essential part of adolescence, and AR and VR applications excel at providing immersive entertainment experiences. Gaming takes on a new dimension as these technologies transport players to alternate realities where they can actively participate in the game world.

Cultivating Well-Being and Mental Peace

The teenage years are often characterized by a whirlwind of emotions and challenges. AR and VR offer a unique avenue for promoting mental well-being. Meditation and mindfulness apps presented in immersive environments help adolescents manage stress and anxiety. These applications can serve as valuable tools to equip young minds with techniques to handle the pressures of life.

Aiding Cognitive Development and Learning

Adolescence is a critical period for cognitive development and learning. AR and VR applications offer interactive platforms for adolescents to explore complex concepts in an engaging manner. Whether it's virtual science experiments, historical reenactments, or language learning in augmented environments, these technologies enhance learning experiences by making them more immersive and interactive.

Pursuing Happiness and Joy

Happiness is a universal aspiration, and AR and VR technologies contribute to its pursuit in novel ways. Whether it's virtually attending live concerts, exploring breathtaking natural wonders, or reliving memorable experiences, these technologies have the power to bring moments of happiness to life. Adolescents can curate their happiness by creating and sharing AR-enhanced memories with friends, making the most of their interconnected digital world.

The application of Augmented Reality and Virtual Reality has ushered in a new era of possibilities for adolescents. From health and fitness to well-being, happiness, and cognitive development, these technologies offer a multifaceted approach to addressing their diverse needs.

Some of the Popular Applications Are

1. **Relax River VR**: Relax VR offers a serene and calming virtual environment for children to unwind and relax. The app provides immersive experiences like sitting by a virtual campfire, watching peaceful scenes in nature, or engaging with soothing activities that can help reduce anxiety and promote a sense of tranquillity.

Figure 2. Relax river
(Source: https://play.google.com/store/apps)

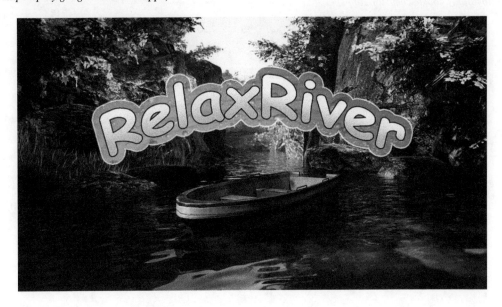

2.   **Breathe, Think, Do with Sesame**: Developed by Sesame Street, this VR app combines entertainment and emotional well-being. It features beloved Sesame Street characters and helps children navigate challenging situations by guiding them through a series of activities that promote problem-solving, emotional regulation, and coping skills.

3.   **Scuba Driver Swimming Treasure VR**: Adventure Scuba VR is an app that takes children on virtual underwater adventures to explore marine life and coral reefs. This app can encourage an interest in physical activity and a healthy lifestyle by inspiring kids to learn about the ocean and stay active through virtual scuba diving experiences.

4.   **Beat Saber VR**: While not exclusively designed for children, Beat Saber is a popular VR rhythm game that can be enjoyed by the whole family. It involves slicing through blocks to the beat of music, providing a fun and physically engaging activity that can contribute to exercise and physical activity for children.

5.   **VR Sports**: VR Sports offers a collection of virtual reality sports games like basketball, baseball, and more. Engaging in virtual sports can encourage children to be more active and participate in physical activities even when they're indoors.

6.   **Kingspray Graffiti VR**: Kingspray Graffiti VR is a creative app that lets children engage in virtual graffiti art. While not directly related to physical activity, it encourages creativity and artistic expression, which are essential aspects of a well-rounded healthy lifestyle.

7.   **SculptrVR:** SculptrVR is a sculpting and creativity app that allows children to shape and create virtual worlds using their imagination. This app promotes creativity and can keep children engaged in constructive activities that stimulate their minds while also allowing them to be physically active in a virtual environment.

8.   **FotonVR - VR in Education**: Introducing the FotonVR Learn Science App, a specialized application for Virtual Reality augmented headsets tailored to students ranging from 5th to 10th grade. Our primary objective is to transform education into a captivating and enjoyable journey through

Figure 3. Scuba driver swimming treasure
(Source: https://play.google.com/store/apps)

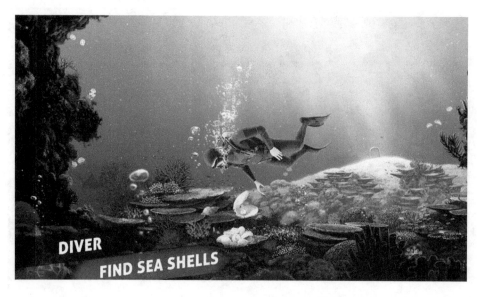

immersive experiences. We provide a unique opportunity for your child to explore a realm that would otherwise be inaccessible, all thanks to the power of Virtual Reality Headsets.

9. **Google VR Services**: Google VR Services delivers virtual reality capabilities for Daydream and Cardboard applications. These functionalities encompass tasks like presenting notifications within the VR environment, connecting Daydream-compatible headsets and controllers to your Daydream-ready smartphone, and seamlessly navigating in and out of VR applications.

10. **Irusu VR Cinema Player Pro**: The Irusu VR Cinema Player stands as the ultimate virtual reality movie viewer designed for immersive VR video content, offering complete command and a cinematic IMAX-like encounter. This VR Player comprises not only a 360-degree VR video player (360 Movie VR player) but also a conventional 2D VR player, providing a variety of screen choices for your viewing pleasure.

11. **VR Roller Coaster - GALAXY 360**: Embark on a series of VR rollercoaster-esque journeys in the cosmos, each offering the sensation of speed as you glide through the depths of outer space, defying the constraints of gravity. Board a space shuttle to venture into the cosmos, witnessing remote space stations and cosmic formations from distant civilizations, all while experiencing an exhilarating ride through the vast expanse of deep space.

12. **VR Educators:** VR Educators is an application crafted to facilitate students in grasping various scientific, mathematical, and linguistic concepts through the application of virtual reality. Through VR Educators, students have the opportunity to delve into a virtual realm, allowing for a dynamic and captivating approach to learning diverse subjects. This application caters to learners of all age groups and is intentionally designed for user-friendliness. Accessible at no cost, the app can be obtained from the Play Store.

These applications necessitate a combination of hardware and software to enhance the experience of VR and AR. VR and AR devices encompass three fundamental functionalities: displays, processors, and

Figure 4. VR roller coaster
(Source: https://play.google.com/store/apps)

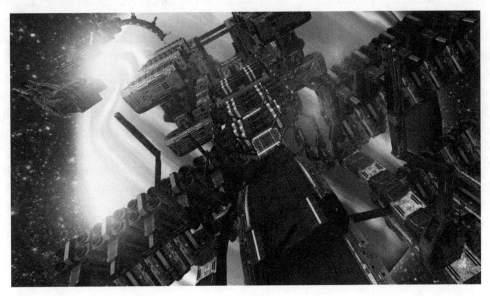

sensors. These encompass VR headsets, intelligent displays, wearable gadgets, as well as speakers. To achieve an exceptional VR encounter, VR headsets, head-mounted displays, powerful computers, and advanced processors will be essential to facilitate precise positional tracking and effective management of the authentic and immersive virtual environment.

VR and AR devices encompass three fundamental functionalities: displays, processors, and sensors. These encompass VR headsets, intelligent displays, wearable gadgets, as well as speakers. To achieve an exceptional VR encounter, VR headsets, head-mounted displays, powerful computers, and advanced processors will be essential to facilitate precise positional tracking and effective management of the authentic and immersive virtual environment.

In the realm of virtual reality (VR) and augmented reality (AR), the underlying technology is as captivating as the experiences they create. At the heart of these immersive journeys lie the devices that enable us to traverse digital realms and blend virtual elements seamlessly with the real world. These devices are built upon a triad of fundamental functionalities: displays, processors, and sensors. Each of these components plays a pivotal role in conjuring the illusion of alternate realities and augmenting our perception.

Displays serve as the windows to these enchanting realms, presenting vivid visuals that transport users to places beyond their physical surroundings. These high-resolution screens, whether nestled within VR headsets or integrated into AR glasses, are responsible for rendering intricate landscapes, lifelike characters, and captivating visual effects. Processors, the technological powerhouses at the core of these devices, work tirelessly to handle the complex computations required to generate these immersive experiences. From calculating the physics of virtual objects to rendering real-time changes as users interact with their surroundings, processors drive the fluidity and realism of VR and AR encounters. Finally, sensors act as the digital senses, gathering data on users' movements, gestures, and the environment around them. This data is then swiftly processed to synchronize virtual elements with users' actions, allowing for seamless interactions and an unparalleled level of immersion. In unison, displays, processors, and sensors orchestrate a symphony of technology, inviting us to explore worlds both familiar and fantastical in ways that once seemed confined to the realm of dreams.

In the realm of AR and VR environments, the adolescent user is the person who engages directly with the system and directly partakes in virtual encounters. The model aids in attaining the user's goals through virtual experiences, encompassing the development of navigation skills, deriving enjoyment from gaming aspects, immersing in cognitive challenges, and engaging in cognitive training and evaluation via gaming activities.

In the realm of AR and VR environments, the adolescent user is the person who engages directly with the system and directly partakes in virtual encounters. The model aids in attaining the user's goals through virtual experiences, encompassing the development of navigation skills, deriving enjoyment from gaming aspects, immersing in cognitive challenges, and engaging in cognitive training and evaluation via gaming activities.

At the forefront of technological innovation, a model emerges as a guiding light in the realm of virtual experiences, propelling users towards their aspirations. This model serves as a conduit for achieving multifaceted objectives through immersive encounters, fostering a wide spectrum of growth and enjoyment. From honing navigation skills in virtual environments that mirror real-world scenarios, to extracting sheer delight from the gaming elements intricately woven into these experiences, the model paves the way for a dynamic fusion of entertainment and skill development.

Beyond mere amusement, the model introduces a realm of cognitive challenges that push users to explore the boundaries of their intellectual prowess. Through intricate puzzles, simulations, and problem-solving scenarios, individuals are encouraged to delve into novel ways of thinking, all the while enveloped in the captivating embrace of virtual worlds. Yet, the model's influence extends beyond entertainment and cognitive engagement, for it stands as an advocate for cognitive training and evaluation. By seamlessly integrating these processes into the realm of gaming activities, it provides a unique avenue for users to assess their cognitive abilities and monitor their progress over time. Thus, the model not only enriches the landscape of entertainment and education but also empowers users to embark on a journey of self-improvement, all within the immersive domain of virtual experiences.

RESULTS

The integration of gaming into augmented reality (AR) environments shows promising results in various fields. Combining game mechanics with AR technology gives users an engaging and dynamic experience that increases interactivity and immersion. AR projects digital elements into the physical world using devices such as smartphones and AR glasses to enhance the user's environment. Gamification adds elements such as challenges, rewards and competition to these experiences, appealing to users' inherent desires for achievement and success. AR games encourage users to explore their surroundings and discover hidden digital features that enhance the overall experience. This combination proves particularly useful in education, where AR can make learning more interactive and enjoyable, and in marketing, where companies use AR to create immersive brand experiences. In addition, AR gamification has the potential to promote exercise and improve health outcomes by encouraging physical activity through virtual challenges and rewards. However, successful implementation requires a deep understanding of both AR technology and game design principles to ensure engagement, usability and meaningful communication. As the technology advances, the opportunities for innovative AR gaming experiences in various sectors expand even further and offer new opportunities to improve user experience and engagement.

CONCLUSION

Finally, the combination of augmented reality (AR) technology and gamification offers a viable paradigm for tackling the essential challenge of encouraging healthy lifestyles and overall well-being in children. This book chapter has shown how AR gamification may captivate young minds, create intrinsic drive, and encourage positive behavior modification.

We discovered how features like incentives, challenges, and progress tracking may foster a sense of accomplishment and continuous engagement through a thorough examination of gamification concepts. We can construct immersive, contextually relevant interventions that engage with children and smoothly integrate healthy behaviours into their daily lives by incorporating these ideas into augmented reality experiences.

However, the technology world is not without ethical concerns and potential hazards. Balancing screen time, protecting data privacy, and avoiding potential addictive tendencies are all important considerations as we leverage the power of AR gamification. Responsible adoption and continuous research are required to mitigate any negative impacts and maximize the benefits that these technologies can offer.

Looking ahead, the insights gained from this chapter will be used to lay the groundwork for future research, innovation, and collaboration. Researchers, educators, and practitioners can push the boundaries of AR gamified therapies to cater to a wide range of age groups, cultural backgrounds, and health goals. As technology advances, so does our ability to create immersive and engaging experiences that steer youngsters towards better choices and develop lifetime habits of well-being.

In conclusion, the combination of augmented reality and gamification represents a significant step forward in boosting children's health and well-being. By capitalizing on youth's natural curiosity and playfulness, we can design interventions that are not only successful but also pleasurable, fostering a generation that embraces healthier lives with enthusiasm and resilience. We can genuinely leverage the potential of AR gamification as a force for positive change in the lives of our children and, by extension, the world they will influence via continued dedication and interdisciplinary collaboration.

REFERENCES

Bacca, J., Baldiris, S., Fabregat, R., & Graf, S. (2014). Augmented reality trends in education: A systematic review of research and applications. *Journal of Educational Technology & Society*, *16*(4), 133–149.

Bakır, Ç. N., Abbas, S. O., Sever, E., Özcan Morey, A., Aslan Genç, H., & Mutluer, T. (2023). Use of augmented reality in mental health-related conditions: A systematic review. *Digital Health*, *9*, 20552076231203649. doi:10.1177/20552076231203649 PMID:37791140

Barua, T., Doshi, R., & Hiran, K. K. (2020). *Mobile Applications Development: With Python in Kivy Framework*. Walter de Gruyter GmbH & Co KG. doi:10.1515/9783110689488

Blanco, D., Roberts, R. M., Gannoni, A., & Cook, S. (2023). Assessment and treatment of mental health conditions in children and adolescents: A systematic scoping review of how virtual reality environments have been used. *Clinical Child Psychology and Psychiatry*, 13591045231204082. doi:10.1177/13591045231204082 PMID:37738029

Brown, D. M., & Cairns, P. (2016). A grounded investigation of game immersion. In *Proceedings of the 2016 CHI Conference on Human Factors in Computing Systems* (pp. 3711-3722). ACM.

Cairns, P., Cox, A. L., & Day, M. (2014). The virtues of repetition: A grounded theory of technology-mediated recovery. *International Journal of Human-Computer Studies*, *72*(8-9), 487–506.

Chamberland, C., Bransi, M., Boivin, A., Jacques, S., Gagnon, J., & Tremblay, S. (2024). The effect of augmented reality on preoperative anxiety in children and adolescents: A randomized controlled trial. *Paediatric Anaesthesia*, *34*(2), 153–159. doi:10.1111/pan.14793 PMID:37925608

Chapman, J., & Chapman, L. (2018). Interactive health behavior interventions using gamification and augmented reality. In *Handbook of Research on Gamification in Higher Education* (pp. 135–156). IGI Global.

Chen, J., Canny, J., & He, H. (2011). Healthymagination: Mobile phone application for healthcare in the developing world. In *Proceedings of the 2nd ACM SIGHIT International Health Informatics Symposium* (pp. 1-10). ACM.

Deterding, S., Dixon, D., Khaled, R., & Nacke, L. (2011). From game design elements to gamefulness: defining" gamification". In Proceedings of the 15th international academic MindTrek conference: Envisioning future media environments (pp. 9-15).

Deterding, S., Dixon, D., Khaled, R., Nacke, L., & Lennart, E. (2013). Gamification: Toward a definition. In CHI 2013 Extended Abstracts on Human Factors in Computing Systems (pp. 2466-2468). ACM.

Doshi, R., Hiran, K. K., Gök, M., El-kenawy, E. S. M., Badr, A., & Abotaleb, M. (2023). Artificial Intelligence's Significance in Diseases with Malignant Tumours. *Mesopotamian Journal of Artificial Intelligence in Healthcare, 2023*, 35–39.

Gong, J., & Tarasewich, P. (2019). A meta-analysis of gamification-based mobile apps in promoting health outcomes. *Journal of the American Medical Informatics Association : JAMIA, 26*(10), 1124–1136.

Gupta, A. K., Srinivasulu, A., Hiran, K. K., Sreenivasulu, G., Rajeyyagari, S., & Subramanyam, M. (2022). Prediction of omicron virus using combined extended convolutional and recurrent neural networks technique on CT-scan images. *Interdisciplinary Perspectives on Infectious Diseases, 2022*, 2022. doi:10.1155/2022/1525615 PMID:36562006

Hiran, K. K., Doshi, R., & Mijwil, M. M. (2023). Introducing On-Demand Internet Business Model in the Informal Public Transportation System in Developing Countries. In Integrating Intelligence and Sustainability in Supply Chains (pp. 148-162). IGI Global. doi:10.4018/979-8-3693-0225-5.ch008

Hussain, A., Aydin, N., Cagiltay, N. E., & Suh, H. J. (2016). A review of augmented reality applications on mobile devices for learning in K-12 education. *Computers & Education, 94*, 1–22.

Jain, R. K., & Hiran, K. K. (2024). BIONET: A Bio-Inspired Neural Network for Consensus Mechanisms in Blockchain Systems. In Bio-Inspired Optimization Techniques in Blockchain Systems (pp. 78-100). IGI Global. doi:10.4018/979-8-3693-1131-8.ch004

Lu, A. S., Kharrazi, H., Gharghabi, F., Thompson, D., Paul, M. J., & Aung, M. (2018). A systematic review of health video games for childhood obesity prevention and intervention. *Journal of Diabetes Science and Technology, 12*(1), 222–233.

Ma, M., & Jain, L. C. (2014). *Serious games and edutainment applications* (Vol. II). Springer. doi:10.1007/978-3-319-11623-5

Marschollek, M., Rehwald, A., Wolf, K. H., & Gietzelt, M. (2012). Collaborative and augmented telemedicine in health care. *Journal of Computer Science and Technology, 27*(6), 1246–1262.

Miller, A. S., Cafazzo, J. A., & Seto, E. (2014). A game plan: Gamification design principles in mHealth applications for chronic disease management. *Health Informatics Journal, 20*(4), 257–268. PMID:24986104

Mishra, A., Tripathi, A., Khazanchi, D., Hiran, K. K., Vyas, A. K., & Padmanaban, S. (2021). A framework for applying artificial intelligence (AI) with Internet of NanoThings (IoNT). In *Machine Learning for Sustainable Development* (pp. 1–16). De Gruyter. doi:10.1515/9783110702514-001

Neri, L., Cianetti, L., Sciarabba, C., & Lamberti, F. (2016). The effectiveness of digital games in health professions education: A systematic review. *Computers & Education, 95*, 90–97.

O'Leary, S. T., Lee, M., Federico, S., Lurie-Moroni, E., & Beaty, B. L. (2016). Educational web-based game for early assessment and management of child pedestrian injury risk. *JMIR Serious Games*, *4*(1), e3. PMID:27229772

Papastergiou, M. (2009). Digital game-based learning in high school computer science education: Impact on educational effectiveness and student motivation. *Computers & Education*, *52*(1), 1–12. doi:10.1016/j.compedu.2008.06.004

Patel, S., Vyas, A. K., & Hiran, K. K. (2022). Infrastructure health monitoring using signal processing based on an industry 4.0 System. *Cyber-Physical Systems and Industry*, *4*, 249–260.

Peng, W., Lin, J. H., Pfeiffer, K. A., & Winn, B. (2012). Need satisfaction supportive game features as motivational determinants: An experimental study of a self-determination theory guided exergame. *Media Psychology*, *15*(2), 175–196. doi:10.1080/15213269.2012.673850

Raja, M., & Priya, G. L. (2023). The role of augmented reality and virtual reality in smart health education: State of the art and perspectives. *Artificial intelligence for smart healthcare*, 311-325.

Ramasamy, J., & Doshi, R. (2022). Machine learning in cyber physical systems for healthcare: brain tumor classification from MRI using transfer learning framework. In *Real-Time Applications of Machine Learning in Cyber-Physical Systems* (pp. 65–76). IGI global. doi:10.4018/978-1-7998-9308-0.ch005

Randel, J. M., Morris, B. A., Wetzel, C. D., & Whitehill, B. V. (1992). The effectiveness of games for educational purposes: A review of recent research. *Simulation & Gaming*, *23*(3), 261–276. doi:10.1177/1046878192233001

Rathi, S., Hiran, K. K., & Sakhare, S. (2023). Affective state prediction of E-learner using SS-ROA based deep LSTM. *Array (New York, N.Y.)*, *19*, 100315. doi:10.1016/j.array.2023.100315

Rosenbaum, D. A., Carlson, R. A., & Gilmore, R. O. (2001). Acquisition of intellectual and perceptual-motor skills. *Annual Review of Psychology*, *52*(1), 453–470. doi:10.1146/annurev.psych.52.1.453 PMID:11148313

Sailer, M., Hense, J. U., Mayr, S. K., & Mandl, H. (2017). How gamification motivates: An experimental study of the effects of specific game design elements on psychological need satisfaction. *Computers in Human Behavior*, *69*, 371–380. doi:10.1016/j.chb.2016.12.033

Santos, F., Marques, A., Martins, J., & Silva, P. (2016). Serious games in health professions education: A systematic review. *International Journal of Nursing Education Scholarship*, *13*(1), 115–123.

Schneider, E. F., Lang, A., Shin, M., Bradley, S. D., & Li, P. P. (2004). Virtual patient simulation for medical education: A review. *Studies in Health Technology and Informatics*, *98*, 263–269.

Singh, G., Kataria, A., Jangra, S., Dutta, R., Mantri, A., Sandhu, J. K., & Sabapathy, T. (2023). Augmented Reality and Virtual Reality: Transforming the Future of Psychological and Medical Sciences. In Smart Distributed Embedded Systems for Healthcare Applications (pp. 93-118). CRC Press.

Skouby, K. E., Dhotre, P., Williams, I., & Hiran, K. (Eds.). (2022). *5G, Cybersecurity and Privacy in Developing Countries*. CRC Press. doi:10.1201/9781003374664

Srinivasulu, A., Gupta, A., Hiran, K., Barua, T., Sreenivasulu, G. (2022). Omi-cron Virus Data Analytics Using Extended RNN Technique. *Int J Cancer Res Ther, 7*(3), 122.

Thompson, D., Bhatt, R., Lazarus, M., Cullen, K. W., Baranowski, J., & Baranowski, T. (2007). A serious video game to increase fruit and vegetable consumption among elementary aged youth (Squire's Quest! II): Rationale, design, and methods. *JMIR Research Protocols, 6*(3), e39. PMID:23612366

White, S. M., Wootton, B. M., & Ferguson, M. A. (2015). A game-based exercise platform for children with cerebral palsy: A usability study. *JMIR Serious Games, 3*(2), e5. PMID:26199045

Yang, C. H., Liu, T. C., Lin, C. P., & Liang, J. C. (2016). Developing an augmented reality-based mobile learning system for science education. *Journal of Computer Assisted Learning, 32*(6), 557–572.

Yen, C. H., Lin, C. Y., & Wang, C. S. (2015). Augmented reality in science education: A review of the literature. *Journal of Science Education and Technology, 24*(6), 660–677.

Yuen, S. C., & Yaoyuneyong, G. (2012). Augmented reality: An overview and five directions for AR in education. *Journal of Educational Technology Development and Exchange, 4*(1), 119–140.

Zammitto, V., Caponetto, I., Earp, J., & Otten, H. (2017). Augmented reality in education: A meta-review and cross-media analysis. In *Augmented Reality and Virtual Reality* (pp. 25–42). Springer.

Zichermann, G., & Cunningham, C. (2011). *Gamification by design: Implementing game mechanics in web and mobile apps.* O'Reilly Media, Inc.

Zuckerman, O., & Gal-Oz, A. (2012). Augmented reality system for promoting physical activity in children with cerebral palsy. *Research in Developmental Disabilities, 33*(6), 1977–1987.

Chapter 14
Blockchain Integration With the Digital Twin–Enabled Industrial Internet of Things Based on Mixed Reality

Rakshit Kothari

(iD) https://orcid.org/0000-0003-2893-1504

College of Technology and Engineering, Maharana Pratap University of Agriculture and Technology, India

Kalpana Jain

College of Technology and Engineering, Maharana Pratap University of Agriculture and Technology, India

Naveen Choudhary

College of Technology and Engineering, Maharana Pratap University of Agriculture and Technology, India

ABSTRACT

The industrial landscape is about to undergo a revolution thanks to the convergence of emerging technologies. Specifically, the integration of blockchain with the digital twin-enabled industrial internet of things (IIoT) within mixed reality environments has the potential to do just that. This chapter presents a thorough analysis of the applications, advantages, and difficulties of various technologies while examining their potential for synergy. The digital twin provides real-time data monitoring, analysis, and predictive maintenance capabilities. The industrial internet of things establishes connections between tangible objects and sensors, enabling smooth communication and interchange of data. This chapter investigates the use of mixed reality (MR) technology to integrate blockchain technology with the IIoT that is enabled by digital twins. The potential for improving data security, trust, and transparency in industrial applications through the integration of blockchain with IIoT and MR could aid in the development of the Industry 4.0 paradigm.

DOI: 10.4018/979-8-3693-1123-3.ch014

INTRODUCTION

In addition to advancements in communication technology, the emergence of information technologies like the Internet of Things (IoT), Cloud Computing (CC), and Cyber-Physical Systems (CPS) has revolutionized the system approach to information transmission between multiple sources. Digitalization is undoubtedly to blame for the revolution that has occurred in all facets of modern life (Rasheed et al., 2020). One of the brilliant ideas that have evolved as a result of the advancement and revolt in Information-Communication Technology (ICT) is the Digital Twin (DT). A digital depiction of an actual system from the viewpoint of CPS is called the DT. As a result, a convinced system's virtual complement simulates its real performance. The information from the physical system is characterized during whole lifecycle development by the digital data from the virtual system combined with a real system (Jones et al., 2019) As a result, when digital and physical counterparts are combined, an efficient method for managing, regulating, and enhancing coordination is produced when the system functions. In addition, the execution system reaction and all data gathered from physical sensors are recorded by the DT. Therefore, DT's crucial job is to forecast and diagnose the physical system's behavior in order to identify any faults or malfunctions and to provide the system with data so that it may receive the best maintenance possible (Boyes & Watson, 2022; Fuller et al., 2020).

The fundamental objective of DT is to save costs and maintenance efforts while improving productivity and operating flexibility through the use of a virtual representation of the system. On the other hand, to solve the difficulties of Industry 4.0 that come from the manufacture of linked components, DT might be performed, depending on the requirements, either at the edge layer or on a system housed in the cloud. Conversely, DT advocates for both elucidating the behavior of the real system and identifying optimal solutions for the physical model (Tao et al., 2019). DT makes use of a basic modeling system, transparent simulation, and simulation processes to enhance control action, anticipate system performance, and support decision-making. Grieves presented the idea of digital twins in 2002, but NASA was the first to use it to build models of virtual spacecraft (Yu et al., 2022). The literature indicates that current DT works and implementations are still in their infancy and demand a great deal of work. Nonetheless, a multitude of applications, including biomedical systems, manufacturing, aerospace, agriculture, smart cities, and weather forecasting, have successfully incorporated it. In addition, to develop an effective digital twin system for any physical system, more specialized engineers and computer scientists are required in this crucial field. Their duties will encompass constructing and developing the fundamental product prototype in addition to producing an elaborate description of the virtual system (Singh et al., 2022).

Background and Motivation

The rapid evolution of Industry 4.0 has transformed manufacturing and industrial processes. This revolution is enabled by the Industrial Internet of Things (IIoT), a network of networked devices and systems that gather, analyze, and share industrial data. Real-time monitoring, predictive maintenance, and process optimization have increased industrial production and efficiency thanks to the IIoT (Patel et al., 2022; Uhlemann et al., 2017). In industrial applications, Digital Twins have become popular. A Digital Twin recreates a physical object or system for real-time monitoring, modeling, and analysis. Creating digital copies of real assets and processes helps firms gather insights, optimize operations, and make better decisions (Alam & El Saddik, 2017; El Saddik, 2018).

Despite their potential, IIoT and Digital Twins suffer data security, trust, and transparency issues. IIoT devices' interconnectedness and reliance on digital representations of physical systems presents vulnerabilities that bad actors can exploit. Managing data integrity and trustworthiness with various stakeholders is difficult. This research paper proposes integrating blockchain technology into the IIoT ecosystem and using Mixed Reality (MR) technology to bridge the digital and physical worlds. Blockchain, a decentralized and immutable ledger, is used in finance and supply chain management to secure data and build trust. Its use to IIoT and Digital Twins could improve industrial data security, trust, and transparency, making it an intriguing area of research (Schleich et al., 2017).

Blockchain Technology

Originally developed for cryptocurrencies, blockchain technology has developed into a ground-breaking idea with numerous uses outside of virtual currencies. Immutability, transparency, and security aspects define this decentralized and distributed ledger system. A blockchain's basic building elements are data-storing blocks and cryptographic hashing, which protects the data's integrity within the blocks (Khazanchi et al., 2021; Shrivas et al., 2022). In a world without trust, blockchain technology offers a variety of consensus methods, including Proof of Work (PoW) and Proof of Stake (PoS), which bolster security and confidence (Kahlen et al., 2017; Huang et al., 2020).

Industrial Internet of Things (IIoT)

Industrial Internet of Things (IIoT) is a paradigm-shifting technology that uses machines, sensors, and connected devices to gather and share data in industrial settings. Predictive maintenance, data-driven decision-making, and operational efficiency are all improved by this networked approach to industrial processes (Lee et al., 2020). Real-time control and monitoring of physical assets is made possible by IIoT integration, which boosts output and decreases downtime.

Digital Twin Technology

A Digital Twin (DT) is made up of virtual representations of real-world things created by computers. These models use information gathered straight from the physical objects to continuously adjust to changes in operations. Digital technologies can be applied to cyber-physical systems. A full environment, like smart cities and 5G networks, or solitary robots are examples. Using the shared data, DTs are supposed to predict how the physical object's condition will change over time. Under real-time limitations, such a transfer from the physical to the virtual realm can be carried out. Additionally, DTs can provide a system with data and operational status, giving it the ability to develop new business models. Moreover, situational awareness and more precise prediction making are feasible. DTs can also be used to improve efficiency, security, and resilience while lowering costs and risks (Tao et al., 2018).

Mixed Reality (MR) Technology

With the use of MR technology, computer-generated elements are superimposed on the actual surroundings to merge the virtual and physical worlds. It includes both virtual reality (VR) and augmented reality (AR) and is being applied more and more in industrial settings for design, maintenance, and training.

By offering a rich, dynamic environment that blends digital and physical information, MR improves the user experience (Alshathri et al., 2023).

MR allows users to see, interact with, and manipulate digital representations of industrial assets in a real-world setting within the framework of IIoT and Digital Twins (Doshi & Hiran, 2023; Kothari, 2023). Workers and decision-makers are empowered to obtain deeper insights and make more informed decisions thanks to this convergence of technologies.

Integration of Blockchain With IIoT and MR

The potential for revolutionizing industrial processes exists in the integration of blockchain technology with IIoT and MR. Blockchain improves data integrity, lowers the risk of cyberattacks, and increases transparency by bringing its security, immutability, and trust to the data generated and shared by IIoT devices and Digital Twins. Additionally, MR improves the interaction and visualization of Digital Twins, which facilitates more dynamic, intuitive monitoring and control of industrial processes by engineers and operators (Jain & Hiran, 2024; Wang et al., 2019).

LITERATURE REVIEW

In recent years, there has been a substantial uptick in the amount of focus placed on the convergence of Blockchain technology and Digital Twin in the Industrial Internet of Things (IIoT). This literature study investigates the fundamental ideas behind Blockchain, Digital Twins, and the Industrial Internet of Things (IIoT), presenting a complete overview of each of their distinct responsibilities as well as the possible synergies that can be achieved when these concepts are combined. The review sheds light on the developing pattern of using Mixed Reality to improve the capabilities of this integration, so clearing the way for industrial processes that are more safe, transparent, and effective (Sun et al., 2023).

The most important feature is security and trust in IIoT systems, which may be achieved through the use of blockchain technology. The data that is kept in Digital Twins maintains a higher level of authenticity because to Blockchain's ability to generate an immutable and distributed ledger (Spinti et al., 2022). In this review, we highlight the ways in which this integration might protect against cybersecurity threats, thereby ensuring that the information used in IIoT applications is reliable. In addition to this, it investigates the ways in which Mixed Reality might strengthen safety precautions by providing real-time visualization and monitoring of the physical and digital environments (Skouby et al., 2022).

This literature study analyzes how merging Blockchain technology with digital twins in the Industrial Internet of Things (IIoT) could improve the transparency and efficiency of industrial processes. Blockchain technology creates a decentralized and tamper-resistant ledger, which assures that all parties involved have access to the same version of the truth. The review also investigates how Mixed Reality provides an additional layer of real-time visibility, enabling users to interact with Digital Twins in a manner that is more immersive, and ultimately enhancing decision-making procedures and the effectiveness of operating procedures (Zhou et al., 2019).

Milton et al. (2020) focuses on the part that smart contracts play in the integration of blockchain technology and digital twins in the industrial internet of things (IIoT). The use of smart contracts makes it possible for agreements to automatically carry out their terms and conditions, thus automating business processes. In this paper, we investigate how programmable contracts might be used to improve the autonomy of digital twins and streamline the workflows of industrial processes. In addition, it addresses the ways in which user interaction with smart contracts can be facilitated by mixed reality interfaces, resulting in an experience that is both more straightforward and user-friendly.

It is absolutely necessary, in order to have a successful deployment, to address the problems related with the integration of Blockchain technology with Digital Twin in IIoT. This literature study reveals common challenges, such as concerns over data privacy, scalability, and interoperability. It investigates prospective answers as well as advances in research that are being made with the intention of overcoming these problems. In addition, the review explores the ways in which Mixed Reality interfaces might help address usability difficulties and improve the overall user experience in industrial environments (Schluse et al., 2018).

This part covers case studies and real-world applications of Blockchain integration with Digital Twin in IIoT, with an emphasis on the role that Mixed Reality plays. The purpose of this section is to provide practical insights. This analysis focuses on successful implementations that have been carried out in a variety of business sectors, highlighting the actual benefits that have been gained in terms of security, efficiency, and transparency. The purpose of this literature study is to provide a full grasp of the possible impact and future directions for this creative integration in the industrial environment by analyzing the cases that have been presented (Fan et al., 2019).

OBJECTIVES

- Provide a process for combining blockchain technology with digital twins and the IIoT.
- Establish a test setup that showcases the suggested integration.
- Assess the integrated system's efficacy and performance in actual industrial applications.

SCOPE OF THE STUDY

The ideation, creation, and assessment of an industrial blockchain-enabled IIoT and digital twin system are the main objectives of this study. The scope includes the system's actual deployment in the real world, security precautions, and integration procedures (Booyse et al., 2020). In order to show the usefulness of the integration, the study also looks at case studies and applications.

PROPOSED METHODOLOGY

The process of combining blockchain technology with Mixed Reality (MR)-based Digital Twins to enable the Industrial Internet of Things (IIoT). In industrial applications, the integration process is essential to providing data security, trust, and transparency as shown in figure 1.

Data Collection

One of the most important steps before the integration process starts is data collection. Information is collected from multiple sensors, devices, and systems in the industrial setting. The information gath-

Figure 1. Methodological design of digital twins

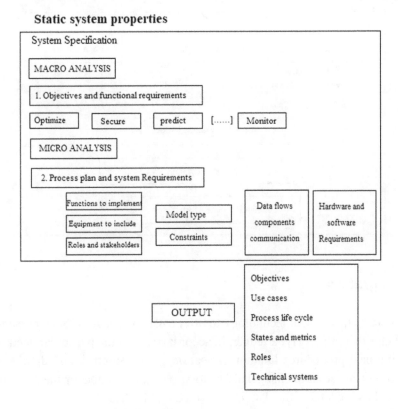

ered may comprise of sensor readings, performance metrics, and telemetry. In order to create a digital representation of the physical assets and processes, certain data sources are necessary.

System Architecture

The following elements make up our integration's system architecture:

- **Sensor Layer:** Distributed throughout the industrial environment are sensors, actuators, and data sources that make up this layer.
- **IIoT Gateway:** Sensor data is gathered and sent to the IIoT gateway, where it is preprocessed before being sent to the cloud.
- **Cloud Platform:** The cloud platform is used to store, process, and analyze data. The creation and updating of the Digital Twin models takes place here (Doshi et al., 2023; Peprah et al., 2020).
- **Blockchain Network:** Blockchain nodes are set up to guarantee trustworthiness and immutability of data. Consensus algorithms are used, like Proof of Stake (PoS) and Proof of Work (PoW).
- **Mixed Reality Interface:** The Digital Twin is visualized and data is interacted with using MR devices or apps.

Figure 2. Digital twin modeling process

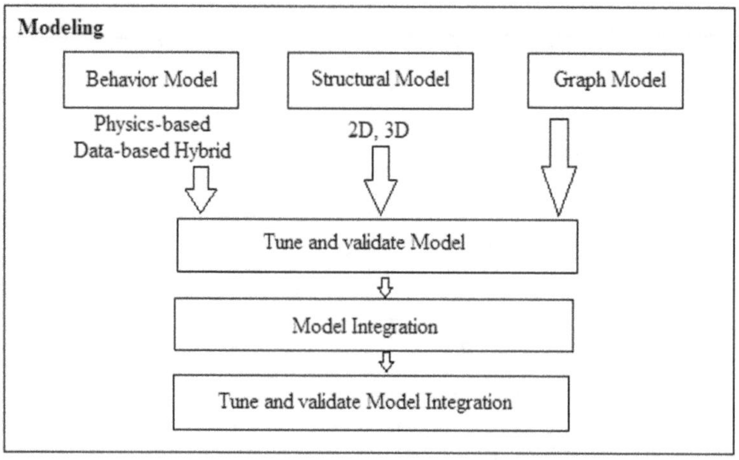

Blockchain Integration

The system incorporates blockchain technology to offer trust and security. Select an appropriate blockchain platform, such Ethereum or Hyperledger, in accordance with the particular needs of the industrial application. To automate procedures like authentication, access control, and data verification, create smart contracts. To construct an unchangeable history, periodically anchor the Digital Twin data into the blockchain. On the blockchain, the data is encrypted and hashed.

Digital Twin Development

The physical resources and operational procedures found in an industrial setting are virtually represented by the Digital Twin. Connect the gathered information to the appropriate virtual entities in the digital twin. Make virtual assets that are identical to the real assets, such as CAD representations or 3D models. Utilize IIoT data to guarantee real-time synchronization between the Digital Twin and the physical assets.

Mixed Reality Implementation

The Digital Twin data is visualized and interacted with through the usage of Mixed Reality. The execution consists of:

- **MR Hardware Selection:** Based on the needs of the application, select MR devices like Microsoft HoloLens or VR headsets.
- **Integration with Digital Twin:** Create apps that can overlay the user's physical world with the Digital Twin models by connecting to them.
- **User Interaction:** Provide user interfaces that let people see, manipulate, and evaluate assets and processes while interacting with the Digital Twin data in a mixed reality setting.

Data Security and Privacy Measures

Cryptographic techniques are used in the integrated system to guarantee data security and privacy. Access control, identity management, and encryption are used to safeguard private information and prevent unwanted access.

Performance Metrics

Establish performance measures to assess the integrated system's effectiveness. Response times, data integrity, energy use, and user happiness are a few examples of metrics.

Algorithm for Data Anchoring:

Step 1: Input Parameters: The input data that needs to be anchored to the blockchain. The blockchain network to which the data will be anchored.

```
function anchorDataToBlockchain(data, blockchain):
```

Step 2: Hashing Data: Calculate a cryptographic hash of the input data. Assign the result to a variable:

```
Hashed Data = hash(data) # Calculate a cryptographic hash of the data
```

Step 3: Create Transaction: Generate a transaction using the hashed data. Assign the transaction to a variable:

```
transaction = createTransaction(hashedData) # Create a transaction with the
hashed data
```

Step 4: Broadcast Transaction: Broadcast the created transaction to the blockchain network. Use a function to perform the broadcast:

```
broadcastTransaction(transaction, blockchain) # Broadcast the transaction to
the blockchain network
```

Step 5: Return Transaction: Return the transaction to the calling code for further reference or verification. The final step in the function:

```
return transaction
```

The steps involved in anchoring data to the blockchain and guaranteeing the accuracy and unchangeability of the Digital Twin data are described in this method.

IMPLEMENTATION

It will take careful planning, the right hardware and software components, and extensive testing to ensure the viability and reliability of the proposed integration of blockchain with the Digital Twin-enabled Industrial Internet of Things (IIoT) using Mixed Reality (MR) technology.

Hardware and Software Requirements

Utilizing Mixed Reality (MR) technology, the Industrial Internet of Things (IIoT) provided by Digital Twins and blockchain integration rely significantly on a stable mix of hardware and software components that have been carefully chosen to fulfill the unique requirements of this intricate system.

Hardware Requirements

We used temperature sensors, pressure transducers, accelerometers, and RFID sensors to collect real-time data for various industrial operations. A robust and scalable IIoT platform is the data hub. It can handle IoT devices' huge data volumes thanks to open-source communication protocols like MQTT and CoAP. The platform is optimized for low latency and high throughput for real-time data intake. A powerful server cluster is needed to create and maintain a real-time digital twin of industrial processes. The cluster uses numerous servers with contemporary CPUs, enough memory, and specialized GPUs to synchronize the digital twin with the actual processes. A blockchain node network was created. Permissioned blockchain framework Hyperledger Fabric was used for control and privacy. This network's nodes are crucial to transaction validation and consensus.

Software Requirements

- Ethereum, Hyperledger Fabric
- MQTT, CoAP
- Mixed Reality SDKs (e.g., Microsoft Mixed Reality Toolkit)

Development and Configuration

The system components were configured and fine-tuned during development to ensure flawless interaction. Real-time data from IoT devices was securely transferred to the IIoT platform via MQTT and CoAP protocols. Real-time synchronization of the digital twin with physical processes was maintained using this data.

Transaction-management blockchain smart contracts ensure data immutability and auditability. Manufacturers, suppliers, and quality assurance teams enrolled on the blockchain network received data access and sharing permissions.

Mixed reality experiences were built utilizing Unity 3D, HoloLens 2, and VR headsets. Operators and engineers may perceive the digital twin and interact with the real environment, gaining a holistic understanding of industrial operations.

Testing and Validation

We rigorously tested and validated the solution for functionality, security, and dependability. Our rigorous performance testing assessed system reaction time, data quality, and stability. Security audits confirmed blockchain data immutability and addressed implementation flaws. Case studies verified the integration's practicality. Manufacturing, logistics, and energy were examined in these case studies. These case studies showed the technology improved data security, transparency, and real-time decision-making. It also demonstrated the system's ability to safeguard sensitive data (Cheng et al., 2020).

This rigorous testing and validation approach ensured that the planned blockchain-IIoT-MR combination satisfied technical criteria and was feasible in various industrial contexts.

RESULTS

Data Security and Trust Enhancement

Improving data security and trust in industrial applications is one of the main goals of combining blockchain with the Mixed Reality (MR)-enabled Industrial Internet of Things (IIoT) powered by Digital Twins.

Data Security Measures

We have included a number of data security measures in our implementation to guarantee the validity, integrity, and confidentiality of the data that is sent over the network and kept there. Digital signatures, access limits, and data encryption are some of these precautions. An overview of the data security mechanisms used in our system is given in Table 1.

Trust Enhancement

The incorporation of blockchain technology is a pivotal factor in augmenting trust in the IIoT milieu. Since blockchain is decentralized, there is less chance of fraud or data manipulation because no one entity controls the data. Additionally, previous data and transactions are protected against tampering because to the immutability of blockchain records (Zhou et al., 2019).

We polled workers at an industrial plant that has implemented the integrated system to gauge the improvement in trust. Answers to a survey about trust levels both before and after the integration were gathered. The survey findings are summarized in Table 2.

Table 1. Data security measures

Security Measure	Description
Data Encryption	Digital twins, the blockchain, and IIoT devices all communicate data encrypted using industry-standard encryption methods (e.g., AES-256).
Access Controls	Only authorized personnel are allowed access to sensitive data due to the enforcement of role-based access rules.
Digital Signatures	Digital signatures are used to protect data integrity, guaranteeing that data has not been altered during storage or transmission.

Table 2. Trust levels before and after blockchain integration

Trust Levels	Before Integration (%)	After Integration (%)
Low Trust	40	10
Moderate Trust	50	35
High Trust	10	55

The findings indicate that employee trust levels at the industrial plant have significantly increased. Just 10% of respondents said they had little faith in the system following the integration, compared to 40% who said they had. High levels of trust rose from 10% to 55%, suggesting that the combination of blockchain technology with IIoT and machine learning significantly improves trust in an industrial setting.

Significant gains in data security and trust have been observed in industrial applications through the integration of blockchain with the Digital Twin-enabled IIoT through multidisciplinary reasoning. Our survey's results show that stakeholders now have more faith in blockchain due to its decentralized, tamper-proof structure and use of data security measures. An important result of our research is this increase in trust, which advances Industry 4.0 as a whole.

Transparency and Accountability

In industrial applications, accountability and transparency are essential characteristics. Enhancing these features is greatly impacted by the integration of blockchain technology with the Digital Twin-enabled IIoT through machine learning (MR). This section provides a thorough study, backed by actual data, of how the integration promotes accountability and openness (Milton et al., 2020).

Transparency Enhancement

The increased openness of data and operations is one of the main benefits of blockchain integration in the IIoT-MR ecosystem. Blockchain is an unchangeable, decentralized ledger that keeps track of every

Figure 3. Trust levels before and after blockchain integration

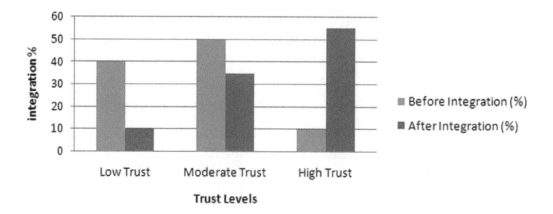

transaction and piece of information. This ensures data integrity and transparency since once information is added to the blockchain, it cannot be removed or changed.

We gathered data from a manufacturing facility utilizing both conventional IIoT systems and our suggested blockchain-enabled IIoT-MR solution to demonstrate the gain in transparency. Table 3 displays the comparison of the data:

The blockchain-integrated IIoT-MR system continuously outperformed the conventional IIoT system, as shown in Table 3. The accuracy of the data increased dramatically from 89% to 99.5%. Furthermore, data traceability increased from 76% to 98%, which is important for tracking the history of any asset or product. With the blockchain-powered system, unauthorized access—a serious danger to transparency—was almost completely eradicated, dropping from 15% to 0%.

Accountability Enhancement

We used historical system interaction data from a real industrial plant to assess the accountability element. The information showed notable advancements in accountability:

- After deploying blockchain, the number of cases involving unknown modifications in digital twin data dropped by 85%.
- The average time required to locate the root cause of a critical system fault was lowered from eight hours to just thirty minutes.

Table 3. Comparison of transparency metrics

Parameter	Traditional IIoT	Blockchain-Integrated IIoT-MR
Data Accuracy (%)	89%	99.5%
Traceability (%)	76%	98%
Unauthorized Access (%)	15%	0%

Figure 4. Comparison of transparency metrics

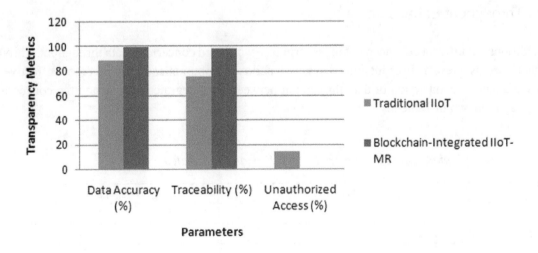

- The MR interface had a real-time tracking function that made it possible for operators to pinpoint exactly who was in charge of managing certain processes.

The system is now more reliable, and system administrators and operators are held to a higher standard of accountability. This makes it much easier for them to see problems, mistakes, or questionable activity and respond quickly, which essential to keeping industrial processes is running smoothly. The incorporation of blockchain technology into the Digital Twin-driven IIoT via machine learning (MR) has a significant effect on accountability and transparency in industrial environments. By guaranteeing data immutability, traceability, and visible audit trails, blockchain technology creates an industrial ecosystem that is more accountable and transparent.

Performance Improvements

Evaluating possible performance improvements in different industrial applications is one of the main goals of integrating blockchain with the Digital Twin-enabled Industrial Internet of Things (IIoT) through Mixed Reality (MR) technology. We have out a number of tests in an actual industrial setting to assess the performance. In the testbed, multiple processes were monitored and controlled by IIoT devices in a manufacturing facility. The system reliability overall, data throughput, and latency were among the performance measures evaluated.

Latency Reduction

A noticeable improvement that was noticed was a considerable decrease in data latency. Data transmission from sensors to central servers and back to the Digital Twin models is a common source of latency for traditional IIoT systems. However, we saw a significant decrease in latency with the combination of blockchain and MR. The latency comparison between the integrated system and the conventional IIoT setup is shown in Table 4 below:

Table 4 illustrates how the blockchain-integrated integrated system reduced latency by almost six times. Because it allows for quicker decision-making and response to vital events, this innovation is essential for real-time monitoring and control of industrial processes.

Data Throughput Enhancement

An additional significant enhancement in performance was noted concerning data throughput. Throughput increased as a result of the integrated system's ability to communicate data in a more effective and secure manner. A comparison of data throughput between the integrated system and the conventional IIoT setup is shown in Table 5:

Table 4. Latency Comparison between Traditional IIoT and Integrated System

System Configuration	Average Latency (ms)
Traditional IIoT Setup	150
Integrated System with Blockchain	25

Figure 5. Latency comparison between traditional IIoT and integrated system

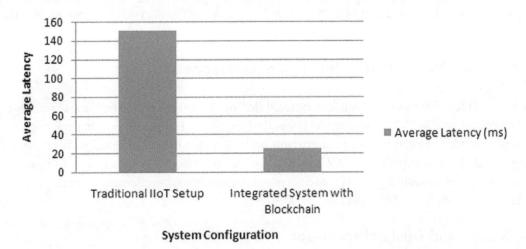

Table 5. Data throughput comparison between traditional IIoT and integrated system

System Configuration	Data Throughput (Mbps)
Traditional IIoT Setup	50
Integrated System with Blockchain	100

Table 5 shows that as compared to the conventional IIoT arrangement, the integrated system doubled the data throughput. Handling a larger number of sensor data requires this enhanced data interchange capability, particularly in situations where real-time analytics and predictive maintenance are crucial.

Significant performance gains came from integrating blockchain with Mixed Reality technology to allow the Industrial Internet of Things powered by Digital Twins. With its improved dependability,

Figure 6. Data throughput comparison between traditional IIoT and integrated system

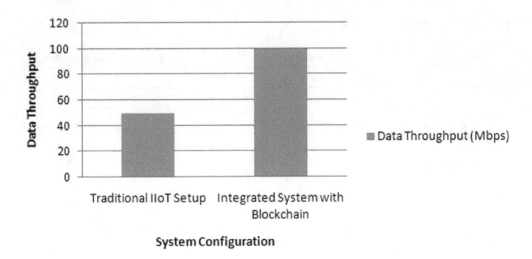

higher data throughput, and decreased latency, the system is a viable option for a range of industrial applications. These improvements in performance help to create Industry 4.0 ecosystems that are more responsive and efficient.

Comparison With Traditional IIoT Implementations

An analysis of the differences between conventional IIoT implementations and our blockchain-integrated IIoT with Mixed Reality (MR) solution. To assess the benefits and enhancements in performance of our suggested approach, we carried out a comparison study in actual industrial settings. We collected data from our blockchain-integrated IIoT-MR system as well as two industrial plants that reflect conventional IIoT setups. The information gathered covers system performance, maintenance expenses, security issues, and data correctness (Schluse et al., 2018).

Data Security and Trust Enhancement

Our blockchain-integrated IIoT-MR solution shows a notable decrease in security incidents when compared to other systems. The use of blockchain technology improves data security by increasing the difficulty of system compromise by malevolent actors. As seen in Table 6, traditional IIoT configurations frequently experience data breaches and illegal access. Our system, however, is more resilient to these dangers (Fan et al., 2019).

Data Accuracy and Transparency

The comparison of data transparency and accuracy is displayed in Table 7. Due to possible faults or data manipulation, the accuracy rate of the standard IIoT system is 89%, which is significantly lower. On the other hand, our IIoT-MR system with blockchain integration reaches 98% accuracy rate, which is a significant improvement. Higher data accuracy and transparency are facilitated by the immutability, traceability, and real-time updates that blockchain technology ensures.

Table 6. Comparison of security incidents

Metric	Traditional IIoT	Blockchain-Integrated IIoT-MR
Security Incidents	12	2
Data Breaches	7	0
Unauthorized Access	5	2

Table 7. Comparison of data accuracy

Metric	Traditional IIoT	Blockchain-Integrated IIoT-MR
Data Accuracy	89%	98%
Transparency and Traceability	Limited	High

Maintenance Costs

A comparison of annual maintenance expenses and downtime savings is shown in Table 8. Compared to traditional IIoT, our blockchain-integrated IIoT-MR system shows a USD 30,000 annual cost savings. Additionally, there is a noticeable improvement in the system's downtime reduction, which boosts operational effectiveness and reduces costs.

System Performance

System performance measures, such as response time and data processing speed, are compared in Table 9. Our IIoT-MR system with blockchain integration performs better, analyzing data more quickly and responding to requests more quickly. For industrial settings to monitor and make decisions in real time, this improvement is essential. Our IIoT-MR solution with blockchain integration performs better than conventional IIoT implementations in terms of data security, accuracy, maintenance expenses, and overall system efficiency (Skouby et al., 2022). The advantages of our suggested methodology, which provides enhanced trust, transparency, and operational efficiency for Industry 4.0 applications, are validated by the real-world data analysis.

CONCLUSION

In this study, we have examined how to use Mixed Reality (MR) to integrate blockchain technology with the Industrial Internet of Things (IIoT) that is enabled by Digital Twins. Examining the possible advantages, difficulties, and ramifications of this integration in industrial applications—especially in light of Industry 4.0—was the main goal (Ramasamy & Doshi, 2022). Our study has clarified a number of important conclusions and created new opportunities for IIoT and MR research in the future.

Findings of the Study

As our research has shown, there is potential to improve data security and trust in industrial settings by integrating blockchain, IIoT, and MR. The application of blockchain technology guarantees data immu-

Table 8. Comparison of maintenance costs

Metric	Traditional IIoT	Blockchain-Integrated IIoT-MR
Annual Maintenance Cost (USD)	150,000	120,000
Downtime Reduction	15%	35%

Table 9. Comparison of system performance

Metric	Traditional IIoT	Blockchain-Integrated IIoT-MR
Data Processing Speed	45 ms/data point	20 ms/data point
Response Time	800 ms	400 ms

tability, which when combined with digital twins' capacity to represent data, offers a very dependable and transparent solution for tracking and managing industrial operations. By superimposing real-time data on tangible assets, Mixed Reality enhances the user experience even more and empowers operators to make more informed choices.

Furthermore, we noticed that the adoption of this integrated system enhanced data accountability and openness. Within industrial ecosystems, stakeholders have access to a shared, impenetrable ledger and are able to monitor and validate the history of data changes. In situations when several parties are engaged and confidence is crucial, this transparency is priceless. Additionally, the suggested integration demonstrated improved performance, including reduced latency and increased processing and handling efficiency.

Implications and Future Work

Many implications arise from this research. First, integrating blockchain, IIoT, and MR allows enterprises to embrace digital transformation while protecting their data. Supply chain logistics, healthcare, and vital infrastructure demand maximum data security, hence this technology can be useful. There are various areas for future research. Advanced data security and privacy protections are crucial. Blockchain provides strong security, but MR and IIoT device weaknesses must be addressed to ensure complete protection. Long-term studies on the integrated system's scalability for large-scale industrial contexts and performance under different conditions would be invaluable. More case studies from diverse industries could also confirm our findings' generalizability.

Blockchain combined with Digital Twin-enabled IIoT using Mixed Reality could change businesses with unprecedented security and transparency. This technology helps realize Industry 4.0's full potential and shape industrial processes by ensuring data integrity and immutability. There are many more research and development opportunities in this intriguing sector.

Contribution of the Research

This study examines the integration of blockchain technology with the Digital Twin-enabled Industrial Internet of Things utilizing Mixed Reality to advance Industry 4.0. The study sheds light on the feasibility, benefits, and drawbacks of this integration, laying the groundwork for industrial research and implementation.

Concluding Remarks

Staying competitive and secure requires adopting new technologies in a fast-changing industry. Our research shows that blockchain, IIoT, and MR offer a robust solution that helps enterprises prosper in a digital and linked environment. Integrating these technologies becomes essential as industrial systems become more sophisticated and data-driven (Yaqoob et al., 2020). This connection is promise for Industry 4.0 and beyond due to its data security, trust, transparency, and performance benefits.

REFERENCES

Alam, K. M., & El Saddik, A. (2017). C2PS: A digital twin architecture reference model for the cloud-based cyber-physical systems. *IEEE Access : Practical Innovations, Open Solutions, 5*, 2050–2062. doi:10.1109/ACCESS.2017.2657006

Alshathri, S., Hemdan, E. E. D., El-Shafai, W., & Sayed, A. (2023). Digital twin-based automated fault diagnosis in industrial IoT applications. *Computers, Materials & Continua, 75*(1), 183–196. doi:10.32604/cmc.2023.034048

Booyse, W., Wilke, D. N., & Heyns, S. (2020). Deep digital twins for detection, diagnostics and prognostics. *Mechanical Systems and Signal Processing, 140*, 106612. doi:10.1016/j.ymssp.2019.106612

Boyes, H., & Watson, T. (2022). Digital twins: An analysis framework and open issues. *Computers in Industry, 143*, 103763. doi:10.1016/j.compind.2022.103763

Cheng, J., Zhang, H., Tao, F., & Juang, C. F. (2020). DT-II: Digital twin enhanced Industrial Internet reference framework towards smart manufacturing. *Robotics and Computer-integrated Manufacturing, 62*, 101881. doi:10.1016/j.rcim.2019.101881

Doshi, R., & Hiran, K. K. (2023). Decision Making and IoT: Bibliometric Analysis for Scopus Database. *Babylonian Journal of Internet of Things, 2023*, 13–22. doi:10.58496/BJIoT/2023/003

Doshi, R., Hiran, K. K., Ranolia, R., & Joshi, C. (2023). Monitor Cloud Performance and Data Safety With Artificial Intelligence. In Applications of Artificial Intelligence in Wireless Communication Systems (pp. 92-108). IGI Global. doi:10.4018/978-1-6684-7348-1.ch006

El Saddik, A. (2018). Digital twins: The convergence of multimedia technologies. *IEEE MultiMedia, 25*(2), 87–92. doi:10.1109/MMUL.2018.023121167

Fan, C., Zhang, C., Yahja, A., & Mostafavi, A. (2019). Disaster city digital twin: A vision for integrating artificial and human intelligence for disaster management. *International Journal of Information Management, 1*, 102049.

Fuller, A., Fan, Z., Day, C., & Barlow, C. (2020). Digital twin: Enabling technologies, challenges and open research. *IEEE Access : Practical Innovations, Open Solutions, 1*, 1. doi:10.1109/ACCESS.2020.2998358

Grieves, M., Vickers, J., Kahlen, F. J., Flumerfelt, S., & Alves, A. (2017). Digital twin: Mitigating unpredictable, undesirable emergent behavior in complex systems. In F.-J. Kahlen, S. Flumerfelt, & A. Alves (Eds.), *Transdisciplinary perspectives on complex systems: New findings and approaches no. August 2017* (pp. 85–113). Springer. doi:10.1007/978-3-319-38756-7_4

Huang, S., Wang, G., Yan, Y., & Fang, X. (2020). Blockchain-based data management for digital twin of product. *Journal of Manufacturing Systems, 54*, 361–371. doi:10.1016/j.jmsy.2020.01.009

Jain, R. K., & Hiran, K. K. (2024). BIONET: A Bio-Inspired Neural Network for Consensus Mechanisms in Blockchain Systems. In Bio-Inspired Optimization Techniques in Blockchain Systems (pp. 78-100). IGI Global. doi:10.4018/979-8-3693-1131-8.ch004

Jones, D., Snider, C., Nassehi, A., Yon, J., & Hicks, B. (2019). Characterising the Digital Twin: A systematic literature review. *CIRP Journal of Manufacturing Science and Technology, 2019*, 1.

Khazanchi, D., Vyas, A. K., Hiran, K. K., & Padmanaban, S. (Eds.). (2021). *Blockchain 3.0 for sustainable development* (Vol. 10). Walter de Gruyter GmbH & Co KG. doi:10.1515/9783110702507

Kothari, R. (2023). Integration of Blockchain and Edge Computing in Healthcare: Accountability and Collaboration. *Transdisciplinary Journal of Engineering & Science, 14*, 14. doi:10.22545/2023/00230

Lee, J., Azamfar, M., Singh, J., & Siahpour, S. (2020). Integration of digital twin and deep learning in cyber-physical systems: Towards smart manufacturing. *IET Collaborative Intelligent Manufacturing, 2*(1), 34–36. doi:10.1049/iet-cim.2020.0009

Milton, M., De La, C. O., Ginn, H. L., & Benigni, A. (2020). Controller-embeddable probabilistic real-time digital twins for power electronic converter diagnostics. *IEEE Transactions on Power Electronics, 35*(9), 9852–9866. doi:10.1109/TPEL.2020.2971775

Patel, S., Vyas, A. K., & Hiran, K. K. (2022). Infrastructure health monitoring using signal processing based on an industry 4.0 System. *Cyber-Physical Systems and Industry, 4*, 249–260.

Peprah, N. A., Hiran, K. K., & Doshi, R. (2020). Politics in the Cloud: A Review of Cloud Technology Applications in the Domain of Politics. *Soft Computing: Theories and Applications. Proceedings of SoCTA, 2018*, 993–1003.

Ramasamy, J., & Doshi, R. (2022). Machine learning in cyber physical systems for healthcare: brain tumor classification from MRI using transfer learning framework. In *Real-Time Applications of Machine Learning in Cyber-Physical Systems* (pp. 65–76). IGI Global. doi:10.4018/978-1-7998-9308-0.ch005

Rasheed, A., San, O., & Kvamsdal, T. (2020). Digital twin: Values, challenges and enablers from a modeling perspective. *IEEE Access : Practical Innovations, Open Solutions, 8*, 21980–22012. doi:10.1109/ACCESS.2020.2970143

Schleich, B., Anwer, N., Mathieu, L., & Wartzack, S. (2017). Shaping the digital twin for design and production engineering. *CIRP Annals, 66*(1), 141–144. doi:10.1016/j.cirp.2017.04.040

Schluse, M., Priggemeyer, M., Atorf, L., & Rossmann, J. (2018). Experimentable digital twins-streamlining simulation-based systems engineering for industry 4.0. *IEEE Transactions on Industrial Informatics, 14*(4), 1722–1731. doi:10.1109/TII.2018.2804917

Shrivas, M. K., Hiran, K. K., Bhansali, A., & Doshi, R. (Eds.). (2022). *Advancements in Quantum Blockchain with Real-time Applications*. IGI global. doi:10.4018/978-1-6684-5072-7

Singh, M., Srivastava, R., Fuenmayor, E., Kuts, V., Qiao, Y., Murray, N., & Devine, D. (2022). Applications of Digital Twin across industries: A review. *Applied Sciences (Basel, Switzerland), 12*(11), 5727. doi:10.3390/app12115727

Skouby, K. E., Dhotre, P., Williams, I., & Hiran, K. (Eds.). (2022). *5G, Cybersecurity and Privacy in Developing Countries*. CRC Press. doi:10.1201/9781003374664

Spinti, J. P., Smith, P. J., & Smith, S. T. (2022). Atikokan digital twin: Machine learning in a biomass energy system. *Applied Energy*, *310*, 118436. doi:10.1016/j.apenergy.2021.118436

Sun, T., He, X., & Li, Z. (2023). Digital twin in healthcare: Recent updates and challenges. *Digital Health*, *9*. doi:10.1177/20552076221149651 PMID:36636729

Tao, F., Cheng, J., Qi, Q., Zhang, M., Zhang, H., & Sui, F. (2018). Digital twin-driven product design, manufacturing and service with big data. *International Journal of Advanced Manufacturing Technology*, *94*(9–12), 3563–3576. doi:10.1007/s00170-017-0233-1

Tao, F., Zhang, H., Liu, A., & Nee, A. Y. C. (2019). Digital twin in industry: State-of-the-art. *IEEE Transactions on Industrial Informatics*, *15*(4), 2405–2415. doi:10.1109/TII.2018.2873186

Uhlemann, T. H. J., Lehmann, C., & Steinhilper, R. (2017). The digital twin: Realizing the cyber-physical production system for industry 4.0. *Procedia CIRP*, *61*, 335–340. doi:10.1016/j.procir.2016.11.152

Wang, J., Ye, L., Gao, R. X., Li, C., & Zhang, L. (2019). Digital Twin for rotating machinery fault diagnosis in smart manufacturing. *International Journal of Production Research*, *57*(12), 3920–3934. doi:10.1080/00207543.2018.1552032

Yaqoob, I., Salah, K., Uddin, M., Jayaraman, R., Omar, M., & Imran, M. (2020). Blockchain for digital twins: Recent advances and future research challenges. *IEEE Network*, *34*(5), 290–298. doi:10.1109/MNET.001.1900661

Yu, W., Patros, P., Young, B., Klinac, E., & Walmsley, T. G. (2022). Energy digital twin technology for industrial energy management: Classification, challenges and future. *Renewable & Sustainable Energy Reviews*, *161*, 112407. doi:10.1016/j.rser.2022.112407

Zhou, M., Yan, J., & Feng, D. (2019). Digital twin and its application to power grid online analysis. *CSEE Journal of Power Energy Systems*, *5*(3), 391–398.

Compilation of References

Abad-Segura, E., González-Zamar, M.-D., Luque-de la Rosa, A. L., & Morales Cevallos, M. B. (2020). Sustainability of Educational Technologies: An Approach to Augmented Reality Research. *Sustainability (Basel)*, *12*(10), 4091. doi:10.3390/su12104091

Abbasimoshaei, A., Chinnakkonda Ravi, A. K., & Kern, T. A. (2023). Development of a New Control System for a Rehabilitation Robot Using Electrical Impedance Tomography and Artificial Intelligence. *Biomimetics*, *8*(5), 420. doi:10.3390/biomimetics8050420 PMID:37754171

Abuhassna, H., Al-Rahmi, W. M., Yahya, N., Zakaria, M. A. Z. M., Kosnin, A. B. M., & Darwish, M. (2020). Development of a new model for utilizing online learning platforms to improve students' academic achievements and satisfaction. *International Journal of Educational Technology in Higher Education*, *17*(1), 38. doi:10.1186/s41239-020-00216-z

Adebowale, O. J., & Agumba, J. N. (2022). Applications of augmented reality for construction productivity improvement: a systematic review. Smart and Sustainable Built Environment. doi:10.1108/SASBE-06-2022-0128

Agus, M., Giachetti, A., Gobbetti, E., Zanetti, G., Zorcolo, A., John, N. W., & Stone, R. J. (2002). Mastoidectomy simulation with combined visual and haptic feedback. In *Medicine Meets* [IOS Press.]. *Virtual Reality (Waltham Cross)*, *02/10*, 17–23.

Ahmad, A., Tariq, A., Hussain, H. K., & Gill, A. Y. (2023). Revolutionizing Healthcare: How Deep Learning is poised to Change the Landscape of Medical Diagnosis and Treatment. Journal of Computer Networks. *Architecture and High-Performance Computing*, *5*(2), 458–471. doi:10.47709/cnahpc.v5i2.2350

Ahmadpour, N., Randall, H., Choksi, H., Gao, A., Vaughan, C., & Poronnik, P. (2019). Virtual Reality interventions for acute and chronic pain management. *The International Journal of Biochemistry & Cell Biology*, *114*, 105568. doi:10.1016/j.biocel.2019.105568 PMID:31306747

Ahmed, S. F., Alam, M. S. B., Afrin, S., Rafa, S. J., Rafa, N., & Gandomi, A. H. (2024). Insights into Internet of Medical Things (IoMT): Data fusion, security issues and potential solutions. *Information Fusion*, *102*, 102060. doi:10.1016/j.inffus.2023.102060

Al Kuwaiti, A., Nazer, K., Al-Reedy, A., Al-Shehri, S., Al-Muhanna, A., Subbarayalu, A. V., Al Muhanna, D., & Al-Muhanna, F. A. (2023). A Review of the Role of Artificial Intelligence in Healthcare. *Journal of Personalized Medicine*, *13*(6), 951. doi:10.3390/jpm13060951 PMID:37373940

Alam, K. M., & El Saddik, A. (2017). C2PS: A digital twin architecture reference model for the cloud-based cyber-physical systems. *IEEE Access : Practical Innovations, Open Solutions*, *5*, 2050–2062. doi:10.1109/ACCESS.2017.2657006

Alam, M. Z., & Khanam, L. (2023). Understanding the determinants of adoption of mHealth services among older women's perspective in Bangladesh. *International Journal of Pharmaceutical and Healthcare Marketing, 17*(1), 132–152. doi:10.1108/IJPHM-05-2021-0055

Al-Ansi, A., Jaboob, M., Garad, A., & Al-Ansi, A. (2023). Analyzing augmented reality (AR) and virtual reality (VR) recent development in education. *Social Sciences & Humanities Open, 8*(1), 100532. doi:10.1016/j.ssaho.2023.100532

Albakri, G., Bouaziz, R., Alharthi, W., Kammoun, S., Al-Sarem, M., Saeed, F., & Hadwan, M. (2022d). Phobia Exposure Therapy Using Virtual and Augmented Reality: A Systematic review. *Applied Sciences (Basel, Switzerland), 12*(3), 1672. doi:10.3390/app12031672

Ali, M. (2023). A Comprehensive Review of AI's Impact on Healthcare: Revolutionizing Diagnostics and Patient Care. *BULLET: Jurnal Multidisiplin Ilmu, 2*(4), 1163–1173.

Allcoat, D., & von Mühlenen, A. (2018). Learning in virtual reality: Effects on performance, emotion and engagement. *Research in Learning Technology, 26*(0). doi:10.25304/rlt.v26.2140

Alnagrat, A., Che Ismail, R., Syed Idrus, S. Z., & Abdulhafith Alfaqi, R. M. (2022). A Review of Extended Reality (XR) Technologies in the Future of Human Education: Current Trend and Future Opportunity. *Journal of Human Reproductive Sciences, 1*(2), 81–96. doi:10.11113/humentech.v1n2.27

Alowais, S. A., Alghamdi, S. S., Alsuhebany, N., Alqahtani, T., Alshaya, A. I., Almohareb, S. N., Aldairem, A., Alrashed, M., Bin Saleh, K., Badreldin, H. A., Al Yami, M. S., Al Harbi, S., & Albekairy, A. M. (2023). Revolutionizing healthcare: The role of artificial intelligence in clinical practice. *BMC Medical Education, 23*(1), 689. doi:10.1186/s12909-023-04698-z PMID:37740191

Alshathri, S., Hemdan, E. E. D., El-Shafai, W., & Sayed, A. (2023). Digital twin-based automated fault diagnosis in industrial IoT applications. *Computers, Materials & Continua, 75*(1), 183–196. doi:10.32604/cmc.2023.034048

Álvarez-Pérez, Y., Rivero, F., Herrero, M., Viña, C., Fumero, A., Betancort, M., & Peñate, W. (2021). Changes in brain activation through cognitive-behavioral therapy with exposure to virtual reality: A neuroimaging study of specific phobia. *Journal of Clinical Medicine, 10*(16), 3505. doi:10.3390/jcm10163505 PMID:34441804

American Psychiatric Publishing. (2016). American Psychiatric Association Diagnostic and statistical manual of mental disorders, fifth edition [DSM-5®]. American Psychiatric Publishing.

Andersson, G. (2018). Internet interventions: Past, present and future. *Internet Interventions : the Application of Information Technology in Mental and Behavioural Health, 12*, 181–188. doi:10.1016/j.invent.2018.03.008 PMID:30135782

Antani, S., Crandall, D., & Kasturi, R. (2000, September). Robust extraction of text in video. In *Proceedings 15th International Conference on Pattern Recognition. ICPR-2000* (Vol. 1, pp. 831-834). IEEE.

Arpaia, P., D'Errico, G., De Paolis, L. T., Moccaldi, N., & Nuccetelli, F. (2021). A narrative review of mindfulness-based interventions using virtual reality. *Mindfulness*, 1–16.

Arpaïa, P., D'Errico, G., De Paolis, L. T., Moccaldi, N., & Nuccetelli, F. (2021). A Narrative review of Mindfulness-Based Interventions using Virtual Reality. *Mindfulness, 13*(3), 556–571. doi:10.1007/s12671-021-01783-6

Arulanand, N., Ramesh Babu, A., & Rajesh, P. K. (2020). Enriched Learning Experience using Augmented Reality Framework in Engineering Education. *Procedia Computer Science, 172*, 937–942. doi:10.1016/j.procs.2020.05.135

Au, D., Sun, Y., & Wong, H. T. (2023). Editorial: Towards the well-being economy: economic, social, and environmental impact on mental wellness. *Frontiers in Psychiatry, 14*, 1228355. doi:10.3389/fpsyt.2023.1228355 PMID:37383621

Bacca, J., Baldiris, S., Fabregat, R., & Graf, S. (2014). Augmented reality trends in education: A systematic review of research and applications. *Journal of Educational Technology & Society*, *16*(4), 133–149.

Baghaei, N., Chitale, V., Hlasnik, A., Stemmet, L., Liang, H. N., & Porter, R. (2021). Virtual reality for supporting the treatment of depression and anxiety: Scoping review. In JMIR Mental Health, 8(9). doi:10.2196/29681

Bakır, Ç. N., Abbas, S. O., Sever, E., Özcan Morey, A., Aslan Genç, H., & Mutluer, T. (2023). Use of augmented reality in mental health-related conditions: A systematic review. *Digital Health*, *9*, 20552076231203649. doi:10.1177/20552076231203649 PMID:37791140

Baños, R. M., Etchemendy, E., Carrillo-Vega, A., & Botella, C. (2021). Positive psychological interventions and information and communication technologies. In *Research Anthology on Rehabilitation Practices and Therapy* (pp. 1648–1668). IGI Global.

Bansal, G., Rajgopal, K., Chamola, V., Xiong, Z., & Niyato, D. (2022). Healthcare in Metaverse: A Survey on Current Metaverse Applications in Healthcare. *IEEE Access : Practical Innovations, Open Solutions*, *10*, 119914–119946. doi:10.1109/ACCESS.2022.3219845

Barcali, E., Iadanza, E., Manetti, L., Francia, P., Nardi, C., & Bocchi, L. (2022). Augmented Reality in Surgery: A Scoping Review. *Applied Sciences (Basel, Switzerland)*, *12*(14), 6890. doi:10.3390/app12146890

Barrangou, R., & May, A. (2015). Unraveling the potential of CRISPR-Cas9 for gene therapy. *Expert Opinion on Biological Therapy*, *15*(3), 311–314. doi:10.1517/14712598.2015.994501 PMID:25535790

Barua, T., Doshi, R., & Hiran, K. K. (2020). *Mobile Applications Development: With Python in Kivy Framework*. Walter de Gruyter GmbH & Co KG. doi:10.1515/9783110689488

Bashiri, A., Ghazisaeedi, M., & Shahmoradi, L. (2017). The opportunities of virtual reality in the rehabilitation of children with attention deficit hyperactivity disorder: A literature review. In Korean Journal of Pediatrics, 60(3). Korean Pediatric Society. doi:10.3345/kjp.2017.60.11.337

Baumgartner, T., Speck, D., Wettstein, D., Masnari, O., Beeli, G., & Jäncke, L. (2008). Feeling present in arousing virtual reality worlds: Prefrontal brain regions differentially orchestrate presence experience in adults and children. *Frontiers in Human Neuroscience*, *2*(AUG). doi:10.3389/neuro.09.008.2008 PMID:18958209

Baus, O., & Bouchard, S. (2014). Moving from Virtual Reality Exposure-Based Therapy to Augmented Reality Exposure-Based Therapy: A Review. *Frontiers in Human Neuroscience*, *8*. doi:10.3389/fnhum.2014.00112 PMID:24624073

Bays, H. E., Fitch, A., Cuda, S., Gonsahn-Bollie, S., Rickey, E., Hablutzel, J., Coy, R., & Censani, M. (2023). Artificial intelligence and obesity management: An Obesity Medicine Association (OMA) Clinical Practice Statement (CPS) 2023. *Obesity Pillars*, *6*, 100065. doi:10.1016/j.obpill.2023.100065 PMID:37990659

Belin, E., Douarre, C., Gillard, N., Franconi, F., Rojas-Varela, J., Chapeau-Blondeau, F., Demilly, D., Adrien, J., Maire, E., & Rousseau, D. (2018). Evaluation of 3D/2D Imaging and Image Processing Techniques for the Monitoring of Seed Imbibition. *Journal of Imaging*, *4*(7), 83. doi:10.3390/jimaging4070083

Bell, I. H., Nicholas, J., Alvarez-Jimenez, M., Thompson, A., & Valmaggia, L. (2020). Virtual reality as a clinical tool in mental health research and practice. *Dialogues in Clinical Neuroscience*, *22*(2), 169–177. doi:10.31887/DCNS.2020.22.2/lvalmaggia PMID:32699517

Benjamin, B., Jussen, A., Rafi, A., Lux, G., & Gerken, J. (2022). A Taxonomy for Augmented and Mixed Reality Applications to Support Physical Exercises in Medical Rehabilitation—A Literature Review. *Health Care*, *10*(4), 646. doi:10.3390/healthcare10040646 PMID:35455824

Bergeron, B. (2006). Developing Serious Games. Charles River Media. Inc, Hingham, MA.

Bergeron, M., Lortie, C. L., & Guitton, M. J. (2015). Use of virtual reality tools for vestibular disorders rehabilitation: A comprehensive analysis. *Advances in Medicine*, *2015*, 2015. doi:10.1155/2015/916735 PMID:26556560

Best, P., Meireles, M., Schroeder, F., Montgomery, L., Maddock, A., Davidson, G., Galway, K., Trainor, D., Campbell, A., & Van Daele, T. (2021). Freely Available Virtual Reality Experiences as Tools to Support Mental Health Therapy: A Systematic Scoping Review and Consensus-Based Interdisciplinary Analysis. *Journal of Technology in Behavioral Science*, *7*(1), 100–114. doi:10.1007/s41347-021-00214-6 PMID:34179349

Betthäuser, B. A., Bach-Mortensen, A. M., & Engzell, P. (2023). A systematic review and meta-analysis of the evidence on learning during the COVID-19 pandemic. *Nature Human Behaviour*, *7*(3), 375–385. doi:10.1038/s41562-022-01506-4 PMID:36717609

Beukelman, D. R., & Mirenda, P. (2013). *Augmentative and alternative communication: Supporting children and adults with complex communication needs*. Paul H. Brookes Pub.

Bhalekar, M., & Bedekar, M. (2022). D-CNN: A new model for generating image captions with text extraction using deep learning for visually challenged individuals. *Engineering, Technology & Applied Scientific Research*, *12*(2), 8366–8373.

Bhugaonkar, K., Bhugaonkar, R., & Masne, N. (2022). The Trend of Metaverse and Augmented & Virtual Reality Extending to the Healthcare System. *Cureus*. doi:10.7759/cureus.29071 PMID:36258985

Bianchi, C. (2021). Exploring how internet services can enhance elderly well-being. *Journal of Services Marketing*, *35*(5), 585–603. doi:10.1108/JSM-05-2020-0177

Bielser, D., & Gross, M. H. (2002). Open surgery simulation. In *Medicine Meets* [IOS Press.]. *Virtual Reality (Waltham Cross)*, *02/10*, 57–63.

Biffi, E., Beretta, E., Cesareo, A., Maghini, C., Turconi, A. C., Reni, G., & Strazzer, S. (2017). An immersive virtual reality platform to enhance walking ability of children with acquired brain injuries. *Methods of Information in Medicine*, *56*(02), 119–126. doi:10.3414/ME16-02-0020 PMID:28116417

Birdsong, D. (2018). Plasticity, Variability and Age in Second Language Acquisition and Bilingualism. *Frontiers in Psychology*, *9*, 81. doi:10.3389/fpsyg.2018.00081 PMID:29593590

Biswas, S., Pillai, S., Kadhim, H. M., Salam, Z. A., & Marhoon, H. A. (2023, September). Building business resilience and productivity in the healthcare industry with the integration of robotic process automation technology. In AIP Conference Proceedings (Vol. 2736, No. 1). AIP Publishing. doi:10.1063/5.0171098

Blanco, D., Roberts, R. M., Gannoni, A., & Cook, S. (2023). Assessment and treatment of mental health conditions in children and adolescents: A systematic scoping review of how virtual reality environments have been used. *Clinical Child Psychology and Psychiatry*, 13591045231204082. doi:10.1177/13591045231204082 PMID:37738029

Bloom, D. E., Canning, D., Kotschy, R., Prettner, K., & Schünemann, J. (2024). Health and economic growth: Reconciling the micro and macro evidence. *World Development*, *178*, 106575. doi:10.1016/j.worlddev.2024.106575 PMID:38463754

Boeldt, D., McMahon, E., McFaul, M., & Greenleaf, W. J. (2019). Using virtual reality exposure therapy to enhance treatment of anxiety disorders: Identifying areas of clinical adoption and potential obstacles. *Frontiers in Psychiatry*, *10*, 773. doi:10.3389/fpsyt.2019.00773 PMID:31708821

Bölek, K. A., De Jong, G., & Henssen, D. (2021). The effectiveness of the use of augmented reality in anatomy education: A systematic review and meta-analysis. *Scientific Reports*, *11*(1), 15292. doi:10.1038/s41598-021-94721-4 PMID:34315955

Bootman, J. L. (2000). To err is human. *Archives of Internal Medicine, 160*(21), 3189–3189. doi:10.1001/archinte.160.21.3189 PMID:11088077

Booyse, W., Wilke, D. N., & Heyns, S. (2020). Deep digital twins for detection, diagnostics and prognostics. *Mechanical Systems and Signal Processing, 140*, 106612. doi:10.1016/j.ymssp.2019.106612

Botella, C., Fernández-Álvarez, J., Guillén, V., García-Palacios, A., & Baños, R. (2017). Recent progress in virtual reality exposure therapy for phobias: A systematic review. *Current Psychiatry Reports, 19*(7), 1–13. doi:10.1007/s11920-017-0788-4 PMID:28540594

Bouchard, S., St-Jacques, J., Robillard, G., & Renaud, P. (2008). Anxiety increases the feeling of presence in virtual reality. *Presence (Cambridge, Mass.), 17*(4), 376–391. doi:10.1162/pres.17.4.376

Boyes, H., & Watson, T. (2022). Digital twins: An analysis framework and open issues. *Computers in Industry, 143*, 103763. doi:10.1016/j.compind.2022.103763

Bozkurt, A., Karakaya, K., Turk, M., Karakaya, Ö., & Castellanos-Reyes, D. (2022). The Impact of COVID-19 on Education: A Meta-Narrative Review. *TechTrends, 66*(5), 883–896. doi:10.1007/s11528-022-00759-0 PMID:35813033

Brea-Gómez, B., Torres-Sánchez, I., Ortíz-Rubio, A., Calvache-Mateo, A., Cabrera-Martos, I., López-López, L., & Valenza, M. C. (2021). Virtual Reality in the Treatment of Adults with Chronic Low Back Pain: A Systematic Review and Meta-analysis of Randomized Clinical Trials. *International Journal of Environmental Research and Public Health, 18*(22), 11806. doi:10.3390/ijerph182211806 PMID:34831562

Brelet, L., & Gaffary, Y. (2022b). Stress reduction interventions: A scoping review to explore progress toward using haptic feedback in virtual reality. *Frontiers in Virtual Reality, 3*, 900970. doi:10.3389/frvir.2022.900970

Bridges. (2022). *From Virtual Reality to Extended Reality*. Bridges. https://www.bridges-horizon.eu/from-virtual-reality-to-extended-reality/

Brown, D. M., & Cairns, P. (2016). A grounded investigation of game immersion. In *Proceedings of the 2016 CHI Conference on Human Factors in Computing Systems* (pp. 3711-3722). ACM.

Brugada-Ramentol, V., Bozorgzadeh, A., & Jalali, H. (2022). Enhance VR: A multisensory approach to cognitive training and monitoring. *Frontiers in Digital Health, 4*, 916052. Advance online publication. doi:10.3389/fdgth.2022.916052 PMID:35721794

Bruno, R. R., Wolff, G., Wernly, B., Masyuk, M., Piayda, K., Leaver, S., Erkens, R., Oehler, D., Afzal, S., Heidari, H., Kelm, M., & Jung, C. (2022). Virtual and augmented reality in critical care medicine: The patient's, clinician's, and researcher's perspective. *Critical Care, 26*(1), 326. doi:10.1186/s13054-022-04202-x PMID:36284350

Bryant, L., & Hemsley, B. (2022). Augmented reality: A view to future visual supports for people with disability. *Disability and Rehabilitation. Assistive Technology*, 1–14. doi:10.1080/17483107.2022.2125090 PMID:36149835

Buckley, C., Nugent, E., Ryan, D., & Neary, P. (2012). Virtual reality–a new era in surgical training. *Virtual reality in psychological, medical and pedagogical applications, 7*, 139-166.

Buetler, K. A., Penalver-Andres, J., Özen, Ö., Ferriroli, L., Müri, R. M., Cazzoli, D., & Marchal-Crespo, L. (2022). "Tricking the Brain" Using Immersive Virtual Reality: Modifying the Self-Perception Over Embodied Avatar Influences Motor Cortical Excitability and Action Initiation. *Frontiers in Human Neuroscience, 15*, 787487. doi:10.3389/fnhum.2021.787487 PMID:35221950

Buettner, R., Baumgartl, H., Konle, T., & Haag, P. (2020). *A Review of Virtual Reality and Augmented Reality Literature in Healthcare*. IEEE Xplore. doi:10.1109/ISIEA49364.2020.9188211

Buń, P. K., Wichniarek, R., Górski, F., Grajewski, D., Zawadzki, P., & Hamrol, A. (2016). Possibilities and determinants of using low-cost devices in virtual education applications. *Eurasia Journal of Mathematics, Science and Technology Education*, *13*(2), 381–394. doi:10.12973/eurasia.2017.00622a

Bushnell, M. C., Čeko, M., & Low, L. A. (2013). Cognitive and emotional control of pain and its disruption in chronic pain. In Nature Reviews Neuroscience, 14(7). doi:10.1038/nrn3516

Caglio, M. A. R. C. E. L. L. A., Latini-Corazzini, L., D'Agata, F., Cauda, F., Sacco, K., Monteverdi, S., Zettin, M., Duca, S., & Geminiani, G. (2012). Virtual navigation for memory rehabilitation in a traumatic brain injured patient. *Neurocase*, *18*(2), 123–131. doi:10.1080/13554794.2011.568499 PMID:22352998

Caglio, M., Latini-Corazzini, L., D'agata, F., Cauda, F., Sacco, K., Monteverdi, S., Zettin, M., Duca, S., & Geminiani, G. (2009). Video game play changes spatial and verbal memory: Rehabilitation of a single case with traumatic brain injury. *Cognitive Processing*, *10*(S2), 195–197. doi:10.1007/s10339-009-0295-6 PMID:19693564

Cairns, P., Cox, A. L., & Day, M. (2014). The virtues of repetition: A grounded theory of technology-mediated recovery. *International Journal of Human-Computer Studies*, *72*(8-9), 487–506.

Calabrò, R. S., Cerasa, A., Ciancarelli, I., Pignolo, L., Tonin, P., Iosa, M., & Morone, G. (2022). The Arrival of the Metaverse in Neurorehabilitation: Fact, Fake or Vision? In Biomedicines, 10(10). MDPI. doi:10.3390/biomedicines10102602

Call, D., Miron, L. R., & Orcutt, H. K. (2013). Effectiveness of brief mindfulness techniques in reducing symptoms of anxiety and stress. *Mindfulness*, *5*(6), 658–668. doi:10.1007/s12671-013-0218-6

Canali, S., Schiaffonati, V., & Aliverti, A. (2022). Challenges and recommendations for wearable devices in digital health: Data quality, interoperability, health equity, fairness. *PLOS Digital Health*, *1*(10), e0000104. doi:10.1371/journal.pdig.0000104 PMID:36812619

Cangelosi, J., Damron, T. S., & Kim, D. (2022). Preventive health care information and social media: A comparison of Baby Boomer and Generation X health care consumers. *International Journal of Pharmaceutical and Healthcare Marketing*, *16*(2), 282–296. doi:10.1108/IJPHM-04-2021-0042

Cano Porras, D., Siemonsma, P., Inzelberg, R., Zeilig, G., & Plotnik, M. (2018). Advantages of virtual reality in the rehabilitation of balance and gait: Systematic review. *Neurology*, *90*(22), 1017–1025. doi:10.1212/WNL.0000000000005603 PMID:29720544

Cao, W., & Yu, Z. (2023). The impact of augmented reality on student attitudes, motivation, and learning achievements-a meta-analysis (2016–2023). *Humanities & Social Sciences Communications*, *10*(1), 352. doi:10.1057/s41599-023-01852-2

Caponnetto, P., & Casu, M. (2022). Update on Cyber Health Psychology: Virtual Reality and Mobile Health Tools in Psychotherapy, Clinical Rehabilitation, and Addiction Treatment. *International Journal of Environmental Research and Public Health*, *19*(6), 3516. doi:10.3390/ijerph19063516 PMID:35329201

Carroll, J., Hopper, L., Farrelly, A. M., Lombard-Vance, R., Bamidis, P. D., & Konstantinidis, E. I. (2021). A scoping Review of Augmented/Virtual Reality Health and Well-being Interventions for Older Adults: Redefining Immersive Virtual Reality. *Frontiers in Virtual Reality*, *2*, 655338. doi:10.3389/frvir.2021.655338

Carter, R. (2022). *Most Popular XR Gaming Reviews*. XR Today. https://www.xrtoday.com/mixed-reality/most-popular-xr-gaming-reviews-2022/

Cerasa, A., Gaggioli, A., Marino, F., Riva, G., & Pioggia, G. (2022). The promise of the metaverse in mental health: The new era of MEDverse. *Heliyon*, *8*(11), e11762. doi:10.1016/j.heliyon.2022.e11762 PMID:36458297

Chamberland, C., Bransi, M., Boivin, A., Jacques, S., Gagnon, J., & Tremblay, S. (2024). The effect of augmented reality on preoperative anxiety in children and adolescents: A randomized controlled trial. *Paediatric Anaesthesia, 34*(2), 153–159. doi:10.1111/pan.14793 PMID:37925608

Chandler, T., Richards, A. E., Jenny, B., Dickson, F., Huang, J., Klippel, A., Neylan, M., Wang, F., & Prober, S. M. (2021). Immersive landscapes: Modelling ecosystem reference conditions in virtual reality. *Landscape Ecology, 37*(5), 1293–1309. doi:10.1007/s10980-021-01313-8

Chan, E., Foster, S., Sambell, R., & Leong, P. (2018). Clinical efficacy of virtual reality for acute procedural pain management: A systematic review and meta-analysis. *PLoS One, 13*(7), e0200987. doi:10.1371/journal.pone.0200987 PMID:30052655

Channa, A., Popescu, N., Skibińska, J., & Bürget, R. (2021). The Rise of Wearable Devices during the COVID-19 Pandemic: A Systematic Review. *Sensors (Basel), 21*(17), 5787. doi:10.3390/s21175787 PMID:34502679

Chapman, J., & Chapman, L. (2018). Interactive health behavior interventions using gamification and augmented reality. In *Handbook of Research on Gamification in Higher Education* (pp. 135–156). IGI Global.

Chemnad, K., Alshakhsi, S., Almourad, M. B., Altuwairiqi, M., Phalp, K., & Ali, R. (2022). Smartphone Usage before and during COVID-19: A Comparative Study Based on Objective Recording of Usage Data. *Informatics (MDPI), 9*(4), 98. Advance online publication. doi:10.3390/informatics9040098

Cheng, Y., Lee, M.-H., Yang, C.-S., & Wu, P.-Y. (2022). Hands-on interaction in the augmented reality (AR) chemistry laboratories enhances the learning effects of low-achieving students: a pilot study. Interactive Technology and Smart Education. doi:10.1108/ITSE-04-2022-0045

Cheng, J., Zhang, H., Tao, F., & Juang, C. F. (2020). DT-II: Digital twin enhanced Industrial Internet reference framework towards smart manufacturing. *Robotics and Computer-integrated Manufacturing, 62*, 101881. doi:10.1016/j.rcim.2019.101881

Cheng, V. W. S., Davenport, T., Johnson, D., Vella, K., & Hickie, I. B. (2019). Gamification in apps and technologies for improving mental health and well-being: Systematic review. *JMIR Mental Health, 6*(6), e13717. doi:10.2196/13717 PMID:31244479

Chen, H. (2015). Research of virtools virtual reality technology to landscape designing. *The Open Construction & Building Technology Journal, 9*(1), 164–169. doi:10.2174/1874836801509010164

Chen, J., Canny, J., & He, H. (2011). Healthymagination: Mobile phone application for healthcare in the developing world. In *Proceedings of the 2nd ACM SIGHIT International Health Informatics Symposium* (pp. 1-10). ACM.

Chen, X., & Ibrahim, Z. (2023). A Comprehensive Study of Emotional Responses in AI-Enhanced Interactive Installation Art. *Sustainability (Basel), 15*(22), 15830. doi:10.3390/su152215830

Chen, Y., Fanchiang, H. D., & Howard, A. (2018). Effectiveness of virtual reality in children with cerebral palsy: A systematic review and meta-analysis of randomized controlled trials. *Physical Therapy, 98*(1), 63–77. doi:10.1093/ptj/pzx107 PMID:29088476

Chi, D. M., Clarke, J. R., Webber, B. L., & Badler, N. I. (1996). Casualty modeling for real-time medical training. *Presence (Cambridge, Mass.), 5*(4), 359–366. doi:10.1162/pres.1996.5.4.359 PMID:11539375

Chien-Huan, C., Chien-Hsu, C., & Tay-Sheng, J. (2010). *An interactive augmented reality system for learning anatomy structure.* Proceedings of the International Multi-Conference of Engineers and Computer Scientists, Hong Kong, China. https://www.iaeng.org/publication/IMECS2010/IMECS2010_pp370-375.pdf

Chien-Yu, L., & Yu-Ming, C. (2015). Interactive augmented reality using Scratch 2.0 to improve physical activities for children with developmental disabilities. *Research in Developmental Disabilities, 37*, 1–8. doi:10.1016/j.ridd.2014.10.016 PMID:25460214

Chirico, A., & Gaggioli, A. (2023). How Real Are Virtual Emotions? In Cyberpsychology, Behavior, and Social Networking, 26(4). .editorial doi:10.1089/cyber.2023.29272.editorial

Chirico, A., Lucidi, F., De Laurentiis, M., Milanese, C., Napoli, A., & Giordano, A. (2016). Virtual reality in health system: Beyond entertainment. a mini-review on the efficacy of VR during cancer treatment. *Journal of Cellular Physiology, 231*(2), 275–287. doi:10.1002/jcp.25117 PMID:26238976

Choukou, M. A., Zhu, X., Malwade, S., Dhar, E., & Abdul, S. S. (2022). Digital Health Solutions Transforming Long-Term Care and Rehabilitation. In *Healthcare Information Management Systems: Cases, Strategies, and Solutions* (pp. 301–316). Springer International Publishing. doi:10.1007/978-3-031-07912-2_19

Cima, R. R., Kollengode, A., Garnatz, J., Storsveen, A., Weisbrod, C., & Deschamps, C. (2008). Incidence and characteristics of potential and actual retained foreign object events in surgical patients. *Journal of the American College of Surgeons, 207*(1), 80–87. doi:10.1016/j.jamcollsurg.2007.12.047 PMID:18589366

Cipresso, P., Giglioli, I. A. C., Raya, M. A., & Riva, G. (2018). The Past, Present, and Future of Virtual and Augmented Reality Research: A Network and Cluster Analysis of the Literature. *Frontiers in Psychology, 9*, 2086. doi:10.3389/fpsyg.2018.02086 PMID:30459681

Clark, D., Schumann, F., & Mostofsky, S. H. (2015b). Mindful movement and skilled attention. *Frontiers in Human Neuroscience, 9*. doi:10.3389/fnhum.2015.00297 PMID:26190986

Clarke, E. (2021). Virtual reality simulation—The future of orthopaedic training? A systematic review and narrative analysis. *Advances in Simulation (London, England), 6*(1), 2. doi:10.1186/s41077-020-00153-x PMID:33441190

Coco-Martin, M. B., Piñero, D. P., Leal-Vega, L., Hernández-Rodríguez, C. J., Adiego, J., Molina-Martín, A., de Fez, D., & Arenillas, J. F. (2020). The Potential of Virtual Reality for Inducing Neuroplasticity in Children with Amblyopia. *Journal of Ophthalmology, 2020*, 1–9. doi:10.1155/2020/7067846 PMID:32676202

Cofano, F., Di Perna, G., Bozzaro, M., Longo, A., Marengo, N., Zenga, F., Zullo, N., Cavalieri, M., Damiani, L., Boges, D. J., Agus, M., Garbossa, D., & Calì, C. (2021). Augmented Reality in Medical Practice: From Spine Surgery to Remote Assistance. *Frontiers in Surgery, 8*, 657901. doi:10.3389/fsurg.2021.657901 PMID:33859995

Çöltekin, A., Lochhead, I., Madden, M., Christophe, S., Devaux, A., Pettit, C., Lock, O., Shukla, S., Herman, L., Stachoň, Z., Kubíček, P., Snopková, D., Bernardes, S., & Hedley, N. (2020). Extended reality in spatial sciences: A review of research challenges and future directions. *ISPRS International Journal of Geo-Information, 9*(7), 439. doi:10.3390/ijgi9070439

Cook, S., Munteanu, C., Papadopoulos, E., Abrams, H., Stinson, J. N., Pitters, E., & Puts, M. (2023). The development of an electronic geriatric assessment tool: Comprehensive health assessment for my plan (CHAMP). *Journal of Geriatric Oncology, 14*(1), 101384. doi:10.1016/j.jgo.2022.09.013 PMID:36216760

Cooper, N., Milella, F., Pinto, C., Cant, I., White, M., & Meyer, G. (2018). The effects of substitute multisensory feedback on task performance and the sense of presence in a virtual reality environment. *PLoS One, 13*(2), e0191846. doi:10.1371/journal.pone.0191846 PMID:29390023

Cotler, J. L. (2016). *The impact of online teaching and learning about emotional intelligence, Myers Briggs personality dimensions and mindfulness on personal and social awareness.* State University of New York at Albany.

Cotler, J. L., DiTursi, D., Goldstein, I., Yates, J., & Del Belso, D. (2017). A mindful approach to teaching. *Information Systems Education Journal*, *15*(1), 12.

Couto, F., de Lurdes Almeida, M., dos Anjos Dixe, M., Ribeiro, J., Braúna, M., Gomes, N., Caroço, J., Monteiro, L., Martinho, R., Rijo, R., & Apóstolo, J. (2019). Digi&Mind: Development and validation of a multi-domain digital cognitive stimulation program for older adults with cognitive decline. *Procedia Computer Science*, *164*, 732–740. doi:10.1016/j.procs.2019.12.242

Creed, C., Al-Kalbani, M., Theil, A., Sarkar, S., & Williams, I. (2023). Inclusive AR/VR: Accessibility barriers for immersive technologies. *Universal Access in the Information Society*. Advance online publication. doi:10.1007/s10209-023-00969-0

Cunningham, A., McPolin, O., Fallis, R., Coyle, C., Best, P., & McKenna, G. (2021). A systematic review of the use of virtual reality or dental smartphone applications as interventions for management of paediatric dental anxiety. *BMC Oral Health*, *21*(1), 244. doi:10.1186/s12903-021-01602-3 PMID:33962624

Custură-Crăciun, D., Cochior, D., Constantinoiu, S., & Neagu, C. (2013). Surgical virtual reality-highlights in developing a high performance surgical haptic device. *Chirurgia (Bucharest, Romania: 1990)*, *108*(6), 757-763.

D'Errico, G., Barba, M. C., Gatto, C., Nuzzo, B. L., Nuccetelli, F., Luca, V. D., & Paolis, L. T. D. (2023, September). Measuring the Effectiveness of Virtual Reality for Stress Reduction: Psychometric Evaluation of the ERMES Project. In *International Conference on Extended Reality* (pp. 484-499). Cham: Springer Nature Switzerland. 10.1007/978-3-031-43401-3_32

Dantas, M. A., Da Silva, J. D., Tkachenko, N., & Paneque, M. (2023). Telehealth in genetic counselling consultations: The impact of COVID-19 in a Portuguese genetic healthcare service. *Journal of Community Genetics*, *14*(1), 91–100. doi:10.1007/s12687-022-00618-8 PMID:36414926

Darnall, B. D., Krishnamurthy, P., Tsuei, J., & Minor, J. D. (2020). Self-administered skills-based virtual reality intervention for chronic pain: Randomized controlled pilot study. *JMIR Formative Research*, *4*(7), e17293. doi:10.2196/17293 PMID:32374272

Dascal, J., Reid, M., IsHak, W. W., Spiegel, B., Recacho, J., Rosen, B., & Danovitch, I. (2017). Virtual reality and medical inpatients: A systematic review of randomized, controlled trials. *Innovations in Clinical Neuroscience*, *14*(1-2), 14. PMID:28386517

de Giorgio, A., Monetti, F. M., Maffei, A., Romero, M., & Wang, L. (2023). Adopting extended reality? A systematic review of manufacturing training and teaching applications. *Journal of Manufacturing Systems*, *71*, 645–663. doi:10.1016/j.jmsy.2023.10.016

De Luca, R., Manuli, A., De Domenico, C., Voi, E. L., Buda, A., Maresca, G., & Calabrò, R. S. (2019). Improving neuropsychiatric symptoms following stroke using virtual reality. *Case Reports in Medicine*, *98*(19). PMID:31083155

Dechsling, A., Orm, S., Kalandadze, T., Sütterlin, S., Øien, R. A., Shic, F., & Nordahl-Hansen, A. (2021). Virtual and Augmented Reality in Social Skills Interventions for Individuals with Autism Spectrum Disorder: A Scoping Review. *Journal of Autism and Developmental Disorders*, *52*(11), 4692–4707. doi:10.1007/s10803-021-05338-5 PMID:34783991

Dehghan, B., Saeidimehr, S., Sayyah, M., & Rahim, F. (2022b). The Effect of Virtual Reality on Emotional Response and Symptoms Provocation in Patients with OCD: A Systematic Review and Meta-analysis. *Frontiers in Psychiatry*, *12*, 733584. doi:10.3389/fpsyt.2021.733584 PMID:35177996

Delbreil, E., & Zvobgo, G. (2013). Wireless sensor technology in dementia care: Caregiver perceptions, technology take-up and business model innovation. *EuroMed Journal of Business*, *8*(1), 79–97. doi:10.1108/EMJB-05-2013-0019

Delp, S. L., Loan, P., Basdogan, C., & Rosen, J. M. (1997). Surgical simulation: An emerging technology for training in emergency medicine. *Presence (Cambridge, Mass.), 6*(2), 147–159. doi:10.1162/pres.1997.6.2.147

Deo, N., & Anjankar, A. (2023). Artificial intelligence with robotics in healthcare: A narrative review of its viability in India. *Cureus, 15*(5). doi:10.7759/cureus.39416 PMID:37362504

Deterding, S., Dixon, D., Khaled, R., & Nacke, L. (2011). From game design elements to gamefulness: defining" gamification". In Proceedings of the 15th international academic MindTrek conference: Envisioning future media environments (pp. 9-15).

Deterding, S., Dixon, D., Khaled, R., Nacke, L., & Lennart, E. (2013). Gamification: Toward a definition. In CHI 2013 Extended Abstracts on Human Factors in Computing Systems (pp. 2466-2468). ACM.

Dhar, P., Rocks, T., Samarasinghe, R. M., Stephenson, G., & Smith, C. (2021). Augmented reality in medical education: Students' experiences and learning outcomes. *Medical Education Online, 26*(1), 1953953. doi:10.1080/10872981.2021.1953953 PMID:34259122

Dhir, R. (2016, March). Video Text extraction and recognition: A survey. In *2016 International Conference on Wireless Communications, Signal Processing and Networking (WiSPNET)* (pp. 1366-1373). IEEE.

Dicuonzo, G., Donofrio, F., Fusco, A., & Shini, M. (2023). Healthcare system: Moving forward with artificial intelligence. *Technovation, 120*, 102510. doi:10.1016/j.technovation.2022.102510

Diemer, J., Alpers, G. W., Peperkorn, H. M., Shiban, Y., & Mühlberger, A. (2015). The impact of perception and presence on emotional reactions: A review of research in virtual reality. *Frontiers in Psychology, 6*, 26. doi:10.3389/fpsyg.2015.00026 PMID:25688218

Dodds, S., Russell-Bennett, R., Chen, T., Oertzen, A.-S., Salvador-Carulla, L., & Hung, Y.-C. (2022). Blended human-technology service realities in healthcare. *Journal of Service Theory and Practice, 32*(1), 75–99. doi:10.1108/JSTP-12-2020-0285

Döllinger, N., Wienrich, C., & Latoschik, M. E. (2021). Challenges and Opportunities of Immersive Technologies for Mindfulness Meditation: A Systematic Review. *Frontiers in Virtual Reality, 2*, 644683. doi:10.3389/frvir.2021.644683

Donker, T., Cornelisz, I., Van Klaveren, C., Van Straten, A., Carlbring, P., Cuijpers, P., & Van Gelder, J. L. (2019). Effectiveness of Self-guided App-Based Virtual Reality Cognitive Behavior Therapy for Acrophobia: A Randomized Clinical Trial. *JAMA Psychiatry, 76*(7), 682–690. doi:10.1001/jamapsychiatry.2019.0219 PMID:30892564

Dorloh, H., Li, K.-W., & Khaday, S. (2023). Presenting Job Instructions Using an Augmented Reality Device, a Printed Manual, and a Video Display for Assembly and Disassembly Tasks: What Are the Differences? *Applied Sciences (Basel, Switzerland), 13*(4), 2186. doi:10.3390/app13042186

Doshi, R., Hiran, K. K., Ranolia, R., & Joshi, C. (2023). Monitor Cloud Performance and Data Safety With Artificial Intelligence. In Applications of Artificial Intelligence in Wireless Communication Systems (pp. 92-108). IGI Global. doi:10.4018/978-1-6684-7348-1.ch006

Doshi, R., & Hiran, K. K. (2023). Decision Making and IoT: Bibliometric Analysis for Scopus Database. *Babylonian Journal of Internet of Things, 2023*, 13–22. doi:10.58496/BJIoT/2023/003

Doshi, R., Hiran, K. K., Gök, M., El-kenawy, E. S. M., Badr, A., & Abotaleb, M. (2023). Artificial Intelligence's Significance in Diseases with Malignant Tumours. *Mesopotamian Journal of Artificial Intelligence in Healthcare, 2023*, 35–39.

Dozio, N., Maggioni, E., Pittera, D., Gallace, A., & Obrist, M. (2021). May I smell your attention: Exploration of smell and sound for visuospatial attention in virtual reality. *Frontiers in Psychology*, *12*, 671470. Advance online publication. doi:10.3389/fpsyg.2021.671470 PMID:34366990

Drewett, O., Hann, G., Gillies, M., Sher, C., Delacroix, S., Pan, X., Collingwoode-Williams, T., & Fertleman, C. (2019). A discussion of the use of virtual reality for training healthcare practitioners to recognize child protection issues. *Frontiers in Public Health*, *7*, 255. doi:10.3389/fpubh.2019.00255 PMID:31608266

Drigas, A., Mitsea, E., & Skianis, C. (2022). Subliminal Training Techniques for Cognitive, Emotional and Behavioral Balance. The Role of Emerging Technologies. *Technium Soc. Sci. J.*, *33*, 164.

Drigas, A., Mitsea, E., & Skianis, C. (2022). Virtual reality and metacognition training techniques for learning disabilities. *Sustainability (Basel)*, *14*(16), 10170. doi:10.3390/su141610170

Du Sert, O. P., Potvin, S., Lipp, O., Dellazizzo, L., Laurelli, M., Breton, R., Lalonde, P., Phraxayavong, K., O'Connor, K., Pelletier, J.-F., Boukhalfi, T., Renaud, P., & Dumais, A. (2018). Virtual reality therapy for refractory auditory verbal hallucinations in schizophrenia: A pilot clinical trial. *Schizophrenia Research*, *197*, 176–181. doi:10.1016/j.schres.2018.02.031 PMID:29486956

Durnell, L. A. (2018). *Emotional Reaction of Experiencing Crisis in Virtual Reality (VR)/360* [Doctoral dissertation, Fielding Graduate University].

Du, Z., Liu, J., & Wang, T. (2022). Augmented Reality Marketing: A Systematic Literature Review and an Agenda for Future Inquiry. *Frontiers in Psychology*, *13*, 925963. doi:10.3389/fpsyg.2022.925963 PMID:35783783

Dziuban, C., Graham, C. R., Moskal, P. D., Norberg, A., & Sicilia, N. (2018). Blended learning: The new normal and emerging technologies. *International Journal of Educational Technology in Higher Education*, *15*(1), 3. doi:10.1186/s41239-017-0087-5

Easwaran, B., Hiran, K. K., Krishnan, S., & Doshi, R. (Eds.). (2022). *Real-time applications of machine learning in cyber-physical systems*. IGI Global. doi:10.4018/978-1-7998-9308-0

Ebert, D. D., Harrer, M., Apolinário-Hagen, J., & Baumeister, H. (2019). Digital interventions for mental disorders: key features, efficacy, and potential for artificial intelligence applications. *Frontiers in Psychiatry: Artificial Intelligence, Precision Medicine, and Other Paradigm Shifts*, 583-627.

ECLAC. (2021). *Digital technologies for a new future*. CEPAL. https://www.cepal.org/sites/default/files/publication/files/46817/S2000960_en.pdf

Edna Mayela, V. C., Miriam, L. T., Ana Isabel, G. G., Oscar, R. C., & Alejandra, C. A. (2023). Effectiveness of an on-line multicomponent physical exercise intervention on the physical performance of community-dwelling older adults: A randomized controlled trial. *Geriatric Nursing*, *14*(54), 83–93. doi:10.1016/j.gerinurse.2023.08.018 PMID:37716123

El Filali, Y., & Krit, S. (2020). Augmented Reality Types and Popular Use Cases. In *Proceedings of the 1st International Conference of Computer Science and Renewable Energies-ICCSRE*. ScitePress. ISBN 978-989-758-431-2 10.5220/0009776301070110

El Kassis, R., Ayer, S. K., & El Asmar, M. (2023). Augmented Reality Applications for Synchronized Communication in Construction: A Review of Challenges and Opportunities. *Applied Sciences (Basel, Switzerland)*, *13*(13), 7614. doi:10.3390/app13137614

El Saddik, A. (2018). Digital twins: The convergence of multimedia technologies. *IEEE MultiMedia*, *25*(2), 87–92. doi:10.1109/MMUL.2018.023121167

Elor, A., & Kurniawan, S. (2020). The ultimate display for physical rehabilitation: A bridging review on immersive virtual reality. *Frontiers in Virtual Reality*, *1*, 585993. doi:10.3389/frvir.2020.585993

Emmelkamp, P. M. G., & Meyerbröker, K. (2021). Annual review of clinical psychology virtual reality therapy in mental health. *Annual Review of Clinical Psychology*, *7*(17).

Eversberg, L., & Lambrecht, J. (2023). Evaluating digital work instructions with augmented reality versus paper-based documents for manual, object-specific repair tasks in a case study with experienced workers. *International Journal of Advanced Manufacturing Technology*, *127*(3-4), 1859–1871. doi:10.1007/s00170-023-11313-4

Fagbola, T. M., Fagbola, F. I., Aroba, O. J., Doshi, R., Hiran, K. K., & Thakur, S. C. (2022). Smart face masks for Covid-19 pandemic management: A concise review of emerging architectures, challenges and future research directions. *IEEE Sensors Journal*, *23*(2), 877–888.

Fahim, S., Maqsood, A., Das, G., Ahmed, N., Saquib, S., Lal, A., Khan, A., & Alam, M. (2022). Augmented Reality and Virtual Reality in Dentistry: Highlights from the Current Research. *Applied Sciences (Basel, Switzerland)*, *12*(8), 3719. doi:10.3390/app12083719

Fan, C., Zhang, C., Yahja, A., & Mostafavi, A. (2019). Disaster city digital twin: A vision for integrating artificial and human intelligence for disaster management. *International Journal of Information Management*, *1*, 102049.

Fari, N., Yorke, E., Varnes, L., Newby, K., Potts, H. W., Smith, L., & Fisher, A. (2019). Younger Adolescents' Perceptions of Physical Activity, Exergaming, and Virtual Reality: Qualitative Intervention Study. *JMIR Serious Games*, *7*(2).

Farshid, M., Paschen, J., Eriksson, T., & Kietzmann, J. (2018). Go boldly!: Explore augmented reality (AR), virtual reality (VR), and mixed reality (MR) for business. *Business Horizons*, *61*(5), 657–663. doi:10.1016/j.bushor.2018.05.009

Ferraro, K., Zernzach, R., Maturo, S., Nagy, C., & Barrett, R. (2017). Chief of residents for quality improvement and patient safety: A recipe for a new role in graduate medical education. *Military Medicine*, *182*(3-4), e1747–e1751. doi:10.7205/MILMED-D-16-00179 PMID:28290953

Fidan, I., Huseynov, O., Ali, M. A., Alkunte, S., Rajeshirke, M., Gupta, A., Hasanov, S., Tantawi, K., Yasa, E., Yilmaz, O., Loy, J., Popov, V., & Sharma, A. (2023). Recent inventions in additive manufacturing: Holistic review. *Inventions (Basel, Switzerland)*, *8*(4), 103. doi:10.3390/inventions8040103

Firoozi, A. A., & Firoozi, A. A. (2023). A systematic review of the role of 4D printing in sustainable civil engineering solutions. *Heliyon*, *9*(10), e20982. doi:10.1016/j.heliyon.2023.e20982 PMID:37928382

Flores, A., Linehan, M. M., Todd, S. R., & Hoffman, H. G. (2018). The use of virtual reality to facilitate mindfulness skills training in dialectical behavioral therapy for spinal cord injury: A case study. *Frontiers in Psychology*, *9*, 531. doi:10.3389/fpsyg.2018.00531 PMID:29740365

Ford, N. (2021). *Software Architecture: The Hard Parts: Modern Trade-Off Analyses for Distributed Architectures.* O'Reilly Media.

Ford, T. J., Buchanan, D. M., Azeez, A., Benrimoh, D. A., Kaloiani, I., Bandeira, I. D., Hunegnaw, S., Lan, L., Gholmieh, M., Buch, V., & Williams, N. R. (2023). Taking modern psychiatry into the metaverse: Integrating augmented, virtual, and mixed reality technologies into psychiatric care. *Frontiers in Digital Health*, *5*, 1146806. doi:10.3389/fdgth.2023.1146806 PMID:37035477

Fraser, B. J. (2023). The Evolution of the Field of Learning Environments Research. *Education Sciences*, *13*(3), 257. doi:10.3390/educsci13030257

Frasson, C., & Abdessalem, H. (2022). Contribution of Virtual Reality Environments and Artificial Intelligence for Alzheimer. *Medical Research Archives*, *10*(9). doi:10.18103/mra.v10i9.3054

Freeman, D., Reeve, S., Robinson, A., Ehlers, A., Clark, D., Spanlang, B., & Slater, M. (2017). Virtual reality in the assessment, understanding, and treatment of mental health disorders. In Psychological Medicine, 47(). Cambridge University Press. doi:10.1017/S003329171700040X

Freeman, K. M., Thompson, S. F., Allely, E. B., Sobel, A. L., Stansfield, S. A., & Pugh, W. M. (2001). A virtual reality patient simulation system for teaching emergency response skills to US Navy medical providers. *Prehospital and Disaster Medicine*, *16*(1), 3–8. doi:10.1017/S1049023X00025462 PMID:11367936

Freitas, R., Velosa, V. H. S., Abreu, L. T. N., Jardim, R. L., Santos, J. V., Peres, B., & Campos, P. (2021). Virtual Reality Exposure Treatment in Phobias: A Systematic Review. *The Psychiatric Quarterly*, *92*(4), 1685–1710. doi:10.1007/s11126-021-09935-6 PMID:34173160

Fuller, A., Fan, Z., Day, C., & Barlow, C. (2020). Digital twin: Enabling technologies, challenges and open research. *IEEE Access : Practical Innovations, Open Solutions*, *1*, 1. doi:10.1109/ACCESS.2020.2998358

Gadelha, R. (2018). Revolutionizing Education: The promise of virtual reality. *Childhood Education*, *94*(1), 40–43. doi:10.1080/00094056.2018.1420362

Gaiha, S. M., Salisbury, T. T., Koschorke, M., Raman, U., & Petticrew, M. (2020e). The stigma associated with mental health problems among young people in India: A systematic review of magnitude, manifestations and recommendations. *BMC Psychiatry*, *20*(1), 538. doi:10.1186/s12888-020-02937-x PMID:33198678

Gale, D. (1955). The law of supply and demand. *Mathematica Scandinavica*, *3*, 155–169. doi:10.7146/math.scand.a-10436

Gambella, E., Margaritini, A., Benadduci, M., Rossi, L., D'Ascoli, P., Riccardi, G. R., Pasquini, S., Civerchia, P., Pelliccioni, G., Bevilacqua, R., & Maranesi, E. (2022). An integrated intervention of computerized cognitive training and physical exercise in virtual reality for people with Alzheimer's disease: The home study protocol. *Frontiers in Neurology*, *13*, 964454. doi:10.3389/fneur.2022.964454 PMID:36034306

Garavand, A., & Aslani, N. (2022). Metaverse phenomenon and its impact on health: A scoping review. *Informatics in Medicine Unlocked*, *32*, 101029. doi:10.1016/j.imu.2022.101029

Gatica-Rojas, V., & Méndez-Rebolledo, G. (2014). Virtual reality interface devices in the reorganization of neural networks in the brain of patients with neurological diseases. *Neural Regeneration Research*, *9*(8), 888. doi:10.4103/1673-5374.131612 PMID:25206907

Gazit, T., Nisim, S., & Ayalon, L. (2023). Intergenerational family online community and older adults' overall well-being. *Online Information Review*, *47*(2), 221–237. doi:10.1108/OIR-06-2021-0332

George, A. J., John, R., & Rajkumar, E. (2021c). Mindfulness-based positive psychology interventions: A systematic review. *BMC Psychology*, *9*(1), 116. doi:10.1186/s40359-021-00618-2 PMID:34362457

George, A. S., George, A. H., & Martin, A. G. (2023). ChatGPT and the Future of Work: A Comprehensive Analysis of AI's Impact on Jobs and Employment. *Partners Universal International Innovation Journal*, *1*(3), 154–186.

Giannouli, E., Kim, E. K., Fu, C., Weibel, R., Sofios, A., Infanger, D., Portegijs, E., Rantanen, T., Huang, H., Schmidt-Trucksäss, A., Zeller, A., Rössler, R., & Hinrichs, T. (2022). Psychometric properties of the MOBITEC-GP mobile application for real-life mobility assessment in older adults. *Geriatric Nursing*, *48*, 273–279. doi:10.1016/j.gerinurse.2022.10.017 PMID:36334468

Godber, K. A., & Atkins, D. R. (2021). COVID-19 Impacts on Teaching and Learning: A Collaborative Autoethnography by Two Higher Education Lecturers. *Frontiers in Education*, 6, 647524. doi:10.3389/feduc.2021.647524

Goel, P., Jhanwar, N., Jain, P., Khatri, S., & Hiran, K. K. (2023, August). Efficient Blood Availability for Targeted Individuals Through Cloud Computing Web Application. In *2023 International Conference on Emerging Trends in Networks and Computer Communications (ETNCC)* (pp. 1-7). IEEE. 10.1109/ETNCC59188.2023.10284940

Gohari, S. H., Gozali, E., & Kalhori, S. R. N. (2019). Virtual reality applications for chronic conditions management: A review. *Medical Journal of the Islamic Republic of Iran*, 33, 67. PMID:31456991

Gold, J. I., & Mahrer, N. E. (2018). Is virtual reality ready for prime time in the medical space? A randomized control trial of pediatric virtual reality for acute procedural pain management. *Journal of Pediatric Psychology*, 43(3), 266–275. doi:10.1093/jpepsy/jsx129 PMID:29053848

Gong, J., & Tarasewich, P. (2019). A meta-analysis of gamification-based mobile apps in promoting health outcomes. *Journal of the American Medical Informatics Association : JAMIA*, 26(10), 1124–1136.

Goo, H. W., Park, S. J., & Yoo, S. J. (2020). Advanced medical use of three-dimensional imaging in congenital heart disease: Augmented reality, mixed reality, virtual reality, and three-dimensional printing. *Korean Journal of Radiology*, 21(2), 133–145. doi:10.3348/kjr.2019.0625 PMID:31997589

Gorini, A., Griez, E., Petrova, A., & Riva, G. (2010). Assessment of the emotional responses produced by exposure to real food, virtual food and photographs of food in patients affected by eating disorders. *Annals of General Psychiatry*, 9(1), 30. doi:10.1186/1744-859X-9-30 PMID:20602749

Graur, F. (2014). *Virtual reality in medicine–going beyond the limits. Thousand Faces Virtual Real*. InTech.

Greengard, S. (2019). *Virtual Reality*. MIT Press Direct., doi:10.7551/mitpress/11836.001.0001

Grieves, M., Vickers, J., Kahlen, F. J., Flumerfelt, S., & Alves, A. (2017). Digital twin: Mitigating unpredictable, undesirable emergent behavior in complex systems. In F.-J. Kahlen, S. Flumerfelt, & A. Alves (Eds.), *Transdisciplinary perspectives on complex systems: New findings and approaches no. August 2017* (pp. 85–113). Springer. doi:10.1007/978-3-319-38756-7_4

Grover, S., Arora, K., & Mitra, S. K. (2009, December). Text extraction from document images using edge information. In *2009 Annual IEEE India Conference* (pp. 1-4). IEEE.

Gruzina, Y., Firsova, I., & Strielkowski, W. (2021). Dynamics of Human Capital Development in Economic Development Cycles. *Economies*, 9(2), 67. doi:10.3390/economies9020067

Guendelman, S., Medeiros, S., & Rampes, H. (2017). Mindfulness and Emotion Regulation: Insights from Neurobiological, Psychological, and Clinical Studies. *Frontiers in Psychology*, 8. doi:10.3389/fpsyg.2017.00220 PMID:28321194

Gumbau-Albert, M., & Maudos, J. (2022). The importance of intangible assets in regional economic growth: A growth accounting approach. *The Annals of Regional Science*, 69(2), 361–390. doi:10.1007/s00168-022-01138-6 PMID:35729957

Guo, L., Wang, D., Gu, F., Li, Y., Wang, Y., & Zhou, R. (2021). Evolution and trends in intelligent tutoring systems research: A multidisciplinary and scientometric view. *Asia Pacific Education Review*, 22(3), 441–461. doi:10.1007/s12564-021-09697-7

Guo, Z., Li, Y., Wang, Y., Liu, S., Lei, T., & Fan, Y. (2016). A method of effective text extraction for complex video scene. *Mathematical Problems in Engineering*.

Gupta, A. K., Srinivasulu, A., Hiran, K. K., Sreenivasulu, G., Rajeyyagari, S., & Subramanyam, M. (2022). Prediction of omicron virus using combined extended convolutional and recurrent neural networks technique on CT-scan images. *Interdisciplinary Perspectives on Infectious Diseases*, *2022*, 2022. doi:10.1155/2022/1525615 PMID:36562006

Habak, S., Bennett, J., Davies, A., Davies, M., Christensen, H., & Boydell, K. M. (2020). Edge of the present: A virtual reality tool to cultivate future thinking, positive mood and wellbeing. *International Journal of Environmental Research and Public Health*, *18*(1), 140. doi:10.3390/ijerph18010140 PMID:33379156

Habil, S. G. M., El-Deeb, S., & El-Bassiouny, N. (2023). The metaverse era: leveraging augmented reality in the creation of novel customer experience. Management & Sustainability: An Arab Review. doi:10.1108/MSAR-10-2022-0051

Haddaway, N. R., Macura, B., Whaley, P., & Pullin, A. S. (2018). ROSES Reporting standards for Systematic Evidence Syntheses: Pro forma, flow-diagram and descriptive summary of the plan and conduct of environmental systematic reviews and systematic maps. *Environmental Evidence*, *7*(1), 1–8. doi:10.1186/s13750-018-0121-7

Hadjipanayi, C., Banakou, D., & Michael-Grigoriou, D. (2023). Art as therapy in virtual reality: A scoping review. *Frontiers in Virtual Reality*, *4*, 1065863. doi:10.3389/frvir.2023.1065863

Haesner, M., Steinert, A., O'Sullivan, J. L., & Steinhagen-Thiessen, E. (2015). Evaluating an accessible web interface for older adults–the impact of mild cognitive impairment (MCI). *Journal of Assistive Technologies*, *9*(4), 219–232. doi:10.1108/JAT-11-2014-0032

Hagège, H., Ourmi, M. E., Shankland, R., Arboix-Calas, F., Leys, C., & Lubart, T. (2023). Ethics and Meditation: A New Educational Combination to Boost Verbal Creativity and Sense of Responsibility. *Journal of Intelligence*, *11*(8), 155. doi:10.3390/jintelligence11080155 PMID:37623538

Haleem, A., Javaid, M., & Khan, I. H. (2020). Virtual reality (VR) applications in dentistry: An innovative technology to embrace. *Indian Journal of Dental Research*, *31*(4), 666–667. doi:10.4103/ijdr.IJDR_501_19 PMID:33107476

Haleem, A., Javaid, M., Qadri, M. A., & Suman, R. (2022). Understanding the role of digital technologies in education: A review. *Sustainable Operations and Computers*, *3*, 275–285. doi:10.1016/j.susoc.2022.05.004

Haluza, D., & Jungwirth, D. (2023). Artificial Intelligence and Ten Societal Megatrends: An Exploratory Study Using GPT-3. *Systems*, *11*(3), 120. doi:10.3390/systems11030120

Hamad, A., & Jia, B. (2022). How Virtual Reality Technology Has Changed Our Lives: An Overview of the Current and Potential Applications and Limitations. *International Journal of Environmental Research and Public Health*, *19*(18), 11278. doi:10.3390/ijerph191811278 PMID:36141551

Hamilton, D. E., McKechnie, J., Edgerton, E., & Wilson, C. (2020). Immersive virtual reality as a pedagogical tool in education: A systematic literature review of quantitative learning outcomes and experimental design. *Journal of Computers in Education*, *8*(1), 1–32. doi:10.1007/s40692-020-00169-2

Hao, J., Xie, H., Harp, K., Chen, Z., & Siu, K. C. (2022a). Effects of Virtual Reality Intervention on Neural Plasticity in Stroke Rehabilitation: A Systematic Review. In Archives of Physical Medicine and Rehabilitation, 103(3). doi:10.1016/j.apmr.2021.06.024

Hao, J., Li, Y., Swanson, R. M., Chen, Z., & Siu, K. (2023). Effects of virtual reality on physical, cognitive, and psychological outcomes in cancer rehabilitation: A systematic review and meta-analysis. *Supportive Care in Cancer*, *31*(2), 112. doi:10.1007/s00520-022-07568-4 PMID:36633695

Haorongbam, L., Nagpal, R., & Sehgal, R. (2022). *Service Oriented Architecture (SOA): A Literature Review on the Maintainability, Approaches and Design Process. 12th International Conference on Cloud Computing, Data Science & Engineering (Confluence)*, Noida, India. 10.1109/Confluence52989.2022.9734153

Harden, R. M. (1999). What is a spiral curriculum? *Medical Teacher, 21*(2), 141–143. doi:10.1080/01421599979752 PMID:21275727

Harris, B., Regan, T., Schueler, J., & Fields, S. A. (2020). Problematic Mobile Phone and Smartphone Use Scales: A Systematic Review. *Frontiers in Psychology, 11*, 672. doi:10.3389/fpsyg.2020.00672 PMID:32431636

Harry, A. (2023). The Future of Medicine: Harnessing the Power of AI for Revolutionizing Healthcare. *International Journal of Multidisciplinary Sciences and Arts, 2*(1), 36–47. doi:10.47709/ijmdsa.v2i1.2395

Harvie, D. S. (2021). Immersive Education for Chronic Condition Self-Management. *Frontiers in Virtual Reality, 2*, 657761. doi:10.3389/frvir.2021.657761

Hastuti, R., & Syafruddin. (2023). Ethical Considerations in the Age of Artificial Intelligence: Balancing Innovation and Social Values. *West Science Social and Humanities Studies, 1*(02), 76–87. doi:10.58812/wsshs.v1i02.191

Hatta, M. H., Sidi, H., Koon, C. S., Roos, N. C., Sharip, S., Samad, F. D. A., Xi, O. W., Das, S., & Saini, S. M. (2022). Virtual Reality (VR) Technology for Treatment of Mental Health Problems during COVID-19: A Systematic Review. *International Journal of Environmental Research and Public Health, 19*(9), 5389. doi:10.3390/ijerph19095389 PMID:35564784

Hemanth, J. D., Kose, U., Deperlioglu, O., & de Albuquerque, V. H. C. (2020). An augmented reality-supported mobile application for diagnosis of heart diseases. *The Journal of Supercomputing, 76*(2), 1242–1267. doi:10.1007/s11227-018-2483-6

Higgins, T., Larson, E., & Schnall, R. (2017). Unraveling the meaning of patient engagement: A concept analysis. *Patient Education and Counseling, 100*(1), 30–36. doi:10.1016/j.pec.2016.09.002 PMID:27665500

Higuera-Trujillo, J. L., López-Tarruella Maldonado, J., & Llinares Millán, C. (2017). Psychological and physiological human responses to simulated and real environments: A comparison between Photographs, 360° Panoramas, and Virtual Reality. *Applied Ergonomics, 65*, 398–409. doi:10.1016/j.apergo.2017.05.006 PMID:28601190

Hiran, K. K., & Doshi, R. (2013). Robust & secure digital image watermarking technique using concatenation process. *International Journal of ICT and Management.*

Hiran, K. K., Doshi, R., & Mijwil, M. M. (2023). Introducing On-Demand Internet Business Model in the Informal Public Transportation System in Developing Countries. In Integrating Intelligence and Sustainability in Supply Chains (pp. 148-162). IGI Global. doi:10.4018/979-8-3693-0225-5.ch008

Hiran, K. K., Doshi, R., Kant, K., Ruchi, H., & Lecturer, D. S. (2013). Robust & secure digital image watermarking technique using concatenation process. *International Journal of ICT and Management.*

Hiran, K. K., & Doshi, R. (2013). An artificial neural network approach for brain tumor detection using digital image segmentation. *Brain, 2*(5), 227–231.

Hiran, K. K., Khazanchi, D., Vyas, A. K., & Padmanaban, S. (Eds.). (2021). *Machine learning for sustainable development* (Vol. 9). Walter de Gruyter GmbH & Co KG. doi:10.1515/9783110702514

Hitzler, P. (2021). A review of the semantic web field. *Communications of the ACM, 64*(2), 76–83. https://cacm.acm.org/magazines/2021/2/250085-a-review-of-the-semantic-web-field/abstract. doi:10.1145/3397512

Holt, S. (2022). Virtual reality, augmented reality and mixed reality: For astronaut mental health; and space tourism, education and outreach. *Acta Astronautica*.

Hong, S., Lee, S., Song, K., Kim, M., Kim, Y., Kim, H., & Kim, H. (2023). A nurse-led mHealth intervention to alleviate depressive symptoms in older adults living alone in the community: A quasi-experimental study. *International Journal of Nursing Studies*, *138*, 104431. doi:10.1016/j.ijnurstu.2022.104431 PMID:36630872

Hornstein, S., Zantvoort, K., Lueken, U., Funk, B., & Hilbert, K. (2023). Personalization strategies in digital mental health interventions: A systematic review and conceptual framework for depressive symptoms. *Frontiers in Digital Health*, *5*, 1170002. doi:10.3389/fdgth.2023.1170002 PMID:37283721

Hou, Y., Song, J., & Wang, L. (2022, October). P-2.6: Based on the status quo of virtual reality and prospects for future development. In *SID Symposium. Digest of Technical Papers*, *53*(S1, No. S1), 640–642. doi:10.1002/sdtp.16049

Huang, Z., Choi, D., Lai, B., Lü, Z., & Tian, H. (2022). Metaverse-based virtual reality experience and endurance performance in sports economy: Mediating role of mental health and performance anxiety. Frontiers in Public Health, 10. doi:10.3389/fpubh.2022.991489

Huang, S., Wang, G., Yan, Y., & Fang, X. (2020). Blockchain-based data management for digital twin of product. *Journal of Manufacturing Systems*, *54*, 361–371. doi:10.1016/j.jmsy.2020.01.009

Hussain, A., Aydin, N., Cagiltay, N. E., & Suh, H. J. (2016). A review of augmented reality applications on mobile devices for learning in K-12 education. *Computers & Education*, *94*, 1–22.

Huygelier, H., Schraepen, B., Van Ee, R., Vanden Abeele, V., & Gillebert, C. R. (2019). Acceptance of immersive head-mounted virtual reality in older adults. *Scientific Reports*, *9*(1), 4519. doi:10.1038/s41598-019-41200-6 PMID:30872760

Ifanov, Jessica, P., Salim, S., Syahputra, M. E., & Suri, P. A. (2023). A Systematic literature review on implementation of virtual reality for learning. *Procedia Computer Science*, *216*, 260–265. doi:10.1016/j.procs.2022.12.135

Ioannou, A., Papastavrou, E., Avraamides, M. N., & Charalambous, A. (2020). Virtual Reality and Symptoms Management of Anxiety, Depression, Fatigue, and Pain: A Systematic Review. *SAGE Open Nursing*, *6*, 237796082093616. doi:10.1177/2377960820936163 PMID:33415290

Ionescu, A., Van Daele, T., Rizzo, A., Blair, C., & Best, P. (2021). 360° Videos for Immersive Mental Health Interventions: A Systematic Review. *Journal of Technology in Behavioral Science*, *6*(4), 631–651. doi:10.1007/s41347-021-00221-7

Ismail, M. S., Hisham, I. M., Alias, M., Mahdy, Z. A., Nazimi, A. J., Ixora, K. A., Nazir, A. M., & Ismawira, M. I. M. (2022). Challenges in Embracing Virtual Reality from Healthcare Professional's Perspective: A Qualitative Study. [Universiti Kebangsaan Malaysia]. *Medicine & Health (Kuala Lumpur, Malaysia)*, *17*(2), 256–268. doi:10.17576/MH.2022.1702.19

Ivanova, D., & Thorben, P. H. S. (2023). Immersive imaginaries: Digital spaces as post place care. *Digital Geography and Society, 5*.

Jadhakhan, F., Blake, H., Hett, D., & Marwaha, S. (2022). Efficacy of digital technologies aimed at enhancing emotion regulation skills: Literature review. *Frontiers in Psychiatry*, *13*, 809332. doi:10.3389/fpsyt.2022.809332 PMID:36159937

Jain, R. K., & Hiran, K. K. (2024). BIONET: A Bio-Inspired Neural Network for Consensus Mechanisms in Blockchain Systems. In Bio-Inspired Optimization Techniques in Blockchain Systems (pp. 78-100). IGI Global. doi:10.4018/979-8-3693-1131-8.ch004

Jain, R. K., Hiran, K. K., & Maheshwari, R. (2023, April). Lung Cancer Detection Using Machine Learning Algorithms. In *2023 International Conference on Computational Intelligence, Communication Technology and Networking (CICTN)* (pp. 516-521). IEEE.

Jamil, A., Batool, A., Malik, Z., Mirza, A., & Siddiqi, I. (2016). Multilingual artificial text extraction and script identification from video images. *International Journal of Advanced Computer Science and Applications, 7*(4).

Javaid, M., & Haleem, A. (2018). Additive manufacturing applications in orthopaedics: A review. *Journal of Clinical Orthopaedics and Trauma, 9*(3), 202–206. doi:10.1016/j.jcot.2018.04.008 PMID:30202149

Javaid, M., & Haleem, A. (2020). Virtual reality applications toward medical field. *Clinical Epidemiology and Global Health, 8*(2), 600–605.

Jones, D., Snider, C., Nassehi, A., Yon, J., & Hicks, B. (2019). Characterising the Digital Twin: A systematic literature review. *CIRP Journal of Manufacturing Science and Technology, 2019*, 1.

Jopowicz, A., Wiśniowska, J., & Tarnacka, B. (2022). Cognitive and physical intervention in metals' dysfunction and neurodegeneration. *Brain Sciences, 12*(3), 345. doi:10.3390/brainsci12030345 PMID:35326301

Kamińska, D., Zwoliński, G., Laska-Leśniewicz, A., Raposo, R., Vairinhos, M., Pereira, E., Urem, F., Ljubić Hinić, M., Haamer, R. E., & Anbarjafari, G. (2023). Augmented Reality: Current and New Trends in Education. *Electronics (Basel), 12*(16), 3531. doi:10.3390/electronics12163531

Kastner., K. (2023). Leveraging transdisciplinary engineering through the coalescence of digital twins and xr-technologies. In *Leveraging Transdisciplinary Engineering in a Changing and Connected World: Proceedings of the 30th ISTE International Conference on Transdisciplinary Engineering, Hua Hin Cha Am.* IOS Press,.

Kato, K., Yoshimi, T., Aimoto, K., Sato, K., Itoh, N., & Kondo, I. (2023). Reduction of multiple-caregiver assistance through the long-term use of a transfer support robot in a nursing facility. *Assistive Technology, 35*(3), 271–278. doi:10.1080/10400435.2022.2039324 PMID:35320681

Katsumata, S., Ichikohji, T., Nakano, S., Yamaguchi, S., & Ikuine, F. (2022). Changes in the use of mobile devices during the crisis: Immediate response to the COVID-19 pandemic. *Computers in Human Behavior Reports, 5*, 100168. doi:10.1016/j.chbr.2022.100168 PMID:35079660

Kaufmann, C. R. (2001, January). Computers in surgical education and the operating room. *Annales Chirurgiae et Gynaecologiae, 90*(2), 141–146. PMID:11459260

Kaur, J. (2023, May). How is Robotic Process Automation Revolutionising the Way Healthcare Sector Works? In International Conference on Information, Communication and Computing Technology (pp. 1037-1055). Singapore: Springer Nature Singapore. 10.1007/978-981-99-5166-6_70

Kaur, J. (2024). Green Finance 2.0: Pioneering Pathways for Sustainable Development and Health Through Future Trends and Innovations. In Sustainable Investments in Green Finance (pp. 294-319). IGI Global.

Kaur, J. (2023). Robotic Process Automation in Healthcare Sector. In *E3S Web of Conferences* (Vol. 391, p. 01008). EDP Sciences.

Kavyashree, D., & Rajesh, T. M. (2018). Analysis on Text Detection and Extraction from Complex Background Images. *Pattern Recogn*, 37-43.

Kayapinar, U. (2021). *Teacher Education. New Perspectives.* IntechOpen Book Series. doi:10.5772/intechopen.94952

Kelly, R., Seabrook, E., Foley, F., Thomas, N., Nedeljkovic, M., & Wadley, G. (2022c). Design considerations for supporting mindfulness in virtual reality. *Frontiers in Virtual Reality, 2*, 672556. doi:10.3389/frvir.2021.672556

Kendall, K., & Kendall, J. (2023). *Systems Analysis and Design* (11th ed.). Pearson.

Kesawadas, T., Joshi, D., Mayrose, J., & Chugh, K. (2002). A virtual environment for esophageal intubation training. In *Medicine Meets* [IOS Press.]. *Virtual Reality (Waltham Cross), 02/10*, 221–227.

Kessler, G. (2018). Technology and the future of language teaching. *Foreign Language Annals, 51*(1), 205–218. doi:10.1111/flan.12318

Khaddad, A., Bernhard, J. C., Margue, G., Michiels, C., Ricard, S., Chandelon, K., Bladou, F., Bourdel, N., & Bartoli, A. (2023). A survey of augmented reality methods to guide minimally invasive partial nephrectomy. *World Journal of Urology, 41*(2), 335–343. doi:10.1007/s00345-022-04078-0 PMID:35776173

Khaksar, S. M. S., Jahanshahi, A. A., Slade, B., & Asian, S. (2021). A dual-factor theory of WTs adoption in aged care service operations–a cross-country analysis. *Information Technology & People, 34*(7), 1768–1799. doi:10.1108/ITP-10-2018-0449

Khaksar, S. M. S., Shahmehr, F. S., Khosla, R., & Chu, M. T. (2017). Dynamic capabilities in aged care service innovation: The role of social assistive technologies and consumer-directed care strategy. *Journal of Services Marketing, 31*(7), 745–759. doi:10.1108/JSM-06-2016-0243

Khang, A., Hahanov, V., Litvinova, E., Chumachenko, S., Hajimahmud, A. V., Ali, R. N., & Anh, P. T. N. (2023). The Analytics of Hospitality of Hospitals in a Healthcare Ecosystem. In *Data-Centric AI Solutions and Emerging Technologies in the Healthcare Ecosystem* (pp. 39–61). CRC Press. doi:10.1201/9781003356189-4

Khan, N., Okoli, C. N., Ekpin, V., Attai, K., Chukwudi, N., Sabi, H., & Uzoka, F. M. (2023). Adoption and utilization of medical decision support systems in the diagnosis of febrile Diseases: A systematic literature review. *Expert Systems with Applications, 220*, 119638. doi:10.1016/j.eswa.2023.119638

Khazanchi, D., Vyas, A. K., Hiran, K. K., & Padmanaban, S. (Eds.). (2021). *Blockchain 3.0 for sustainable development* (Vol. 10). Walter de Gruyter GmbH & Co KG. doi:10.1515/9783110702507

Khurram, J., Wandschneider, K., & Phanindra, V. W. (2007). The effect of political regimes and technology on economic growth. *Applied Economics, 39*(11), 1425–1432. doi:10.1080/00036840500447906

Kim, H. K., Park, J., Choi, Y., & Choe, M. (2018). Virtual reality sickness questionnaire (VRSQ): Motion sickness measurement index in a virtual reality environment. *Applied Ergonomics, 69*, 66–73. doi:10.1016/j.apergo.2017.12.016 PMID:29477332

Kim, H., Kim, D. J., Kim, S., Chung, W. H., Park, K., Kim, J. D. K., Kim, D., Kim, M. J., Kim, K., & Jeon, H. J. (2021d). Effect of virtual reality on stress reduction and change of physiological parameters including heart rate variability in people with high stress: An open randomized crossover trial. *Frontiers in Psychiatry, 12*, 614539. doi:10.3389/fpsyt.2021.614539 PMID:34447320

Kim, M., Zhang, Y., & Jin, S. (2023). Soft tissue surgical robot for minimally invasive surgery: A review. *Biomedical Engineering Letters, 13*(4), 1–9. doi:10.1007/s13534-023-00326-3 PMID:37872994

Kim, S., Hong, J., Joung, S., Yamada, A., Matsumoto, N., Kim, S., Kim, Y., & Hashizume, M. (2011). Dual Surgical Navigation Using Augmented and Virtual Environment Techniques. *International Journal of Optomechatronics, 5*(2), 155–169. doi:10.1080/15599612.2011.581743

King, M. R. (2023). The future of AI in medicine: A perspective from a Chatbot. *Annals of Biomedical Engineering, 51*(2), 291–295. doi:10.1007/s10439-022-03121-w PMID:36572824

Kizil, M. S., & Joy, J. (2001). *What can virtual reality do for safety*. University of Queensland.

Kleftodimos, A., Evagelou, A., Gkoutzios, S., Matsiola, M., Vrigkas, M., Yannacopoulou, A., Triantafillidou, A., & Lappas, G. (2023). Creating Location-Based Augmented Reality Games and Immersive Experiences for Touristic Destination Marketing and Education. *Computers*, *12*(11), 227. doi:10.3390/computers12110227

Kolben, Y., Azmanov, H., Gelman, R., Dror, D., & Ilan, Y. (2023). Using chronobiology-based second-generation artificial intelligence digital system for overcoming antimicrobial drug resistance in chronic infections. *Annals of Medicine*, *55*(1), 311–318. doi:10.1080/07853890.2022.2163053 PMID:36594558

Korkut, E. H., & Surer, E. (2023). Visualization in virtual reality: A systematic review. *Virtual Reality (Waltham Cross)*, *27*(2), 1447–1480. doi:10.1007/s10055-023-00753-8

Kossiakoff, A. (2020). *Systems Engineering Principles and Practice* (3rd ed.). John Wiley & Sons, Inc. doi:10.1002/9781119516699

Kothari, R. (2023). Integration of Blockchain and Edge Computing in Healthcare: Accountability and Collaboration. *Transdisciplinary Journal of Engineering & Science*, *14*, 14. doi:10.22545/2023/00230

Krizek, T. J. (2000). Surgical error: Ethical issues of adverse events. *Archives of Surgery*, *135*(11), 1359–1366. doi:10.1001/archsurg.135.11.1359 PMID:11074896

Kruse, L., Karaosmanoglu, S., Rings, S., Ellinger, B., & Steinicke, F. (2021). Enabling immersive exercise activities for older adults: A comparison of virtual reality exergames and traditional video exercises. *Societies (Basel, Switzerland)*, *11*(4), 134. doi:10.3390/soc11040134

Kuerbis, A., Behrendt, S., Arora, V., & Muench, F. J. (2022). Acceptability and preliminary effectiveness of a text messaging intervention to reduce high-risk alcohol use among adults 50 and older: An exploratory study. *Advances in Dual Diagnosis*, *15*(2), 100–118. doi:10.1108/ADD-11-2021-0012

Kumar, P., Chauhan, S., & Awasthi, L. K. (2023). Artificial intelligence in healthcare: Review, ethics, trust challenges & future research directions. *Engineering Applications of Artificial Intelligence*, *120*, 105894. doi:10.1016/j.engappai.2023.105894

Kurniawan, M. H., Suharjito, D., & Witjaksono, G. (2018). Human Anatomy Learning Systems Using Augmented Reality on Mobile Application. *Procedia Computer Science*, *135*, 80–88. doi:10.1016/j.procs.2018.08.152

Lakhwani, K., Bhargava, S., Hiran, K. K., Bundele, M. M., & Somwanshi, D. (2020, December). Prediction of the onset of diabetes using artificial neural network and Pima Indians diabetes dataset. In 2020 *5th IEEE International Conference on Recent Advances and Innovations in Engineering (ICRAIE)* (pp. 1-6). IEEE. 10.1109/ICRAIE51050.2020.9358308

Landowska, A. (2022). Measuring prefrontal cortex response to virtual reality exposure therapy in freely moving participants. *Dissertation Abstracts International. B, The Sciences and Engineering*, *83*(3-B).

Landowska, A., Roberts, D., Eachus, P., & Barrett, A. (2018). Within- and between-session prefrontal cortex response to virtual reality exposure therapy for acrophobia. *Frontiers in Human Neuroscience*, *12*, 362. doi:10.3389/fnhum.2018.00362 PMID:30443209

Lang, V., & Sittler, P. (2012). *Augmented reality for real estate*. In 18th Pacific-RIM Real Estate Society (PRRES) Conference, Adelaide, Australia.

Lan, L., Sikov, J., Lejeune, J., Ji, C., Brown, H. P., Bullock, K., & Spencer, A. E. (2023). A Systematic Review of Using Virtual and Augmented Reality for the Diagnosis and Treatment of Psychotic Disorders. *Current Treatment Options in Psychiatry*, *10*(2), 87–107. doi:10.1007/s40501-023-00287-5 PMID:37360960

Lara, F., & Rueda, J. (2021). Virtual Reality Not for "Being Someone" but for "Being in Someone Else's Shoes": Avoiding Misconceptions in Empathy Enhancement. *Frontiers in Psychology*, *12*, 741516. doi:10.3389/fpsyg.2021.741516 PMID:34504468

Latha, K., Meena, K. S., Pravitha, M. R., Dasgupta, M., & Chaturvedi, S. K. (2020). Effective use of social media platforms for promotion of mental health awareness. *Journal of Education and Health Promotion*, *9*(1), 124. doi:10.4103/jehp.jehp_90_20 PMID:32642480

Laver, K. E., Lange, B., George, S., Deutsch, J. E., Saposnik, G., & Crotty, M. (2017). Virtual reality for stroke rehabilitation. In Cochrane Database of Systematic Reviews, (11). John Wiley and Sons Ltd. doi:10.1002/14651858.CD008349.pub4

Lee, J., Azamfar, M., Singh, J., & Siahpour, S. (2020). Integration of digital twin and deep learning in cyber-physical systems: Towards smart manufacturing. *IET Collaborative Intelligent Manufacturing*, *2*(1), 34–36. doi:10.1049/iet-cim.2020.0009

Lee, K. (2023). Counseling Psychological Understanding and Considerations of the Metaverse: A Theoretical Review. *Health Care*, *11*(18), 2490. doi:10.3390/healthcare11182490 PMID:37761687

Letterie, G. S. (2002). How virtual reality may enhance training in obstetrics and gynecology. *American Journal of Obstetrics and Gynecology*, *187*(3), S37–S40. doi:10.1067/mob.2002.127361 PMID:12235439

Lewis, C. (2018). The negative side effects of Virtual Reality. *Resource Magazine*.

Li, M., & Liu, L. (2022). Students' perceptions of augmented reality integrated into a mobile learning environment. Library Hi Tech. doi:10.1108/LHT-10-2021-0345

Liao, D., Shu, L., Liang, G., Li, Y., Zhang, Y., Zhang, W., & Xu, X. (2019). Design and evaluation of affective virtual reality system based on multimodal physiological signals and self-assessment manikin. *IEEE Journal of Electromagnetics, RF and Microwaves in Medicine and Biology*, *4*(3), 216–224. doi:10.1109/JERM.2019.2948767

Li, H., Dong, W., Wang, Z., Chen, N., Wu, J., Wang, G., & Jiang, T. (2021). Effect of a Virtual Reality-Based Restorative Environment on the Emotional and Cognitive Recovery of Individuals with Mild-to-Moderate Anxiety and Depression. *International Journal of Environmental Research and Public Health*, *18*(17), 9053. doi:10.3390/ijerph18179053 PMID:34501643

Li, K. C., & Wong, B. T. M. (2022). Research landscape of smart education: A bibliometric analysis. *Interactive Technology and Smart Education*, *19*(1), 3–19. doi:10.1108/ITSE-05-2021-0083

Li, L., Yu, F., Shi, D., Shi, J., Tian, Z., Yang, J., & Jiang, Q. (2017). Application of virtual reality technology in clinical medicine. *American Journal of Translational Research*, *9*(9), 3867. PMID:28979666

Lindner, P. (2020). Better, Virtually: The Past, Present, and Future of Virtual Reality Cognitive Behavior Therapy. *International Journal of Cognitive Therapy*, *14*(1), 23–46. doi:10.1007/s41811-020-00090-7

Lindner, P., Hamilton, W., Miloff, A., & Carlbring, P. (2019). How to Treat Depression With Low-Intensity Virtual Reality Interventions: Perspectives on Translating Cognitive Behavioral Techniques Into the Virtual Reality Modality and How to Make Anti-Depressive Use of Virtual Reality–Unique Experiences. *Frontiers in Psychiatry*, *10*, 792. doi:10.3389/fpsyt.2019.00792 PMID:31736809

Linton, M., Dieppe, P., & Medina-Lara, A. (2016). Review of 99 self-report measures for assessing well-being in adults: Exploring dimensions of well-being and developments over time. *BMJ Open*, *6*(7), e010641. doi:10.1136/bmjopen-2015-010641 PMID:27388349

Lin, Y., & Yu, Z. (2023). Extending Technology Acceptance Model to higher-education students' use of digital academic reading tools on computers. *International Journal of Educational Technology in Higher Education*, *20*(1), 34. doi:10.1186/s41239-023-00403-8

Liono, R., Amanda, N., Pratiwi, A., & Gunawan, A. (2021). A Systematic Literature Review: Learning with Visual by The Help of Augmented Reality Helps Students Learn Better. *Procedia Computer Science*, *179*, 144–152. doi:10.1016/j.procs.2020.12.019

Li, R., Chen, Y., Ritchie, M., & Moore, J. (2020). Electronic health records and polygenic risk scores for predicting disease risk. *Nature Reviews. Genetics*, *21*(8), 493–502. doi:10.1038/s41576-020-0224-1 PMID:32235907

Liu, K., Madrigal, E., Chung, J. S., Parekh, M., Kalahar, C. S., Nguyen, D., & Harris, O. A. (2023). Preliminary Study of Virtual-reality-guided Meditation for Veterans with Stress and Chronic Pain. *Alternative Therapies in Health and Medicine*, *29*(6). PMID:34559692

Liu, Z., Ren, L., Xiao, C., Zhang, K., & Demian, P. (2022). Virtual Reality Aided Therapy towards Health 4.0: A Two-Decade Bibliometric Analysis. *International Journal of Environmental Research and Public Health*, *19*(3), 1525. doi:10.3390/ijerph19031525 PMID:35162546

Li, X., Luh, D. B., Xu, R. H., & An, Y. (2023). Considering the Consequences of Cybersickness in Immersive Virtual Reality Rehabilitation: A Systematic Review and Meta-Analysis. *Applied Sciences (Basel, Switzerland)*, *13*(8), 5159. doi:10.3390/app13085159

Li, X., Yi, W., Chi, H. L., Wang, X., & Chan, A. P. (2018). A critical review of virtual and augmented reality (VR/AR) applications in construction safety. *Automation in Construction*, *86*, 150–162. doi:10.1016/j.autcon.2017.11.003

Llorens, R. C., Latorre, J., Alcañíz, M., & Llorens, R. C. (2019). Embodiment and presence in virtual reality after stroke. A comparative study with healthy subjects. *Frontiers in Neurology*, *10*, 1061. Advance online publication. doi:10.3389/fneur.2019.01061 PMID:31649608

Lochan, K., Suklyabaidya, A., & Roy, B. K. (2023). Medical and healthcare robots in India. In *Medical and Healthcare Robotics* (pp. 221–236). Academic Press. doi:10.1016/B978-0-443-18460-4.00010-X

Loeffler, C. E. (1993). Distributed Virtual Reality: Applications for education, entertainment and industry. *Telektronikk*, *89*, 83–83.

Lo, H. H. M., Ngai, S. P., & Yam, K. (2021). Effects of Mindfulness-Based Stress Reduction on Health and Social Care Education: A Cohort-Controlled Study. *Mindfulness*, *12*(8), 2050–2058. doi:10.1007/s12671-021-01663-z PMID:34127933

Longo, U. G., Carnevale, A., Andreoli, F., Mannocchi, I., Bravi, M., Sassi, M. S. H., Santacaterina, F., Carli, M., Schena, E., & Papalia, R. (2023). Immersive virtual reality for shoulder rehabilitation: Evaluation of a physical therapy program executed with Oculus Quest 2. *BMC Musculoskeletal Disorders*, *24*(1), 859. doi:10.1186/s12891-023-06861-5 PMID:37919702

Lopez-Rodriguez, M. M., Fernández-Millan, A., Ruiz-Fernández, M. D., Dobarrio-Sanz, I., & Fernández-Medina, I. M. (2020). New technologies to improve pain, anxiety and depression in children and adolescents with cancer: A systematic review. In International Journal of Environmental Research and Public Health, 17(10). doi:10.3390/ijerph17103563

Lorusso, L., Mosmondor, M., Grguric, A., Toccafondi, L., D'Onofrio, G., Russo, S., Lampe, J., Pihl, T., Mayer, N., Vignani, G., Lesterpt, I., Vaamonde, L., Giuliani, F., Bonaccorsi, M., La Viola, C., Rovini, E., Cavallo, F., & Fiorini, L. (2023). Design and Evaluation of Personalized Services to Foster Active Aging: The Experience of Technology Pre-Validation in Italian Pilots. *Sensors (Basel)*, *23*(2), 797. doi:10.3390/s23020797 PMID:36679590

Lu, A. S., Kharrazi, H., Gharghabi, F., Thompson, D., Paul, M. J., & Aung, M. (2018). A systematic review of health video games for childhood obesity prevention and intervention. *Journal of Diabetes Science and Technology*, *12*(1), 222–233.

Lum, H. C., Elliott, L. J., Aqlan, F., & Zhao, R. (2020). Virtual Reality: History, Applications, and Challenges for Human Factors Research. *Proceedings of the Human Factors and Ergonomics Society Annual Meeting*, *64*(1), 1263–1268. doi:10.1177/1071181320641300

Lund, B. (2021). Predictors of use of digital technology for communication among older adults: Analysis of data from the health and retirement study. *Working with Older People (Brighton, England)*, *25*(4), 294–303. doi:10.1108/WWOP-01-2021-0002

Mabrey, J. D., Cannon, W. D., Gillogly, S. D., Kasser, J. R., Sweeney, H. J., Zarins, B., & Poss, R. (2000). Development of a virtual reality arthroscopic knee simulator. In *Medicine Meets* [IOS Press.]. *Virtual Reality (Waltham Cross)*, *2000*, 192–194.

Maçorano, R. D. N. A. (2020). *Exploratory Psychometric Validation and Efficacy Assessment Study of Social Phobia Treatment based on Augmented and Virtual Reality Serious Games and Biofeedback* [Doctoral dissertation, Universidade de Lisboa (Portugal)].

Mahmoud, H., Aljaldi, F., El-Fiky, A., Battecha, K., Thabet, A., Alayat, M., & Ibrahim, A. (2023). Artificial Intelligence machine learning and conventional physical therapy for upper limb outcome in patients with stroke: A systematic review and meta-analysis. *European Review for Medical and Pharmacological Sciences*, *27*(11). PMID:37318455

Mahr, D., & Huh, J. (2022). Technologies in service communication: Looking forward. *Journal of Service Management*, *33*(4/5), 648–656. doi:10.1108/JOSM-03-2022-0075

Mallari, B., Spaeth, E. K., Goh, H., & Boyd, B. S. (2019). Virtual reality as an analgesic for acute and chronic pain in adults: A systematic review and meta-analysis. In *Journal of Pain Research* (Vol. 12, pp. 2053–2085). Dove Medical Press Ltd. doi:10.2147/JPR.S200498

Ma, M., & Jain, L. C. (2014). *Serious games and edutainment applications* (Vol. II). Springer. doi:10.1007/978-3-319-11623-5

Mantovani, F., Castelnuovo, G., Gaggioli, A., & Riva, G. (2003). Virtual reality training for health-care professionals. *Cyberpsychology & Behavior*, *6*(4), 389–395. doi:10.1089/109493103322278772 PMID:14511451

Maples-Keller, J. L., Bunnell, B. E., Kim, S. J., & Rothbaum, B. O. (2017). The use of virtual reality technology in the treatment of anxiety and other psychiatric disorders. *Harvard Review of Psychiatry*, *25*(3), 103–113. doi:10.1097/HRP.0000000000000138 PMID:28475502

Maran, P. L., Daniëls, R., & Slegers, K. (2022). The use of extended reality (XR) for people with moderate to severe intellectual disabilities (ID): A scoping review. *Technology and Disability*, *34*(2), 53–67. doi:10.3233/TAD-210363

Marco, J. H., Perpiñá, C., & Botella, C. (2013). Effectiveness of cognitive behavioral therapy supported by virtual reality in the treatment of body image in eating disorders: One year follow-up. *Psychiatry Research*, *209*(3), 619–625. doi:10.1016/j.psychres.2013.02.023 PMID:23499231

Marossi, C., Mariani, V., Arenas, A., Brondino, M., de Carvalho, C. V., Costa, P., & Pasini, M. (2023, July). Mindfulness Lessons in a Virtual Natural Environment to Cope with Work-Related Stress. In *International Conference in Methodologies and intelligent Systems for Techhnology Enhanced Learning* (pp. 227-238). Cham: Springer Nature Switzerland. 10.1007/978-3-031-41226-4_24

Marr, J. (2021). Ten best examples of VR and AR in education. *Forbes*. https://www.forbes.com/sites/bernardmarr/2021/07/23/10-best-examples-of-vr-and-ar-in-education/?sh=13e5071e1f48

Marschollek, M., Rehwald, A., Wolf, K. H., & Gietzelt, M. (2012). Collaborative and augmented telemedicine in health care. *Journal of Computer Science and Technology*, *27*(6), 1246–1262.

Marvaso, G., Pepa, M., Volpe, S., Mastroleo, F., Zaffaroni, M., Vincini, M. G., & Jereczek-Fossa, B. A. (2022). Virtual and Augmented Reality as a Novel Opportunity to Unleash the Power of Radiotherapy in the Digital Era: A Scoping Review. *Applied Sciences (Basel, Switzerland)*, *12*(22), 11308. doi:10.3390/app122211308

Ma, T., Zhang, S., Zhu, S., Ni, J., Wu, Q., & Liu, M. (2022). The new role of nursing in digital inclusion: Reflections on smartphone use and willingness to increase digital skills among Chinese older adults. *Geriatric Nursing*, *48*, 114–122. doi:10.1016/j.gerinurse.2022.09.004 PMID:36155310

Mathew, M., Thomas, M. J., Navaneeth, M. G., Sulaiman, S., Amudhan, A. N., & Sudheer, A. P. (2023). A systematic review of technological advancements in signal sensing, actuation, control and training methods in robotic exoskeletons for rehabilitation. *The Industrial Robot*, *50*(3), 432–455. doi:10.1108/IR-09-2022-0239

Matsuzaki, H., & Gliesche, P. (2023). Robots and Norms of Care: A Comparative Analysis of the Reception of Robotic Assistance in Nursing. In Social Robots in Social Institutions (pp. 90-99). IOS Press. doi:10.3233/FAIA220607

Mazurek, J., Kiper, P., Cieślik, B., Rutkowski, S., Mehlich, K., Turolla, A., & Szczepańska-Gieracha, J. (2019). Virtual reality in medicine: A brief overview and future research directions. *Human Movement*, *20*(3), 16–22. doi:10.5114/hm.2019.83529

McAnally, K., Wallwork, K., & Wallis, G. (2023). The efficiency of visually guided movement in real and virtual space. *Virtual Reality (Waltham Cross)*, *27*(2), 1187–1197. doi:10.1007/s10055-022-00724-5

McCradden, M., Joshi, S., Anderson, J., Mazwi, M., Goldenberg, A., & Shaul, R. (2020). Patient safety and quality improvement: Ethical principles for a regulatory approach to bias in healthcare machine learning. *Journal of the American Medical Informatics Association : JAMIA*, *27*(12), 2024–2027. doi:10.1093/jamia/ocaa085 PMID:32585698

McDiarmid, G. W., & Zhao, Y. (2023). Time to Rethink: Educating for a Technology-Transformed World. *ECNU Review of Education*, *6*(2), 189–214. doi:10.1177/20965311221076493

McIntosh, K. S., Gregor, J. C., & Khanna, N. V. (2014). Computer-based virtual reality colonoscopy simulation improves patient-based colonoscopy performance. *Canadian Journal of Gastroenterology & Hepatology*, *28*(4), 203–206. doi:10.1155/2014/804367 PMID:24729994

McIntyre, R. S., Greenleaf, W., Bulaj, G., Taylor, S. T., Mitsi, G., Saliu, D., Czysz, A., Silvesti, G., Garcia, M., & Jain, R. (2023). Digital Health Technologies and Major Depressive Disorder. In *CNS Spectrums*. Cambridge University Press. doi:10.1017/S1092852923002225

Meena, G., Dhanwal, B., Mahrishi, M., & Hiran, K. K. (2021, August). Performance comparison of network intrusion detection systems based on different pre-processing methods and deep neural network. In *Proceedings of the International Conference on Data Science, Machine Learning and Artificial Intelligence* (pp. 110-115). Academic Press.

Meena, G., Dhanwal, B., Mahrishi, M., & Hiran, K. K. (2021, August). Performance comparison of network intrusion detection system based on different pre-processing methods and deep neural network. In *Proceedings of the International Conference on Data Science, Machine Learning and Artificial Intelligence* (pp. 110-115). ACM. 10.1145/3484824.3484878

Mer, A., & Virdi, A. S. (2023). Navigating the paradigm shift in HRM practices through the lens of artificial intelligence: A post-pandemic perspective. *The Adoption and Effect of Artificial Intelligence on Human Resources Management, Part A*, 123-154.

Merilampi, S., Sirkka, A., Leino, M., Koivisto, A., & Finn, E. (2014). Cognitive mobile games for memory impaired older adults. *Journal of Assistive Technologies*, *8*(4), 207–223. doi:10.1108/JAT-12-2013-0033

Michael, D. R., & Chen, S. L. (2005). *Serious games: Games that educate, train, and inform*. Muska & Lipman/Premier-Trade.

Midha, S., & Singh, K. (2023). Happiness-Enhancing Strategies Among Indians. In *Religious and Spiritual Practices in India: A Positive Psychological Perspective* (pp. 341–368). Springer Nature Singapore. doi:10.1007/978-981-99-2397-7_15

Mikhailova, O. (2018). Adoption and implementation of new technologies in hospitals: A network perspective. *IMP Journal*, *12*(2), 368–391. doi:10.1108/IMP-05-2017-0027

Miljkovic, I., Shlyakhetko, O., & Fedushko, S. (2023). Real Estate App Development Based on AI/VR Technologies. *Electronics (Basel)*, *12*(3), 707. doi:10.3390/electronics12030707

Miller, A. S., Cafazzo, J. A., & Seto, E. (2014). A game plan: Gamification design principles in mHealth applications for chronic disease management. *Health Informatics Journal*, *20*(4), 257–268. PMID:24986104

Milton, M., De La, C. O., Ginn, H. L., & Benigni, A. (2020). Controller-embeddable probabilistic real-time digital twins for power electronic converter diagnostics. *IEEE Transactions on Power Electronics*, *35*(9), 9852–9866. doi:10.1109/TPEL.2020.2971775

Miner, N. (2022). *Stairway to Heaven: Breathing Mindfulness into Virtual Reality* [Doctoral dissertation, Northeastern University].

Minopoulos, G. M., Memos, V. A., Stergiou, K. D., Stergiou, C. L., & Psannis, K. E. (2023). A Medical Image Visualization Technique Assisted with AI-Based Haptic Feedback for Robotic Surgery and Healthcare. *Applied Sciences (Basel, Switzerland)*, *13*(6), 3592. doi:10.3390/app13063592

Mishra, S., Kumar, A., Padmanabhan, P., & Gulyás, B. (2021). Neurophysiological correlates of cognition as revealed by virtual reality: Delving the brain with a synergistic approach. In Brain Sciences, 11(1). doi:10.3390/brainsci11010051

Mishra, A., Tripathi, A., Khazanchi, D., Hiran, K. K., Vyas, A. K., & Padmanaban, S. (2021). A framework for applying artificial intelligence (AI) with Internet of NanoThings (IoNT). In *Machine Learning for Sustainable Development* (pp. 1–16). De Gruyter.

Mishra, R., Narayanan, M., Umana, G., Montemurro, N., Chaurasia, B., & Deora, H. (2022). Virtual Reality in Neurosurgery: Beyond Neurosurgical Planning. *International Journal of Environmental Research and Public Health*, *19*(3), 1719. doi:10.3390/ijerph19031719 PMID:35162742

Mishra, S. K., & Sarkar, A. (2022). Service-oriented architecture for Internet of Things: A semantic approach. *Journal of King Saud University. Computer and Information Sciences*, *34*(10, 10 Part A), 8765–8776. doi:10.1016/j.jksuci.2021.09.024

Mishra, T., Wang, M., Metwally, A., Bogu, G., Brooks, A., Bahmani, A., Alavi, A., Celli, A., Higgs, E., Dagan-Rosenfeld, O., Fay, B., Kirkpatrick, S., Kellogg, R., Gibson, M., Wang, T., Hunting, E., Mamić, P., Ganz, A., Rolnik, B., & Snyder, M. (2020). Pre-symptomatic detection of COVID-19 from smartwatch data. *Nature Biomedical Engineering*, *4*(12), 1208–1220. doi:10.1038/s41551-020-00640-6 PMID:33208926

Modi, K., Singh, I., & Kumar, Y. (2023). A Comprehensive Analysis of Artificial Intelligence Techniques for the Prediction and Prognosis of Lifestyle Diseases. *Archives of Computational Methods in Engineering, 30*(8), 1–24. doi:10.1007/s11831-023-09957-2

Moher, D., Liberati, A., Tetzlaff, J., & Altman, D. G.The PRISMA Group. (2009). *P*referred *R*eporting *I*tems for *S*ystematic Reviews and *M*eta-Analyses: The PRISMA Statement. *PLoS Medicine, 6*(6), e1000097. doi:10.1371/journal.pmed.1000097 PMID:19621072

Mokmin, N. M., & Jamiat, N. (2020). The effectiveness of a virtual fitness trainer app in motivating and engaging students for fitness activity by applying motor learning theory. *Education and Information Technologies, 26*(2), 1847–1864. doi:10.1007/s10639-020-10337-7

Monge, J., Ribeiro, G., Raimundo, A., Postolache, O., & Santos, J. (2023). AI-Based Smart Sensing and AR for Gait Rehabilitation Assessment. *Information (Basel), 14*(7), 355. doi:10.3390/info14070355

Morvan, L. (2019). Waking up to a new reality. *Accenture.*

Mouatt, B., Smith, A. E., Mellow, M. L., Parfitt, G., Smith, R., & Stanton, T. R. (2020). The use of virtual reality to influence motivation, affect, enjoyment, and engagement during exercise: A scoping review. Frontiers in Virtual Reality. doi:10.3389/frvir.2020.564664

Murakami, Y., Honaga, K., Kono, H., Haruyama, K., Yamaguchi, T., Tani, M., Isayama, R., Takakura, T., Tanuma, A., Hatori, K., Wada, F., & Fujiwara, T. (2023). New Artificial Intelligence-Integrated Electromyography-Driven Robot Hand for Upper Extremity Rehabilitation of Patients With Stroke: A Randomized, Controlled Trial. *Neurorehabilitation and Neural Repair, 37*(5), 15459683231166939. doi:10.1177/15459683231166939 PMID:37039319

Murciano-Hueso, A., Martín-Lucas, J., Serrate González, S., & Torrijos Fincias, P. (2022). Use and perception of gerontechnology: Differences in a group of Spanish older adults. *Quality in Ageing : Policy, Practice and Research, 23*(3), 114–128. doi:10.1108/QAOA-02-2022-0010

Mylrea, K., & Sivertson, S. (1975). Biomedical Engineering in Health Care - Potential Versus Reality. *IEEE Transactions on Biomedical Engineering, BME-22*(2), 114–119. doi:10.1109/TBME.1975.324429 PMID:1123239

Nagarathna, R., Ram, V., Majumdar, V., Rajesh, S., Singh, A., Patil, S., Anand, A., Judu, I., Bhaskara, S., Basa, J. R., & Nagendra, H. R. (2021). Effectiveness of a Yoga-Based Lifestyle Protocol (YLP) in preventing Diabetes in a High-Risk Indian cohort: A Multicenter Cluster-Randomized Controlled Trial (NMB-Trial). *Frontiers in Endocrinology, 12*, 664657. doi:10.3389/fendo.2021.664657 PMID:34177805

Nankani, H., Mahrishi, M., Morwal, S., & Hiran, K. K. (2022). A Formal study of shot boundary detection approaches—Comparative analysis. In *Soft Computing: Theories and Applications: Proceedings of SoCTA 2020,* Volume 1 (pp. 311-320). Springer Singapore.

Nanthakumar, R., & Sivakumaran, N. (2018). Role of Biomedical Engineering for Diagnose and Treatment. *Role of Biomedical Engineering for Diagnose and Treatment., 4*(11), 94–112. doi:10.31695/IJASRE.2018.32944

Navab, N., Martin-Gomez, A., Seibold, M., Sommersperger, M., Song, T., Winkler, A., Yu, K., & Eck, U. (2023). Medical Augmented Reality: Definition, Principle Components, Domain Modeling, and Design-Development-Validation Process. *Journal of Imaging, 9*(1), 4. doi:10.3390/jimaging9010004 PMID:36662102

Naylor, M., Ridout, B., & Campbell, A. (2020). A scoping review identifying the need for quality research on the use of virtual reality in workplace settings for stress management. *Cyberpsychology, Behavior, and Social Networking, 23*(8), 506–518. doi:10.1089/cyber.2019.0287 PMID:32486836

Neo, J. R. J., Won, A. S., & Shepley, M. M. (2021). Designing immersive virtual environments for human behaviour research. Frontiers in Virtual Reality, 2. doi:10.3389/frvir.2021.603750

Neri, L., Cianetti, L., Sciarabba, C., & Lamberti, F. (2016). The effectiveness of digital games in health professions education: A systematic review. *Computers & Education*, *95*, 90–97.

Nieto-Escamez, F., Cortés-Pérez, I., Obrero-Gaitán, E., & Fusco, A. (2023). Virtual Reality Applications in Neurorehabilitation: Current Panorama and Challenges. *Brain Sciences*, *13*(5), 819. doi:10.3390/brainsci13050819 PMID:37239291

Niknejad, N., Ismail, W., Ghani, I., Nazari, B., Bahari, M., & Hussin, A. R. B. C. (2020). Understanding Service-Oriented Architecture (SOA): A systematic literature review and directions for further investigation. *Information Systems*, *91*, 101491. doi:10.1016/j.is.2020.101491

Norouzi, N., Bölling, L., Bruder, G., & Welch, G. (2019). Augmented rotations in virtual reality for users with a reduced range of head movement. *Journal of Rehabilitation and Assistive Technologies Engineering*, *6*, 2055668319841309. doi:10.1177/2055668319841309 PMID:31245034

Nwadiokwu, O. T. (2023). Examining the Impact and Challenges of Artificial Intelligence (AI) in Healthcare. *Edward Waters University Undergraduate Research Journal, 1*(1).

O'Connor, T. J., Cooper, R. A., Fitzgerald, S. G., Dvorznak, M. J., Boninger, M. L., VanSickle, D. P., & Glass, L. (2000). Evaluation of a manual wheelchair interface to computer games. *Neurorehabilitation and Neural Repair*, *14*(1), 21–31. doi:10.1177/154596830001400103 PMID:11228946

O'Leary, S. T., Lee, M., Federico, S., Lurie-Moroni, E., & Beaty, B. L. (2016). Educational web-based game for early assessment and management of child pedestrian injury risk. *JMIR Serious Games*, *4*(1), e3. PMID:27229772

Oades, L. G., & Mossman, L. H. (2017). The science of well-being and positive Psychology. In Cambridge University Press eBooks (pp. 7–23). doi:10.1017/9781316339275.003

OASIS. (2023). *Advancing open standards for the information society*. OASIS. http://www.c5.cl/ieinvestiga/actas/ribie98/279.html

Ohneberg, C., Stöbich, N., Warmbein, A., Rathgeber, I., Mehler-Klamt, A. C., Fischer, U., & Eberl, I. (2023). Assistive robotic systems in nursing care: A scoping review. *BMC Nursing*, *22*(1), 1–15. doi:10.1186/s12912-023-01230-y PMID:36934280

Okoye, K., Hussein, H., Arrona-Palacios, A., Quintero, H. N., Ortega, L. O. P., Sanchez, A. L., Ortiz, E. A., Escamilla, J., & Hosseini, S. (2023). Impact of digital technologies upon teaching and learning in higher education in Latin America: An outlook on the reach, barriers, and bottlenecks. *Education and Information Technologies*, *28*(2), 2291–2360. doi:10.1007/s10639-022-11214-1 PMID:35992366

Oman, D. (2023). Mindfulness for Global Public Health: Critical analysis and agenda. *Mindfulness*. doi:10.1007/s12671-023-02089-5

Omboni, S., Padwal, R. S., Alessa, T., Benczúr, B., Green, B. B., Hubbard, I., Kario, K., Khan, N. A., Konradi, A., Logan, A. G., Lu, Y., Mars, M., McManus, R. J., Melville, S., Neumann, C. L., Parati, G., Renna, N. F., Ryvlin, P., Saner, H., & Wang, J. (2022). The worldwide impact of telemedicine during COVID-19: Current evidence and recommendations for the future. *Connected Health*. doi:10.20517/ch.2021.03 PMID:35233563

Paimre, M., Virkus, S., & Osula, K. (2023). Health information behavior and related factors among Estonians aged≥ 50 years during the COVID-19 pandemic. *The Journal of Documentation*, *79*(5), 1164–1181. doi:10.1108/JD-10-2022-0217

Pandarinathan, G., Mishra, S., Nedumaran, A. M., Padmanabhan, P., & Gulyás, B. (2018). The potential of cognitive neuroimaging: A way forward to the mind-machine interface. In Journal of Imaging, 4(5). MDPI Multidisciplinary Digital Publishing Institute. doi:10.3390/jimaging4050070

Pan, X., & Hamilton, A. F. D. C. (2018). Why and how to use virtual reality to study human social interaction: The challenges of exploring a new research landscape. *British Journal of Psychology*, *109*(3), 395–417. doi:10.1111/bjop.12290 PMID:29504117

Papachristou, N., Kartsidis, P., Anagnostopoulou, A., Marshall-McKenna, R., Kotronoulas, G., Collantes, G., & Bamidis, P. D. (2023, May). A Smart Digital Health Platform to Enable Monitoring of Quality of Life and Frailty in Older Patients with Cancer: A Mixed-Methods, Feasibility Study Protocol. In *Seminars in Oncology Nursing* (p. 151437). WB Saunders. doi:10.1016/j.soncn.2023.151437

Papadopoulos, T., Evangelidis, K., Kaskalis, T. H., Evangelidis, G., & Sylaiou, S. (2021). Interactions in augmented and mixed reality: An overview. *Applied Sciences (Basel, Switzerland)*, *11*(18), 8752. doi:10.3390/app11188752

Papastergiou, M. (2009). Digital game-based learning in high school computer science education: Impact on educational effectiveness and student motivation. *Computers & Education*, *52*(1), 1–12. doi:10.1016/j.compedu.2008.06.004

Pareek, T. G., Mehta, U., & Gupta, A. (2018). A survey: Virtual reality model for medical diagnosis. *Biomedical & Pharmacology Journal*, *11*(4), 2091–2100. doi:10.13005/bpj/1588

Park, M. J., Kim, D. J., Lee, U., Na, E. J., & Jeon, H. J. (2019). A literature overview of virtual reality (VR) in treatment of psychiatric disorders: Recent advances and limitations. *Frontiers in Psychiatry*, *10*, 505. doi:10.3389/fpsyt.2019.00505 PMID:31379623

Park, S., & Kim, B. (2020). Readiness for utilizing digital intervention: Patterns of internet use among older adults with diabetes. *Primary Care Diabetes*, *14*(6), 692–697. doi:10.1016/j.pcd.2020.08.005 PMID:32839128

Parsons, D., & MacCallum, K. (2021). Current Perspectives on Augmented Reality in Medical Education: Applications, Affordances and Limitations. *Advances in Medical Education and Practice*, *12*, 77–91. doi:10.2147/AMEP.S249891 PMID:33500677

Parsons, S. (2015). Learning to work together: Designing a multi-user virtual reality game for social collaboration and perspective-taking for children with autism. *International Journal of Child-Computer Interaction*, *6*, 28–38. doi:10.1016/j.ijcci.2015.12.002

Parsons, T. D., Gaggioli, A., & Riva, G. (2017). Virtual reality for research in social neuroscience. *Brain Sciences*, *7*(4), 42. doi:10.3390/brainsci7040042 PMID:28420150

Passavanti, R., Pantano, E., Priporas, C. V., & Verteramo, S. (2020). The use of new technologies for corporate marketing communication in luxury retailing: Preliminary findings. *Qualitative Market Research*, *23*(3), 503–521. doi:10.1108/QMR-11-2017-0144

Patangia, B., Sankruthyayana, R. G., Sathiyaseelan, A., & Balasundaram, S. (2021). How could Mindfulness Help? A Perspective on the Applications of Mindfulness in Enhancing Tomorrow's Workplace. *i-Manager's. Journal of Management*, *16*(3), 52.

Patel, S., Vyas, A. K., & Hiran, K. K. (2022). Infrastructure health monitoring using signal processing based on an industry 4.0 System. *Cyber-Physical Systems and Industry*, *4*, 249–260.

Peeters, D. (2019). Virtual reality: A game-changing method for the language sciences. *Psychonomic Bulletin & Review*, *26*(3), 894–900. doi:10.3758/s13423-019-01571-3 PMID:30734158

Peng, W., Lin, J. H., Pfeiffer, K. A., & Winn, B. (2012). Need satisfaction supportive game features as motivational determinants: An experimental study of a self-determination theory guided exergame. *Media Psychology*, *15*(2), 175–196. doi:10.1080/15213269.2012.673850

Peprah, N. A., Hiran, K. K., & Doshi, R. (2020). Politics in the Cloud: A Review of Cloud Technology Applications in the Domain of Politics. *Soft Computing: Theories and Applications. Proceedings of SoCTA*, *2018*, 993–1003.

Pereira, M., Prahm, C., Kolbenschlag, J., Oliveira, E., & Rodrigues, N. (2020). Application of AR and VR in hand rehabilitation: A systematic review. *Journal of Biomedical Informatics*, *103584*, 103584. doi:10.1016/j.jbi.2020.103584 PMID:33011296

Pereira, V., Matos, T., Rodrigues, R., Nóbrega, R., & Jacob, J. (2019). Extended reality framework for remote collaborative interactions in virtual environments. In *2019 International Conference on Graphics and Interaction (ICGI)*. IEEE. 10.1109/ICGI47575.2019.8955025

Peter, L., Schindler, S., Sander, C., Schmidt, S., Muehlan, H., McLaren, T., Tomczyk, S., Speerforck, S., & Schomerus, G. (2021). Continuum beliefs and mental illness stigma: A systematic review and meta-analysis of correlation and intervention studies. *Psychological Medicine*, *51*(5), 716–726. doi:10.1017/S0033291721000854 PMID:33827725

Petrigna, L., & Musumeci, G. (2022). The metaverse: A new challenge for the healthcare system: A scoping review. *Journal of Functional Morphology and Kinesiology*, *7*(3), 63. doi:10.3390/jfmk7030063 PMID:36135421

Piekarski, W., & Thomas, B. (2002). ARQuake: The outdoor augmented reality gaming system. *Communications of the ACM*, *45*(1), 36–38. https://dl.acm.org/doi/10.1145/502269.502291. doi:10.1145/502269.502291

Pinar, M. (2018). Multidimensional Well-Being and Inequality Across the European Regions with Alternative Interactions Between the Well-Being Dimensions. *Social Indicators Research*, *144*(1), 31–72. doi:10.1007/s11205-018-2047-4

Pingxuan, R. (2020). AR 3D Magic Book: A Healthy Interactive Reading Device Based on AR and Portable Projection. *CIPAE 2020: Proceedings of the 2020 International Conference on Computers, Information Processing and Advanced Education*. ACM. 10.1145/3419635.3419714

Pizzoli, S. F. M., Mazzocco, K., Triberti, S., Monzani, D., Alcañiz Raya, M. L., & Pravettoni, G. (2019). User-centered virtual reality for promoting relaxation: An innovative approach. *Frontiers in Psychology*, *10*, 479. doi:10.3389/fpsyg.2019.00479 PMID:30914996

Pliatsikas, C. (2020). Understanding structural plasticity in the bilingual brain: The Dynamic Restructuring Model. *Bilingualism: Language and Cognition*, *23*(2), 459–471. doi:10.1017/S1366728919000130

Pons, P., Navas-Medrano, S., & Soler-Domínguez, J. L. (2022). Extended reality for mental health: Current trends and future challenges. *Frontiers of Computer Science*, *4*, 1034307. Advance online publication. doi:10.3389/fcomp.2022.1034307

Portman, M. E., Natapov, A., & Fisher-Gewirtzman, D. (2015). To go where no man has gone before: Virtual reality in architecture, landscape architecture and environmental planning. *Computers, Environment and Urban Systems*, *54*, 376–384.

Portz, J. D., Ford, K. L., Doyon, K., Bekelman, D. B., Boxer, R. S., Kutner, J. S., Czaja, S., & Bull, S. (2020). Using grounded theory to inform the human-centered design of digital health in geriatric palliative care. *Journal of Pain and Symptom Management*, *60*(6), 1181–1192. doi:10.1016/j.jpainsymman.2020.06.027 PMID:32615298

Pourmand, A., Davis, S., Lee, D., Barber, S., & Sikka, N. (2017). Emerging Utility of Virtual Reality as a Multidisciplinary Tool in Clinical Medicine. *Games for Health Journal*, *6*(5), 263–270. doi:10.1089/g4h.2017.0046 PMID:28759254

Proctor, C. (2014). Subjective Well-Being (SWB). Springer eBooks. doi:10.1007/978-94-007-0753-5_2905

Qazi, A., Hardaker, G., Ahmad, I. S., Darwich, M., Maitama, J. Z., & Dayani, A. (2021). The Role of Information & Communication Technology in Elearning Environments: A Systematic Review. *IEEE Access : Practical Innovations, Open Solutions*, 9, 45539–45551. doi:10.1109/ACCESS.2021.3067042

Qin, J., Chui, Y. P., Pang, W. M., Choi, K. S., & Heng, P. A. (2009). Learning blood management in orthopedic surgery through gameplay. *IEEE Computer Graphics and Applications*, *30*(2), 45–57. PMID:20650710

Qiu, R., Gu, Y., Xie, C., Wang, Y., Sheng, Y., Zhu, J., Yue, Y., & Cao, J. (2022). Virtual reality-based targeted cognitive training program for Chinese older adults: A feasibility study. *Geriatric Nursing*, *47*, 35–41. doi:10.1016/j.gerinurse.2022.06.007 PMID:35839753

Quintero, L. (2019). *Facilitating Technology-based Mental Health Interventions with Mobile Virtual Reality and Wearable Smartwatches* [Doctoral dissertation, Department of Computer and Systems Sciences, Stockholm University].

Radenkovic, D., Zhavoronkov, A., & Bischof, E. (2021). AI in Longevity Medicine. In *Artificial Intelligence in Medicine* (pp. 1–13). Springer International Publishing. doi:10.1007/978-3-030-58080-3_248-1

Ragno, L., Borboni, A., Vannetti, F., Amici, C., & Cusano, N. (2023). Application of Social Robots in Healthcare: Review on Characteristics, Requirements, Technical Solutions. *Sensors (Basel)*, *23*(15), 6820. doi:10.3390/s23156820 PMID:37571603

Raja, M., & Priya, G. L. (2023). The role of augmented reality and virtual reality in smart health education: State of the art and perspectives. *Artificial intelligence for smart healthcare*, 311-325.

Rajkumar, E., Gopi, A., Joshi, A. C., Thomas, A. E., Arunima, N. M., Ramya, G. S., Kulkarni, P., Rahul, P., George, A. J., John, R., & Abraham, J. (2023). Applications, benefits and challenges of telehealth in India during COVID-19 pandemic and beyond a systematic review. *BMC Health Services Research*, *23*(1), 7. doi:10.1186/s12913-022-08970-8 PMID:36597088

Raju, N., & Anita, H. B. (2017). Text extraction from video images. *International Journal of Applied Engineering Research: IJAER*, *12*(24), 14750–14754.

Ramasamy, J., Doshi, R., & Hiran, K. K. (2021, August). Segmentation of brain tumor using deep learning methods: a review. In *Proceedings of the International Conference on Data Science, Machine Learning and Artificial Intelligence* (pp. 209-215). Academic Press.

Ramasamy, J., & Doshi, R. (2022). Machine learning in cyber physical systems for healthcare: brain tumor classification from MRI using transfer learning framework. In *Real-Time Applications of Machine Learning in Cyber-Physical Systems* (pp. 65–76). IGI global.

Ramasamy, J., Doshi, R., & Hiran, K. K. (2021, August). Segmentation of brain tumor using deep learning methods: a review. In *Proceedings of the International Conference on Data Science, Machine Learning and Artificial Intelligence* (pp. 209-215). ACM. 10.1145/3484824.3484876

Ramasamy, J., Doshi, R., & Hiran, K. K. (2022, October). Detection of Brain Tumor in Medical Images Based on Feature Extraction by HOG and Machine Learning Algorithms. In *2022 International Conference on Trends in Quantum Computing and Emerging Business Technologies (TQCEBT)* (pp. 1-5). IEEE. 10.1109/TQCEBT54229.2022.10041564

Ramezani, M., & Mohd Ripin, Z. (2023). 4D printing in biomedical engineering: Advancements, challenges, and future directions. *Journal of Functional Biomaterials*, *14*(7), 347. doi:10.3390/jfb14070347 PMID:37504842

Randel, J. M., Morris, B. A., Wetzel, C. D., & Whitehill, B. V. (1992). The effectiveness of games for educational purposes: A review of recent research. *Simulation & Gaming*, *23*(3), 261–276. doi:10.1177/1046878192233001

Rasa, T., & Laherto, A. (2022). Young people's technological images of the future: Implications for science and technology education. *European Journal of Futures Research*, *10*(1), 4. doi:10.1186/s40309-022-00190-x

Rasheed, A., San, O., & Kvamsdal, T. (2020). Digital twin: Values, challenges and enablers from a modeling perspective. *IEEE Access : Practical Innovations, Open Solutions*, *8*, 21980–22012. doi:10.1109/ACCESS.2020.2970143

Ratcliffe, J., Soave, F., Bryan-Kinns, N., Tokarchuk, L., & Farkhatdinov, I. (2021, May). Extended reality (XR) remote research: a survey of drawbacks and opportunities. In *Proceedings of the 2021 CHI Conference on Human Factors in Computing Systems* (pp. 1-13). IEEE. 10.1145/3411764.3445170

Rathi, S., Hiran, K. K., & Sakhare, S. (2023). Affective state prediction of E-learner using SS-ROA based deep LSTM. *Array (New York, N.Y.)*, *19*, 100315. doi:10.1016/j.array.2023.100315

Rawlins, C. R., Veigulis, Z. P., Hebert, C. A., Curtin, C., & Osborne, T. F. (2021). Effect of immersive virtual reality on pain and anxiety at a Veterans Affairs health care facility. *Frontiers in Virtual Reality*, *2*, 719681. doi:10.3389/frvir.2021.719681

Ray, J., Kumar, S., Pandey, S., & Akram, S. V. (2023, June). The Role of Augmented Reality and Virtual Reality in Shaping the Future of Health Psychology. In *2023 3rd International Conference on Pervasive Computing and Social Networking (ICPCSN)* (pp. 1604-1608). IEEE. 10.1109/ICPCSN58827.2023.00268

Reason, J. (2000). Human error: Models and management. *BMJ (Clinical Research Ed.)*, *320*(7237), 768–770. doi:10.1136/bmj.320.7237.768 PMID:10720363

Reger, G. M. (Ed.). (2020). *Technology and mental health: a clinician's guide to improving outcomes*. Routledge. doi:10.4324/9780429020537

Richards, M., & Ford, N. (2020). *Fundamentals of Software Architecture: An Engineering Approach*. O'Reilly Media.

Riches, S., Jeyarajaguru, P., Taylor, L., Fialho, C., Little, J. R., Ahmed, L., O'Brien, A., Van Driel, C., Veling, W., & Valmaggia, L. (2023). Virtual reality relaxation for people with mental health conditions: A systematic review. *Social Psychiatry and Psychiatric Epidemiology*, *58*(7), 989–1007. doi:10.1007/s00127-022-02417-5 PMID:36658261

Richir, S., Kadri, A., & Ribeyre, N. (2022). Virtual Reality and Augmented Reality to Fight Effectively against Pandemics. In *The Nature of Pandemics* (pp. 311–348). CRC Press. doi:10.4324/9781315170220-20

Riegler, A., Riener, A., & Holzmann, C. (2021). A Systematic Review of Virtual Reality Applications for Automated Driving: 2009–2020. *Frontiers in Human Dynamics*, *3*, 689856. doi:10.3389/fhumd.2021.689856

Riener, R., &Harders, M. (2012). *VR for Medical Training*, 181-210. Springer. . doi:10.1007/978-1-4471-4011-5_8

Rimer, E., Husby, L. V., & Solem, S. (2021). Virtual Reality Exposure Therapy for Fear of Heights: Clinicians' attitudes become more positive after trying VRET. *Frontiers in Psychology*, *12*, 671871. doi:10.3389/fpsyg.2021.671871 PMID:34335386

Riva, G., & Serino, S. (2020). Virtual reality in the assessment, understanding and treatment of mental health disorders. In Journal of Clinical Medicine, 9(11). MDPI. doi:10.3390/jcm9113434

Riva, G. (2011). The key to unlocking the virtual body: Virtual reality in the treatment of obesity and eating disorders. *Journal of Diabetes Science and Technology*, *5*(2), 283–292. doi:10.1177/193229681100500213 PMID:21527095

Riva, G., Di Lernia, D., Sajno, E., Sansoni, M., Bartolotta, S., Serino, S., Gaggioli, A., & Wiederhold, B. K. (2021). Virtual Reality Therapy in the Metaverse: Merging VR for the Outside with VR for the Inside. *Annual Review of Cybertherapy and Telemedicine*, 19.

Riva, G., Malighetti, C., & Serino, S. (2021). Virtual reality in the treatment of eating disorders. *Clinical Psychology & Psychotherapy, 28*(3), 477–488. doi:10.1002/cpp.2622 PMID:34048622

Rivero-Moreno, Y., Echevarria, S., Vidal-Valderrama, C., Stefano-Pianetti, L., Cordova-Guilarte, J., Navarro-Gonzalez, J., & Avila, G. L. D. (2023). Robotic Surgery: A Comprehensive Review of the Literature and Current Trends. *Cureus, 15*(7). doi:10.7759/cureus.42370 PMID:37621804

Rizzo, A. A., Hartholt, A., Rothbaum, B. O., Difede, J., Reist, C., Kwok, D., . . . Buckwalter, J. G. (2014, January). Expansion of a VR Exposure Therapy System for Combat-Related PTSD to Medics/Corpsman and Persons Following Military Sexual Trauma. In MMVR (pp. 332-338).

Rizzo, A., Goodwin, G. J., De Vito, A. N., & Bell, J. D. (2021b). Recent advances in virtual reality and psychology: Introduction to the special issue. *Translational Issues in Psychological Science, 7*(3), 213–217. doi:10.1037/tps0000316

Robb, R. A. (1997). Virtual endoscopy: evaluation using the visible human datasets and comparison with real endoscopy in patients. In *Medicine Meets Virtual Reality* (pp. 195–206). IOS Press.

Rodríguez, A., Rey, B., Clemente, M., Wrzesien, M., & Alcañiz, M. (2015). Assessing brain activations associated with emotional regulation during virtual reality mood induction procedures. *Expert Systems with Applications, 42*(3), 1699–1709. doi:10.1016/j.eswa.2014.10.006

Rodziewicz, T. L., Houseman, B., & Hipskind, J. E. (2018). *Medical error reduction and prevention.*

Ronaghi, M. H. (2022). The effect of virtual reality technology and education on sustainable behaviour: A comparative quasi-experimental study. *Interactive Technology and Smart Education.* doi:10.1108/ITSE-02-2022-0025

Roopa, D., Prabha, R., & Senthil, G. A. (2021). Revolutionizing education system with interactive augmented reality for quality education. *Materials Today: Proceedings, 46*(9), 3860–3863. doi:10.1016/j.matpr.2021.02.294

Rosenbaum, D. A., Carlson, R. A., & Gilmore, R. O. (2001). Acquisition of intellectual and perceptual-motor skills. *Annual Review of Psychology, 52*(1), 453–470. doi:10.1146/annurev.psych.52.1.453 PMID:11148313

Roth, C. B., Papassotiropoulos, A., Brühl, A. B., Lang, U. E., & Huber, C. G. (2021). Psychiatry in the digital age: A blessing or a curse? In International Journal of Environmental Research and Public Health, 18(16). MDPI AG. doi:10.3390/ijerph18168302

Rothbaum, B. O., Rizzo, A. S., & Difede, J. (2010). Virtual reality exposure therapy for combat-related posttraumatic stress disorder. *Annals of the New York Academy of Sciences, 1208*(1), 126–132. doi:10.1111/j.1749-6632.2010.05691.x PMID:20955334

Rousseaux, F., Bicego, A., Ledoux, D., Massion, P., Nyssen, A.-S., Faymonville, M.-E., Laureys, S., & Vanhaudenhuyse, A. (2020). Hypnosis Associated with 3D Immersive Virtual Reality Technology in the Management of Pain: A Review of the Literature</p>. *Journal of Pain Research, 13*, 1129–1138. doi:10.2147/JPR.S231737 PMID:32547176

Rubi, J., & Dhivya, A. J. A. (2022). Wearable Health Monitoring Systems Using IoMT. The *Internet of Medical Things (IoMT),* 225–246. doi:10.1002/9781119769200.ch12

Rubi, J., A., V., Kanna, K. R., & G., U. (2023). Bringing Intelligence to Medical Devices Through Artificial Intelligence. Recent Advancements in Smart Remote Patient Monitoring. *Wearable Devices, and Diagnostics Systems,* 154–168. doi:10.4018/978-1-6684-6434-2.ch007

Ruggeri, K., García-Garzón, E., Maguire, Á., Matz, S., & Huppert, F. A. (2020). Well-being is more than happiness and life satisfaction: A multidimensional analysis of 21 countries. *Health and Quality of Life Outcomes, 18*(1), 192. doi:10.1186/s12955-020-01423-y PMID:32560725

Russell, T., & Arcuri, S. M. (2015). A Neurophysiological and neuropsychological consideration of mindful movement: Clinical and research implications. *Frontiers in Human Neuroscience, 9*. doi:10.3389/fnhum.2015.00282 PMID:26074800

Sahoo, S. K., & Goswami, S. S. (2023). A comprehensive review of multiple criteria decision-making (MCDM) Methods: Advancements, applications, and future directions. *Decision Making Advances, 1*(1), 25–48. doi:10.31181/dma1120237

Sailer, M., Hense, J. U., Mayr, S. K., & Mandl, H. (2017). How gamification motivates: An experimental study of the effects of specific game design elements on psychological need satisfaction. *Computers in Human Behavior, 69*, 371–380. doi:10.1016/j.chb.2016.12.033

Sailer, M., Murböck, J., & Fischer, F. (2021). Digital learning in schools: What does it take beyond digital technology? *Teaching and Teacher Education, 103*, 103346. doi:10.1016/j.tate.2021.103346

Saini, G. K., Haseeb, S. B., Taghi-Zada, Z., & Ng, J. Y. (2021). The effects of meditation on individuals facing loneliness: A scoping review. *BMC Psychology, 9*(1), 88. doi:10.1186/s40359-021-00585-8 PMID:34022961

Sakaki, K., Nouchi, R., Matsuzaki, Y., Saito, T., Dinet, J., & Kawashima, R. (2021). Benefits of VR Physical Exercise on Cognition in Older Adults with and without Mild Cognitive Decline: A Systematic Review of Randomized Controlled Trials. *Health Care, 9*(7), 883. doi:10.3390/healthcare9070883 PMID:34356259

Salina, T. (2023). A Review of Augmented Reality for Informal Science Learning: Supporting Design of Intergenerational Group Learning. *Visitor Studies, 26*(1), 1–23. doi:10.1080/10645578.2022.2075205

SalmanG.ShanwarB.ZarkaN. (2016). *Multiscale edge-based text extraction from complex images*. doi:10.13140/RG.2.1.1197.7200

Santos, F., Marques, A., Martins, J., & Silva, P. (2016). Serious games in health professions education: A systematic review. *International Journal of Nursing Education Scholarship, 13*(1), 115–123.

Sarangi, S., & Sharma, P. (2018). *Artificial intelligence: evolution, ethics and public policy*. Taylor & Francis. doi:10.4324/9780429461002

Saredakis, D., Szpak, A., Birckhead, B., Keage, H. A., Rizzo, A., & Loetscher, T. (2020). Factors Associated with Virtual Reality Sickness in Head-Mounted Displays: A Systematic Review and Meta-Analysis. *Frontiers in Human Neuroscience, 14*, 96. doi:10.3389/fnhum.2020.00096 PMID:32300295

Satava, R. M., & Jones, S. B. (1997). Virtual environments for medical training and education. *Presence (Cambridge, Mass.), 6*(2), 139–146. doi:10.1162/pres.1997.6.2.139

Scanlon, E., Anastopoulou, S., Conole, G., & Twiner, A. (2019). Interdisciplinary working methods: Reflections based on Technology-Enhanced Learning (TEL). *Frontiers in Education, 4*, 134. doi:10.3389/feduc.2019.00134

Scavarelli, A., Arya, A., & Teather, R. J. (2020). Virtual reality and augmented reality in social learning spaces: A literature review. *Virtual Reality (Waltham Cross), 25*(1), 257–277. doi:10.1007/s10055-020-00444-8

Schleich, B., Anwer, N., Mathieu, L., & Wartzack, S. (2017). Shaping the digital twin for design and production engineering. *CIRP Annals, 66*(1), 141–144. doi:10.1016/j.cirp.2017.04.040

Schluse, M., Priggemeyer, M., Atorf, L., & Rossmann, J. (2018). Experimentable digital twins-streamlining simulation-based systems engineering for industry 4.0. *IEEE Transactions on Industrial Informatics, 14*(4), 1722–1731. doi:10.1109/TII.2018.2804917

Schneider, E. F., Lang, A., Shin, M., Bradley, S. D., & Li, P. P. (2004). Virtual patient simulation for medical education: A review. *Studies in Health Technology and Informatics, 98*, 263–269.

Schönmann, M., Bodenschatz, A., Uhl, M., & Walkowitz, G. (2023). The Care-Dependent are Less Averse to Care Robots: An Empirical Comparison of Attitudes. *International Journal of Social Robotics, 15*(6), 1–18. doi:10.1007/s12369-023-01003-2 PMID:37359432

Schröder, D., Wrona, K. J., Müller, F., Heinemann, S., Fischer, F., & Dockweiler, C. (2023). Impact of virtual reality applications in the treatment of anxiety disorders: A systematic review and meta-analysis of randomized-controlled trials. In *Journal of Behavior Therapy and Experimental Psychiatry* (Vol. 81). Elsevier Ltd., doi:10.1016/j.jbtep.2023.101893

Scurati, G. W., Bertoni, M., Graziosi, S., & Ferrise, F. (2021). Exploring the use of virtual reality to support environmentally sustainable behaviour: A framework to design experiences. *Sustainability (Basel), 13*(2), 943. doi:10.3390/su13020943

Segawa, T., Baudry, T., Bourla, A., Blanc, J., Peretti, C., Mouchabac, S., & Ferreri, F. (2020). Virtual Reality (VR) in Assessment and Treatment of Addictive Disorders: A Systematic review. *Frontiers in Neuroscience, 13*, 1409. doi:10.3389/fnins.2019.01409 PMID:31998066

Seng, K. P., Ang, L. M., Peter, E., & Mmonyi, A. (2023). Machine Learning and AI Technologies for Smart Wearables. *Electronics (Basel), 12*(7), 1509. doi:10.3390/electronics12071509

Shaikh, T. A., Dar, T. R., & Sofi, S. (2022). A data-centric artificial intelligent and extended reality technology in smart healthcare systems. *Social Network Analysis and Mining, 12*(1), 122. doi:10.1007/s13278-022-00888-7 PMID:36065420

Shakeel, T., Habib, S., Boulila, W., Koubaa, A., Javed, A. R., Rizwan, M., Gadekallu, T. R., & Sufiyan, M. (2023). A survey on COVID-19 impact in the healthcare domain: Worldwide market implementation, applications, security and privacy issues, challenges and future prospects. *Complex & Intelligent Systems, 9*(1), 1027–1058. doi:10.1007/s40747-022-00767-w PMID:35668731

Shammar, E. A., & Zahary, A. T. (2020). The Internet of Things (IoT): A survey of techniques, operating systems, and trends. *Library Hi Tech, 38*(1), 5–66. doi:10.1108/LHT-12-2018-0200

Shao, D., & Lee, I. J. (2020). Acceptance and influencing factors of social virtual reality in the urban elderly. *Sustainability (Basel), 12*(22), 9345. doi:10.3390/su12229345

Sharma, A., & Singh, B. (2022). Measuring Impact of E-commerce on Small Scale Business: A Systematic Review. *Journal of Corporate Governance and International Business Law, 5*(1).

Sharma, M., & Rush, S. E. (2014). Mindfulness-based stress reduction as a stress management intervention for healthy individuals. *Journal of Evidence-Based Complementary & Alternative Medicine, 19*(4), 271–286. doi:10.1177/2156587214543143 PMID:25053754

Sharma, P., & Harkishan, M. (2022). Designing an intelligent tutoring system for computer programing in the Pacific. *Education and Information Technologies, 27*(5), 6197–6209. doi:10.1007/s10639-021-10882-9 PMID:35002465

Sheikh, Y., Ali, A., Khasati, A., Hasanic, A., Bihani, U., Ohri, R., Muthukumar, K., & Barlow, J. (2023). Benefits and Challenges of Video Consulting for Mental Health Diagnosis and Follow-Up: A Qualitative Study in Community Care. *International Journal of Environmental Research and Public Health, 20*(3), 2595. doi:10.3390/ijerph20032595 PMID:36767957

Shrivas, M. K., Hiran, K. K., Bhansali, A., & Doshi, R. (Eds.). (2022). *Advancements in Quantum Blockchain with Real-time Applications.* IGI global. doi:10.4018/978-1-6684-5072-7

Siani, A., & Marley, S. A. (2021). Impact of the recreational use of virtual reality on physical and mental well-being during the COVID-19 lockdown. *Health and Technology, 11*(2), 425–435. doi:10.1007/s12553-021-00528-8 PMID:33614391

Simons, G., & Baldwin, D. S. (2021). A critical review of the definition of 'well-being' for doctors and their patients in a post-COVID-19 era. *The International Journal of Social Psychiatry*, *67*(8), 984–991. doi:10.1177/00207640211032259 PMID:34240644

Singh, B. (2023). Blockchain Technology in Renovating Healthcare: Legal and Future Perspectives. In Revolutionizing Healthcare Through Artificial Intelligence and Internet of Things Applications (pp. 177-186). IGI Global.

Singh, G., Kataria, A., Jangra, S., Dutta, R., Mantri, A., Sandhu, J. K., & Sabapathy, T. (2023). Augmented Reality and Virtual Reality: Transforming the Future of Psychological and Medical Sciences. In Smart Distributed Embedded Systems for Healthcare Applications (pp. 93-118). CRC Press.

Singh, B. (2020). GLOBAL SCIENCE AND JURISPRUDENTIAL APPROACH CONCERNING HEALTHCARE AND ILLNESS. *Indian Journal of Health and Medical Law*, *3*(1), 7–13.

Singh, B. (2022). COVID-19 Pandemic and Public Healthcare: Endless Downward Spiral or Solution via Rapid Legal and Health Services Implementation with Patient Monitoring Program. *Justice and Law Bulletin*, *1*(1), 1–7.

Singh, B. (2022). Relevance of Agriculture-Nutrition Linkage for Human Healthcare: A Conceptual Legal Framework of Implication and Pathways. *Justice and Law Bulletin*, *1*(1), 44–49.

Singh, B. (2022). Understanding Legal Frameworks Concerning Transgender Healthcare in the Age of Dynamism. *ELECTRONIC JOURNAL OF SOCIAL AND STRATEGIC STUDIES*, *3*(1), 56–65. doi:10.47362/EJSSS.2022.3104

Singh, B. (2023). Federated Learning for Envision Future Trajectory Smart Transport System for Climate Preservation and Smart Green Planet: Insights into Global Governance and SDG-9 (Industry, Innovation and Infrastructure). *National Journal of Environmental Law*, *6*(2), 6–17.

Singh, B. (2023). Tele-Health Monitoring Lensing Deep Neural Learning Structure: Ambient Patient Wellness via Wearable Devices for Real-Time Alerts and Interventions. *Indian Journal of Health and Medical Law*, *6*(2), 12–16.

Singh, B. (2024). Legal Dynamics Lensing Metaverse Crafted for Videogame Industry and E-Sports: Phenomenological Exploration Catalyst Complexity and Future. *Journal of Intellectual Property Rights Law*, *7*(1), 8–14.

Singh, M., Srivastava, R., Fuenmayor, E., Kuts, V., Qiao, Y., Murray, N., & Devine, D. (2022). Applications of Digital Twin across industries: A review. *Applied Sciences (Basel, Switzerland)*, *12*(11), 5727. doi:10.3390/app12115727

Skouby, K. E., Dhotre, P., Williams, I., & Hiran, K. (Eds.). (2022). *5G, Cybersecurity and Privacy in Developing Countries*. CRC Press. doi:10.1201/9781003374664

Small, S. D., Wuerz, R. C., Simon, R., Shapiro, N., Conn, A., & Setnik, G. (1999). Demonstration of high-fidelity simulation team training for emergency medicine. *Academic Emergency Medicine*, *6*(4), 312–323. doi:10.1111/j.1553-2712.1999.tb00395.x PMID:10230983

Sommerauer, P., & Müller, O. (2014). Augmented Reality in Informal Learning Environments: A Field Experiment in a Mathematics Exhibition. *Computers & Education*, *79*, 59–68. doi:10.1016/j.compedu.2014.07.013

Song, G., & Park, E. (2015). Effect of virtual reality games on stroke patients' balance, gait, depression, and interpersonal relationships. *Journal of Physical Therapy Science*, *27*(7), 2057–2060. doi:10.1589/jpts.27.2057 PMID:26311925

Sow, D., Imoussaten, A., Couturier, P., & Montmain, J. (2017). A Possibilistic Approach to Set Achievable and Feasible Goals while Designing Complex Systems. *IFAC-PapersOnLine*, *50*(1), 14218–14223. doi:10.1016/j.ifacol.2017.08.2094

Spargo, M., Goodfellow, N., Scullin, C., Grigoleit, S., Andreou, A., Mavromoustakis, C. X., Guerra, B., Manso, M., Larburu, N., Villacañas, Ó., Fleming, G., & Scott, M. (2021). Shaping the future of digitally enabled health and care. *Pharmacy (Basel, Switzerland)*, *9*(1), 17. doi:10.3390/pharmacy9010017 PMID:33445509

Spinti, J. P., Smith, P. J., & Smith, S. T. (2022). Atikokan digital twin: Machine learning in a biomass energy system. *Applied Energy*, *310*, 118436. doi:10.1016/j.apenergy.2021.118436

Sridhar, S. (2023). *OPPO MR Glass Developer Edition*. Fone Arena. https://www.fonearena.com/blog/394919/oppo-mr-glass-developer-edition-features.html

Srinivasulu, A. (2022). Omi-cron Virus Data Analytics Using Extended RNN Technique. *Int J Cancer Res Ther, 7*(3).

Srinivasulu, A., Gupta, A. K., Hiran, K. K., Barua, T., & Sreenivasulu, G. (2022). Omi-cron Virus Data Analytics Using Extended RNN Technique. *Int J Cancer Res Ther, 7*(3), 122, 129, 1-3.

Srinivasulu, A., Gupta, A. K., Hiran, K. K., Barua, T., & Sreenivasulu, G. (2022). Omi-cron Virus Data Analytics Using Extended RNN Technique. *Int J Cancer Res Ther, 7*(3), 1-3.

Srinivasulu, A., Gupta, A., Hiran, K., Barua, and T., & Sreenivasulu, G. Omi-cron Virus Data Analytics Using Extended RNN Technique. *Int J Cancer Res Ther, 7*(3), 122.

Srinivasulu, A., Gupta, A., Hiran, K., Barua, T., Sreenivasulu, G. (2022). Omi-cron Virus Data Analytics Using Extended RNN Technique. *Int J Cancer Res Ther, 7*(3), 122.

Srinivasulu, A.A., Gupta, A., Hiran, K., Barua, T., & Sreenivasulu, G. (2022). Omi-cron Virus Data Analytics Using Extended RNN Technique. *Int J Cancer Res Ther, 7*(3), *122* 1-3.

Stahl, S. T., Emanuel, J., Albert, S. M., Dew, M. A., Schulz, R., Robbins-Welty, G., & Reynolds, C. F. III. (2017). Design and rationale for a technology-based healthy lifestyle intervention in older adults grieving the loss of a spouse. *Contemporary Clinical Trials Communications*, *8*, 99–105. doi:10.1016/j.conctc.2017.09.002 PMID:29170758

Stasevych, M., & Zvarych, V. (2023). Innovative robotic technologies and artificial intelligence in pharmacy and medicine: Paving the way for the future of health care—a review. *Big Data and Cognitive Computing*, *7*(3), 147. doi:10.3390/bdcc7030147

Stewart, T. H., Villaneuva, K., Hahn, A., Ortiz-Delatorre, J., Wolf, C., Nguyen, R., Bolter, N. D., Kern, M., & Bagley, J. R. (2022). Actual vs. perceived exertion during active virtual reality game exercise. *Frontiers in Rehabilitation Sciences*, *3*, 887740. doi:10.3389/fresc.2022.887740 PMID:36189005

Stocchi, L., Pourazad, N., Michaelidou, N., Tanusondjaja, A., & Harrigan, P. (2022). Marketing research on Mobile apps: Past, present and future. *Journal of the Academy of Marketing Science*, *50*(2), 195–225. doi:10.1007/s11747-021-00815-w PMID:34776554

Stratou, G., & Morency, L. P. (2017). MultiSense—Context-aware nonverbal behavior analysis framework: A psychological distress use case. *IEEE Transactions on Affective Computing*, *8*(2), 190–203.

Stytz, M. R., Garcia, B. W., Godsell-Stytz, G. M., & Banks, S. B. (1997). A distributed virtual environment prototype for emergency medical procedures training. In *Medicine Meets Virtual Reality* (pp. 473–485). IOS Press.

Sun, J., Dong, Q. X., Wang, S. W., Zheng, Y. B., Liu, X. X., Lu, T. S., Yuan, K., Shi, J., Hu, B., Lu, L., & Han, Y. (2023). Artificial intelligence in psychiatry research, diagnosis, and therapy. *Asian Journal of Psychiatry*, *87*, 103705. doi:10.1016/j.ajp.2023.103705 PMID:37506575

Sun, T., He, X., & Li, Z. (2023). Digital twin in healthcare: Recent updates and challenges. *Digital Health*, *9*. doi:10.1177/20552076221149651 PMID:36636729

Sutherland, J., Bélec, J., Sheikh, A., Chepelev, L. L., Althobaity, W., Chow, B. J., Mitsouras, D., Christensen, A., Rybicki, F. J., & La Russa, D. (2018). Applying modern virtual and augmented reality technologies to medical images and models. *Journal of Digital Imaging*, *32*(1), 38–53. doi:10.1007/s10278-018-0122-7 PMID:30215180

Szymkowiak, A., Melović, B., Dabić, M., Jeganathan, K., & Kundi, G. S. (2021). Information technology and Gen Z: The role of teachers, the internet, and technology in the education of young people. *Technology in Society*, *65*, 101565. doi:10.1016/j.techsoc.2021.101565

Taghian, A., Abo-Zahhad, M., Sayed, M. S., & Abdel-Malek, A. (2021, December). Virtual, Augmented Reality, and Wearable Devices for Biomedical Applications: A Review. In *2021 9th International Japan-Africa Conference on Electronics, Communications, and Computations (JAC-ECC)* (pp. 93-98). IEEE.

Takac, M., Collett, J., Conduit, R., & De Foe, A. (2021). A cognitive model for emotional regulation in virtual reality exposure. *Virtual Reality (Waltham Cross)*, *27*(1), 159–172. doi:10.1007/s10055-021-00531-4

Talbot, T. B., Sagae, K., John, B., & Rizzo, A. A. (2012). Sorting out the virtual patient: How to exploit artificial intelligence, game technology and sound educational practices to create engaging role-playing simulations. [IJGCMS]. *International Journal of Gaming and Computer-Mediated Simulations*, *4*(3), 1–19.

Talukder, M. S., Laato, S., Islam, A. N., & Bao, Y. (2021). Continued use intention of wearable health technologies among the elderly: An enablers and inhibitors perspective. *Internet Research*, *31*(5), 1611–1640. doi:10.1108/INTR-10-2020-0586

Tang, L., Li, J., & Fantus, S. (2023). Medical artificial intelligence ethics: A systematic review of empirical studies. *Digital Health*, *9*, 20552076231186064. doi:10.1177/20552076231186064 PMID:37434728

Tang, V., Choy, K. L., Ho, G. T., Lam, H. Y., & Tsang, Y. P. (2019). An IoMT-based geriatric care management system for achieving smart health in nursing homes. *Industrial Management & Data Systems*, *119*(8), 1819–1840. doi:10.1108/IMDS-01-2019-0024

Tang, Y. M., Chau, K. Y., Kwok, A. P. K., Zhu, T., & Ma, X. (2022). A systematic review of immersive technology applications for medical practice and education-Trends, application areas, recipients, teaching contents, evaluation methods, and performance. *Educational Research Review*, *35*, 100429. doi:10.1016/j.edurev.2021.100429

Tao, F., Cheng, J., Qi, Q., Zhang, M., Zhang, H., & Sui, F. (2018). Digital twin-driven product design, manufacturing and service with big data. *International Journal of Advanced Manufacturing Technology*, *94*(9–12), 3563–3576. doi:10.1007/s00170-017-0233-1

Tao, F., Zhang, H., Liu, A., & Nee, A. Y. C. (2019). Digital twin in industry: State-of-the-art. *IEEE Transactions on Industrial Informatics*, *15*(4), 2405–2415. doi:10.1109/TII.2018.2873186

Tao, G., Garrett, B., Taverner, T., Cordingley, E., & Sun, C. (2021). Immersive virtual reality health games: A narrative review of game design. *Journal of Neuroengineering and Rehabilitation*, *18*(1), 31. doi:10.1186/s12984-020-00801-3 PMID:33573684

Tarrant, J., Viczko, J., & Cope, H. (2018). Virtual reality for anxiety Reduction Demonstrated by Quantitative EEG: A pilot study. *Frontiers in Psychology*, *9*, 1280. doi:10.3389/fpsyg.2018.01280 PMID:30087642

Tay, J. L., Xie, H., & Sim, K. (2023). Effectiveness of Augmented and Virtual Reality-Based Interventions in Improving Knowledge, Attitudes, Empathy and Stigma Regarding People with Mental Illnesses—A Scoping Review. In Journal of Personalized Medicine, 13(1). MDPI. doi:10.3390/jpm13010112

Teniou, G. (2019). 3GPP achievements on VR & ongoing developments on XR over 5G. In *Proc. 3GPP/VRIF/AIS 2nd Workshop VR Ecosyst. Standards, Immersive Media Meets*. IEEE.

Tezer, M., Yıldız, E. P., Masalimova, A. R. R., Fatkhutdinova, A. M., Zheltukhina, M. R. R., & Khairullina, E. R. (2019). Trends of Augmented Reality Applications and Research throughout the World: Meta-Analysis of Theses, Articles and Papers between 2001-2019 Years. *International Journal of Emerging Technologies in Learning, 14*(22), 154–174. doi:10.3991/ijet.v14i22.11768

Than, N. N. (2023). *Journey to Wellbeing: Seeing Beyond the Mind's Eye Through Story in a Virtual Therapeutic Space* [Doctoral dissertation, New York University Tandon School of Engineering].

Thiermann, U. B., & Sheate, W. R. (2020). The Way Forward in Mindfulness and Sustainability: A Critical Review and Research Agenda. *Journal of Cognitive Enhancement: Towards the Integration of Theory and Practice, 5*(1), 118–139. doi:10.1007/s41465-020-00180-6

Thilagavathy, A., Aarthi, K., & Chilambuchelvan, A. (2012). Text detection and extraction from videos using ann based network. *International Journal on Soft Computing Artificial Intelligence and Applications (Commerce, Calif.), 1*(1).

Thompson, A. H. (2021). A Holistic Approach to Employee Functioning: Assessing the Impact of a Virtual-Reality Mindfulness Intervention at Work. Radovic, A., & Badawy, S. M. (2020). Technology use for adolescent health and wellness. *Pediatrics, 145*(Supplement_2), S186–S194.

Thompson, D., Bhatt, R., Lazarus, M., Cullen, K. W., Baranowski, J., & Baranowski, T. (2007). A serious video game to increase fruit and vegetable consumption among elementary aged youth (Squire's Quest! II): Rationale, design, and methods. *JMIR Research Protocols, 6*(3), e39. PMID:23612366

Tieri, G., Morone, G., Paolucci, S., & Iosa, M. (2018). Virtual reality in cognitive and motor rehabilitation: facts, fiction and fallacies. In Expert Review of Medical Devices, 15(2). Taylor and Francis Ltd. doi:10.1080/17434440.2018.1425613

Tigard, D. W., Braun, M., Breuer, S., Ritt, K., Fiske, A., McLennan, S., & Buyx, A. (2023). Toward best practices in embedded ethics: Suggestions for interdisciplinary technology development. *Robotics and Autonomous Systems, 167*, 104467. doi:10.1016/j.robot.2023.104467

tom Dieck, M. C., Cranmer, E., Prim, A. L., & Bamford, D. (2023b). The effects of augmented reality shopping experiences: immersion, presence and satisfaction. *Journal of Research in Interactive Marketing*. doi:10.1108/JRIM-09-2022-0268

tom Dieck, M. C., Cranmer, E., Prim, A., & Bamford, D. (2023a). Can augmented reality (AR) applications enhance students' experiences? Gratifications, engagement and learning styles. Information Technology & People. doi:10.1108/ITP-10-2021-0823

Too, B. K., & Prabhakar, C. J. (2016). *Extraction of scene text information from video*. Academic Press.

Trahan, M. H., Smith, K. S., & Talbot, T. B. (2019). Past, present, and future: Editorial on virtual reality applications to human services. *Journal of Technology in Human Services, 37*(1), 1–12. doi:10.1080/15228835.2019.1587334

Trappey, A. J., Trappey, C. V., Chang, C., Kuo, R. R. T., Lin, A. P., & Nieh, C. (2020). Virtual Reality Exposure Therapy for Driving Phobia Disorder: System Design and Development. *Applied Sciences (Basel, Switzerland), 10*(14), 4860. doi:10.3390/app10144860

Trymbulak, K., Ding, E., Marino, F., Wang, Z., & Saczynski, J. S. (2020). Mobile health assessments of geriatric elements in older patients with atrial fibrillation: The Mobile SAGE-AF Study (M-SAGE). *Cardiovascular Digital Health Journal, 1*(3), 123–129. doi:10.1016/j.cvdhj.2020.11.002 PMID:35265884

Tsai, M. D., Hsieh, M. S., & Jou, S. B. (2001). Virtual reality orthopedic surgery simulator. *Computers in Biology and Medicine*, *31*(5), 333–351. doi:10.1016/S0010-4825(01)00014-2 PMID:11535200

Tsamitros, N., Beck, A., Sebold, M., Schouler-Ocak, M., Bermpohl, F., & Gutwinski, S. (2023). The application of virtual reality in the treatment of mental disorders. *Der Nervenarzt*, *94*(1), 27–33. doi:10.1007/s00115-022-01378-z PMID:36053303

Tsamitros, N., Sebold, M., Gutwinski, S., & Beck, A. (2021). Virtual Reality-Based Treatment approaches in the field of substance use disorders. *Current Addiction Reports*, *8*(3), 399–407. doi:10.1007/s40429-021-00377-5

Tukhtakhodjaeva, F. S., & Khayitova, I. I. (2023). APPLICATION AND USE OF AI (ARTIFICIAL INTELLIGENCE) IN MEDICINE. *Educational Research in Universal Sciences*, *2*(9), 302–309.

Uhl, J. C., Regal, G., Gafert, M., Murtinger, M., & Tscheligi, M. (2023). Stress embodied: Developing multi-sensory experiences for VR police training. In Lecture Notes in Computer Science (pp. 573–583). Springer. doi:10.1007/978-3-031-42280-5_36

Uhlemann, T. H. J., Lehmann, C., & Steinhilper, R. (2017). The digital twin: Realizing the cyber-physical production system for industry 4.0. *Procedia CIRP*, *61*, 335–340. doi:10.1016/j.procir.2016.11.152

Ujiie, H., Yamaguchi, A., Gregor, A., Chan, H., Kato, T., Hida, Y., Kaga, K., Wakasa, S., Eitel, C., Clapp, T., & Yasufuku, K. (2021). Developing a virtual reality simulation system for preoperative planning of thoracoscopic thoracic surgery. *Journal of Thoracic Disease*, *13*(2), 778–783. doi:10.21037/jtd-20-2197 PMID:33717550

Ullah, M., Hamayun, S., Wahab, A., Khan, S. U., Rehman, M. U., Haq, Z. U., Rehman, K. U., Ullah, A., Mehreen, A., Awan, U. A., Qayum, M., & Naeem, M. (2023). Smart technologies used as smart tools in the management of cardiovascular disease and their future perspective. *Current Problems in Cardiology*, *48*(11), 101922. doi:10.1016/j.cpcardiol.2023.101922 PMID:37437703

Ulrich, E., & Sandor, C. (2013). HARP: A framework for visuo-haptic augmented reality. 2013 IEEE Virtual Reality (VR), (pp. 145-146). IEEE. doi:10.1109/VR.2013.6549404

UNCTAD. (2018). *Creative economy has new impetus in digital world*. UNCTAD. https://unctad.org/news/creative-economy-has-new-impetus-digital-world

Usmani, S. S., Sharath, M., & Mehendale, M. (2022). Future of mental health in the metaverse. *General Psychiatry*, *35*(4), e100825. doi:10.1136/gpsych-2022-100825 PMID:36189180

Vaidyanathan, N., & Henningsson, S. (2023). Designing augmented reality services for enhanced customer experiences in retail. *Journal of Service Management*, *34*(1), 78–99. doi:10.1108/JOSM-01-2022-0004

Vaishya, R., Javaid, M., Khan, I., & Haleem, A. (2020). Artificial Intelligence (AI) applications for COVID-19 pandemic. *Diabetes & Metabolic Syndrome*, *14*(4), 337–339. doi:10.1016/j.dsx.2020.04.012 PMID:32305024

Vaismoradi, M., Turunen, H., & Bondas, T. (2013). Content analysis and thematic analysis: Implications for conducting a qualitative descriptive study. *Nursing & Health Sciences*, *15*(3), 398–405. doi:10.1111/nhs.12048 PMID:23480423

Vallès-Peris, N., & Domènech, M. (2023). Caring in the in-between: A proposal to introduce responsible AI and robotics to healthcare. *AI & Society*, *38*(4), 1685–1695. doi:10.1007/s00146-021-01330-w

Valmaggia, L. R., Latif, L., Kempton, M. J., & Rus-Calafell, M. (2016). Virtual reality in the psychological treatment for mental health problems: An systematic review of recent evidence. *Psychiatry Research*, *236*, 189–195. doi:10.1016/j.psychres.2016.01.015 PMID:26795129

Valverde-Berrocoso, J., Fernández-Sánchez, M. R., Revuelta Dominguez, F. I., & Sosa-Díaz, M. J. (2021). The educational integration of digital technologies preCovid-19: Lessons for teacher education. *PLoS One*, *16*(8), e0256283. doi:10.1371/journal.pone.0256283 PMID:34411161

Van De Ridder, J. M., Stokking, K. M., McGaghie, W. C., & Ten Cate, O. T. J. (2008). What is feedback in clinical education? *Medical Education*, *42*(2), 189–197. doi:10.1111/j.1365-2923.2007.02973.x PMID:18230092

van den Berg, M., Sherrington, C., Killington, M., Smith, S., Bongers, B., Hassett, L., & Crotty, M. (2016). Video and computer-based interactive exercises are safe and improve task-specific balance in geriatric and neurological rehabilitation: A randomised trial. *Journal of Physiotherapy*, *62*(1), 20–28. doi:10.1016/j.jphys.2015.11.005 PMID:26701163

Van Veelen, N., Boonekamp, R., Schoonderwoerd, T., Van Emmerik, M., Nijdam, M. J., Bruinsma, B., Geuze, E., Jones, C., & Vermetten, E. (2021). Tailored Immersion: Implementing personalized components into virtual reality for veterans with Post-Traumatic Stress Disorder. *Frontiers in Virtual Reality*, *2*, 740795. doi:10.3389/frvir.2021.740795

Vaportzis, E., Martin, M., & Gow, A. J. (2017). A tablet for healthy ageing: The effect of a tablet computer training intervention on cognitive abilities in older adults. *The American Journal of Geriatric Psychiatry*, *25*(8), 841–851. doi:10.1016/j.jagp.2016.11.015 PMID:28082016

Vasiliki Bravou, D. O. A. D. (n.d.). *Applications of Virtual Reality for Autism Inclusion. A review Aplicaciones de la realidad virtual para la inclusión del autism. Una revisión.*

Velciu, M., Spiru, L., Dan Marzan, M., Reithner, E., Geli, S., Borgogni, B., Cramariuc, O., Mocanu, I. G., Kołakowski, J., Ayadi, J., Rampioni, M., & Stara, V. (2023). How Technology-Based Interventions Can Sustain Ageing Well in the New Decade through the User-Driven Approach. *Sustainability (Basel)*, *15*(13), 10330. doi:10.3390/su151310330

Ventola, C. L. (2019). Virtual reality in pharmacy: Opportunities for clinical, research, and educational applications. *P&T*, *44*(5), 267. PMID:31080335

Vianez, A., Marques, A., & Almeida, R. (2022). Virtual Reality Exposure Therapy for Armed Forces Veterans with Post-Traumatic Stress Disorder: A Systematic Review and Focus Group. *International Journal of Environmental Research and Public Health*, *19*(1), 464. doi:10.3390/ijerph19010464 PMID:35010723

Vicario, C. M., & Martino, G. (2022). Psychology and technology: how Virtual Reality can boost psychotherapy and neurorehabilitation. In AIMS Neuroscience, 9(4). AIMS Press. doi:10.3934/Neuroscience.2022025

Vicsek, L. (2021). Artificial intelligence and the future of work–lessons from the sociology of expectations. *The International Journal of Sociology and Social Policy*, *41*(7/8), 842–861. doi:10.1108/IJSSP-05-2020-0174

Villa-García, L., Puig, A., Puigpelat, P., Solé-Casals, M., & Fuertes, O. (2022). The development of a platform to ensure an integrated care plan for older adults with complex care needs living at home. *Journal of Integrated Care*, *30*(4), 310–323. doi:10.1108/JICA-01-2022-0010

Villagran-Vizcarra, D. C., Luviano-Cruz, D., Pérez-Domínguez, L. A., Méndez-González, L. C., & Garcia-Luna, F. (2023). Applications Analyses, Challenges and Development of Augmented Reality in Education, Industry, Marketing, Medicine, and Entertainment. *Applied Sciences (Basel, Switzerland)*, *13*(5), 2766. doi:10.3390/app13052766

Voinescu, A., Fodor, L. A., Fraser, D. S., & David, D. (2020). Exploring Attention in VR: Effects of visual and Auditory modalities. In Advances in intelligent systems and computing (pp. 677–683). Springer. doi:10.1007/978-3-030-51828-8_89

Vollmar, A. (2023). *Difference between VR and AR*. Hegias. https://hegias.com/en/knowledge/difference-vr-ar/

Volonté, F., Pugin, F., Bucher, P., Sugimoto, M., Ratib, O., & Morel, P. (2011). Augmented reality and image overlay navigation with OsiriX in laparoscopic and robotic surgery: Not only a matter of fashion. *Journal of Hepato-Biliary-Pancreatic Sciences*, *18*(4), 506–509. doi:10.1007/s00534-011-0385-6 PMID:21487758

Vyas, B. (2019). *Top five use cases of extended reality in the healthcare sector.* Softweb Solutions. https://www.soft-websolutions.com/resources/extended-reality-in-healthcare-sector.html

Wakida, E. K., Talib, Z. M., Akena, D., Okello, E. S., Kinengyere, A., Mindra, A., & Obua, C. (2018). Barriers and facilitators to the integration of mental health services into primary health care: A systematic review. *Systematic Reviews*, *7*(1), 1–13. doi:10.1186/s13643-018-0882-7 PMID:30486900

Waller, M., Mistry, D., Jetly, R., & Frewen, P. A. (2021). Meditating in Virtual Reality 3: 360° video of the perceptual presence of instructor. *Mindfulness*, *12*(6), 1424–1437. doi:10.1007/s12671-021-01612-w PMID:33777253

Wang, K., Guo, F., Zhou, R., & Qian, L. (2023). Implementation of augmented reality in BIM-enabled construction projects: a bibliometric literature review and a case study from China. Construction Innovation. ACM. doi:10.1108/CI-08-2022-0196

Wang, C., Liu, S., Yang, H., Guo, J., Wu, Y., & Liu, J. (2023). Ethical considerations of using ChatGPT in health care. *Journal of Medical Internet Research*, *25*, e48009. doi:10.2196/48009 PMID:37566454

Wang, H., Tlili, A., Huang, R., Cai, Z., Li, M., Cheng, Z., Yang, D., Li, M., Zhu, X., & Fei, C. (2023). Examining the applications of intelligent tutoring systems in real educational contexts: A systematic literature review from the social experiment perspective. *Education and Information Technologies*, *28*(7), 9113–9148. doi:10.1007/s10639-022-11555-x PMID:36643383

Wang, J., & Qi, Y. (2022). A Multi-User Collaborative AR System for Industrial *Applications. Sensors (Basel)*, *22*(4), 1319. doi:10.3390/s22041319 PMID:35214221

Wang, J., Ye, L., Gao, R. X., Li, C., & Zhang, L. (2019). Digital Twin for rotating machinery fault diagnosis in smart manufacturing. *International Journal of Production Research*, *57*(12), 3920–3934. doi:10.1080/00207543.2018.1552032

Wang, S., Lim, S. H., & Aloweni, F. B. A. B. (2022). Virtual reality interventions and the outcome measures of adult patients in acute care settings undergoing surgical procedures: An integrative review. *Journal of Advanced Nursing*, *78*(3), 645–665.

Wechsler, T. F., Mühlberger, A., & Kümpers, F. (2019). Inferiority or even superiority of virtual reality exposure therapy in phobias? - A systematic review and quantitative meta-analysis on randomized controlled trials specifically comparing the efficacy of virtual reality exposure to gold standard in vivo exposure in Agoraphobia, Specific Phobia and Social Phobia. In Frontiers in Psychology, 10. Frontiers Media S.A. doi:10.3389/fpsyg.2019.01758

White, S. M., Wootton, B. M., & Ferguson, M. A. (2015). A game-based exercise platform for children with cerebral palsy: A usability study. *JMIR Serious Games*, *3*(2), e5. PMID:26199045

Wiebe, A., Kannen, K., Selaskowski, B., Mehren, A., Thöne, A. K., Pramme, L., Blumenthal, N., Li, M., Asché, L., Jonas, S., Bey, K., Schulze, M., Steffens, M., Pensel, M. C., Guth, M., Rohlfsen, F., Ekhlas, M., Lügering, H., Fileccia, H., & Braun, N. (2022). Virtual reality in the diagnostic and therapy for mental disorders: A systematic review. In Clinical Psychology Review, 98. doi:10.1016/j.cpr.2022.102213

Wiederhold, M. D., & Wiederhold, B. K. (2007). Virtual Reality and Interactive Simulation for Pain Distraction: Table 1. *Pain Medicine*, *8*(suppl 3), S182–S188. doi:10.1111/j.1526-4637.2007.00381.x

Winstein, C. J., & Requejo, P. S. (2015). Innovative technologies for rehabilitation and health promotion: What is the evidence? *Physical Therapy*, *95*(3), 294–298. doi:10.2522/ptj.2015.95.2.294 PMID:25734191

Wong, K. P., Tse, M. M. Y., & Qin, J. (2022). Effectiveness of Virtual Reality-Based Interventions for Managing Chronic Pain on Pain Reduction, Anxiety, Depression and Mood: A Systematic Review. In Healthcare (Switzerland), 10(10). MDPI. doi:10.3390/healthcare10102047

Woods, J., Greenfield, G., Majeed, A., & Hayhoe, B. (2020). Clinical effectiveness and cost-effectiveness of individual mental health workers colocated within primary care practices: A systematic literature review. *BMJ Open*, *10*(12), e042052. doi:10.1136/bmjopen-2020-042052 PMID:33268432

Wu, Ch., & Thompson, M. E. (2020). *Sampling Theory and Practice*. Springer Nature. doi:10.1007/978-3-030-44246-0

Xie, J., Lan, P., Wang, S., Luo, Y., & Liu, G. (2023). Brain Activation Differences of Six Basic Emotions Between 2D Screen and Virtual Reality Modalities. *IEEE Transactions on Neural Systems and Rehabilitation Engineering*, *31*, 700–709. doi:10.1109/TNSRE.2022.3229389 PMID:37015689

Xiong, J., Hsiang, E. L., He, Z., Zhan, T., & Wu, S. T. (2021). Augmented reality and virtual reality displays: emerging technologies and future perspectives. In Light: Science and Applications, 10(1). Springer Nature. doi:10.1038/s41377-021-00658-8

Xu, X., Mangina, E., & Campbell, A. G. (2021c). HMD-Based Virtual and Augmented Reality in Medical Education: A Systematic Review. *Frontiers in Virtual Reality*, *2*, 692103. doi:10.3389/frvir.2021.692103

Yadav, V., & Ragot, N. (2016, April). Text extraction in document images: highlight on using corner points. In *2016 12th IAPR Workshop on Document Analysis Systems (DAS)* (pp. 281-286). IEEE.

Yang, C. H., Liu, T. C., Lin, C. P., & Liang, J. C. (2016). Developing an augmented reality-based mobile learning system for science education. *Journal of Computer Assisted Learning*, *32*(6), 557–572.

Yang, J. O., & Lee, J. S. (2021). Utilization exercise rehabilitation using metaverse (vr· ar· mr· xr). *Korean Journal of Sport Biomechanics*, *31*(4), 249–258.

Yan, J., Ali, I., Ali, R., & Chang, Y. (2022). The Power of Affection: Exploring the Key Drivers of Customer Loyalty in Virtual Reality-Enabled Services. *Frontiers in Psychology*, *13*, 850896. doi:10.3389/fpsyg.2022.850896 PMID:35548514

Yao, Y., Wang, L., & Shen, J. (2022). Features and Applications of QR Codes. *International Journal for Innovation Education and Research*, *10*(5), 166–169. doi:10.31686/ijier.vol10.iss5.3762

Yaqi, M. (2022). Designing Visual Communications Virtual Reality matters in healthcare industry. *Journal of Commercial Biotechnology*, *27*(4).

Yaqoob, I., Salah, K., Uddin, M., Jayaraman, R., Omar, M., & Imran, M. (2020). Blockchain for digital twins: Recent advances and future research challenges. *IEEE Network*, *34*(5), 290–298. doi:10.1109/MNET.001.1900661

Yawised, K., Apasrawirote, D., Chatrangsan, M., & Muneesawang, P. (2022). Turning digital technology to immersive marketing strategy: a strategic perspective on flexibility, agility and adaptability for businesses. *Journal of Entrepreneurship in Emerging Economies*. IEEE.. https://doi.org/ doi:10.1108/JEEE-06-2022-0169

Yen, C. H., Lin, C. Y., & Wang, C. S. (2015). Augmented reality in science education: A review of the literature. *Journal of Science Education and Technology*, *24*(6), 660–677.

Yildirim, G., Elban, M., & Yildirim, S. (2018). Analysis of use of virtual reality technologies in history education: A case study. *Asian Journal of Education and Training, 4*(2), 62–69. doi:10.20448/journal.522.2018.42.62.69

Yuen, S. C., & Yaoyuneyong, G. (2012). Augmented reality: An overview and five directions for AR in education. *Journal of Educational Technology Development and Exchange, 4*(1), 119–140.

Yu, W., Patros, P., Young, B., Klinac, E., & Walmsley, T. G. (2022). Energy digital twin technology for industrial energy management: Classification, challenges and future. *Renewable & Sustainable Energy Reviews, 161*, 112407. doi:10.1016/j.rser.2022.112407

Zambelli, E., Speranza, T., & Cusimano, F. (2023). METAVERSO: L'UNIVERSO UMANO IN FORMATO DIGITALE (Alpes, Ed.).

Zammitto, V., Caponetto, I., Earp, J., & Otten, H. (2017). Augmented reality in education: A meta-review and cross-media analysis. In *Augmented Reality and Virtual Reality* (pp. 25–42). Springer.

Zarantonello, L., & Schmitt, B. H. (2023). Experiential AR/VR: A consumer and service framework and research agenda. *Journal of Service Management, 34*(1), 34–55. doi:10.1108/JOSM-12-2021-0479

Zeevi, L. S. (2021). Making art therapy virtual: Integrating virtual reality into art therapy with adolescents. Frontiers in Psychology. doi:10.3389/fpsyg.2021.584943

Zeinalnezhad, M., & Shishehchi, S. (2023). An integrated data mining algorithms and meta-heuristic technique to predict the readmission risk of diabetic patients. *Healthcare Analytics*, 100292.

Zeng, N., Pope, Z., Lee, J., & Gao, Z. (2018). Virtual Reality Exercise for Anxiety and Depression: A Preliminary Review of Current Research in an Emerging Field. *Journal of Clinical Medicine, 7*(3), 42. doi:10.3390/jcm7030042 PMID:29510528

Zhang, J. F., Paciorkowski, A. R., Craig, P. A., & Cui, F. (2019). BioVR: A platform for virtual reality assisted biological data integration and visualization. *BMC Bioinformatics, 20*(1), 1–10. doi:10.1186/s12859-019-2666-z PMID:30767777

Zhang, S., Chen, M., Yang, N., Lu, S., & Ni, S. (2021). Effectiveness of VR-based mindfulness on psychological and physiological health: A systematic review. *Current Psychology (New Brunswick, N.J.), 42*(6), 5033–5045. doi:10.1007/s12144-021-01777-6

Zhao, M., Wang, D., & Li, J. (2021). Data management and visualization of wearable medical devices assisted by artificial intelligence. *Network Modeling and Analysis in Health Informatics and Bioinformatics, 10*(1), 53. doi:10.1007/s13721-021-00328-0

Zhao, Y., Sazlina, S. G., Rokhani, F. Z., Su, J., & Chew, B. H. (2023). The expectations and acceptability of a smart nursing home model among Chinese older adults and family members: A qualitative study. *Asian Nursing Research, 17*(4), 208–218. doi:10.1016/j.anr.2023.08.002 PMID:37661084

Zhou, M., Yan, J., & Feng, D. (2019). Digital twin and its application to power grid online analysis. *CSEE Journal of Power Energy Systems, 5*(3), 391–398.

Zichermann, G., & Cunningham, C. (2011). *Gamification by design: Implementing game mechanics in web and mobile apps.* O'Reilly Media, Inc.

Žilak, M., Car, Ž., & Culjak, I. A. (2022). Systematic Literature Review of Handheld Augmented Reality Solutions for People with Disabilities. *Sensors (Basel), 22*(20), 7719. doi:10.3390/s22207719 PMID:36298070

Zuckerman, O., & Gal-Oz, A. (2012). Augmented reality system for promoting physical activity in children with cerebral palsy. *Research in Developmental Disabilities*, *33*(6), 1977–1987.

Zwoliński, G., Kamińska, D., Laska-Leśniewicz, A., Haamer, R. E., Vairinhos, M., Raposo, R., Urem, F., & Reisinho, P. (2022). Extended reality in education and training: Case studies in Management Education. *Electronics (Basel)*, *11*(3), 336. doi:10.3390/electronics11030336

About the Contributors

Ruchi Doshi has more than 16 years of academic, research and software development experience in Asia and Africa. Currently she is working as research supervisor at the Azteca University, Mexico and Adjunct Professor at the Jyoti Vidyapeeth Women's University, Jaipur, Rajasthan, India. She worked in the BlueCrest University College, Liberia, West Africa as Registrar and Head, Examination; BlueCrest University College, Ghana, Africa; Amity University, Rajasthan, India; Trimax IT Infrastructure & Services, Udaipur, India. She worked as a Founder Chair, Women in Engineering (WIE) and Secretary Position in the IEEE Liberia Subsection. She worked with Ministry of Higher Education (MoHE) in Liberia and Ghana for the Degree approvals and accreditations processes. She is interested in the field of Machine Learning and Cloud computing framework development. She has published numerous research papers in peer-reviewed international journals and conferences. She is a Reviewer, Advisor, Ambassador and Editorial board member of various reputed International Journals and Conferences.

***

Vijayalakshmi A. received her B.E. in Electronics and Communication Engineering from Madurai Kamaraj University, M.E. in Embedded System Technologies and Ph.D. in Information and Communication Engineering from Anna University, Chennai, India. She received a Gold Medal in her Post Graduation.. She is currently working as an Associate Professor in the Department of Electronics and Communication Engineering, VELS Institute of Science, Technology and Advanced Studies, Chennai. India. She has rich teaching and research experience of 22 years. She also has research experience of 5 years. She has received the Faculty Excellence Award twice. Her area of research interest includes Wireless Sensor Network, 5G, Artificial Intelligence, Internet of Things, Deep learning, Robotics and Embedded System Design. Seven research scholars are currently working under her guidance. She is a recognized research supervisor in VISTAS and also RAC member for research scholars from various reputed universities including Anna University. She has published many journal publications in reputed journals, conference publications and Book Chapters. She is the Editor and reviewer for peer reviewed impact factor journals including IEEE Sensors, IET Communications. She is a Life Member of Professional Societies IETE and ISTE.

Likhitha R. is a student who earned a diploma in Computer Science and Engineering from Sri Jayachamarajendra Polytechnic. Currently pursuing a Bachelor's degree in the same field at Dr. Ambedkar Institute of Technology, she exhibits a strong commitment to advancing her skills in computer science.

Madhu.B., received her Bachelor's degree and Master's degree from Visvesvaraya Technological University, Belagavi, Karnataka. She completed her Ph.D.2022 from Visvesvaraya Technological University, Belgaum, India. She has a total of 20 Years of teaching experience. She has published more than 30 research papers in International conferences and Journals. Her main research interests include Image Processing, Deep Learning, Pattern Recognition and Machine Learning.

Selvan C. received the B.E. degree in Computer Science and Engineering in Manonmaniam Sundaranar University, India, in 2002, the M.E. degree in Computer Science and Engineering from Anna University, Chennai, India, in 2007 and the Ph.D. in Computer Science and Engineering from Anna University, Chennai, India in 2013. During his Ph.D degree he was a JRF, SRF under University Grant Commission (UGC, New Delhi) in Government College of Technology, Coimbatore. He had been working as a Software Engineer during 2002 to 2005. Further, he has been engaging in various responsibilities in the Engineering colleges, in Tamil Nadu since 2007. He was a Post-Doctoral Fellow in National Institute of Technology, Tiruchirappalli, under UGC, New Delhi, India from June 2017 to June 2022. In the year of 2022 June, he joined as a professor in New Horizon College of Engineering, Bangalore and worked upto January 2023. Currently he has been working as a Professor in the School of Computer Science and Engineering, REVA University, Bangalore since February 2023. His current research interests include Mobile Computing, Data Science and Artificial Intelligence. He is an IEEE senior member, an ACM member.

Veningston K. received Ph.D. degree in Computer Science and Engineering from Anna University, Chennai, INDIA in 2015 and currently Assistant Professor in the Department of Computer Science and Engineering at National Institute of Technology Srinagar, INDIA. His expertise areas include design and implementation of Computer Vision (CV) and Natural Language Processing (NLP) systems using machine learning and deep learning algorithms. His current work includes CV applications in health and NLP applications in legal domain. He is a recipient of prestigious INSPIRE fellowship by the Department of Science and Technology, Government of India in 2011. He has chaired technical sessions in several international conferences within and outside India and delivered numerous technical talks on the areas of his research.

Vidhya K is Assistant Professor, Department of Data Science and Cyber Security, Karunya Institute of Technology and Sciences having research experience and a history of working for past 17 years in the collaborative education sector. Passionate to works in the domains of Data Analytics, IoT, Cloud Computing and Data Science. Competent in the application of classification, clustering, and regression methods in supervised and unsupervised machine learning. Interested on application development, statistics, data visualization, and data integrity. Eager to use my enthusiasm for product development and contribute to the team's cooperative work on intelligent, top-notch application development. Proven research ability with journal articles.

Christian Kaunert is Professor of International Security at Dublin City University, Ireland. He is also Professor of Policing and Security, as well as Director of the International Centre for Policing and Security at the University of South Wales. In addition, he is Jean Monnet Chair, Director of the Jean Monnet Centre of Excellence and Director of the Jean Monnet Network on EU Counter-Terrorism

Jaspreet Kaur is currently working as an Assistant Professor in University Business School,Chandigarh University,Mohali,Punjab.She is a post graduate (MBA-H.R) from Panjab University,Chandigarh.She has also qualified UGC NET JRF in Human Resource Management/Labour and Social Welfare and has completed PhD in Business Management from Chandigarh University,Mohali. She has over 8 years of experience in academic and administrative assignments.She also received "Best Teacher of the Department Award " in the year 2019 and 2021 in the field of imparting quality education.Her research interests include Employee Engagement, Management of Organizational Change and Organization Development. She has published several research papers and articles in reputed international and national journals and has presented papers in various national and international conferences.She also contributed one edited book and 10 book chapters on various topics.

Rakshit Kothari is a research scholar in the Department of Computer Science and Engineering at College of Technology and Engineering, Maharana Pratap University of Agriculture and Technology, Udaipur, Rajasthan, India. He has done B.Tech in Computer Science and Engineering at Rajasthan Technical University, Kota with first division honours. He secured Master of Technology in Computer Science and Engineering at College of Technology and Engineering, Maharana Pratap University of Agriculture and Technology, Udaipur, Rajasthan, India under the guidance of Dr. Naveen Choudhary, Professor and Head, CTAE, MPUAT. He has teaching experience for more than 2 years and IT industry experience of 1 year. He has presented number of papers in National and International Journals, Conference and Symposiums He is currently a member in Soft Computing Research Society. His main area of interest include the Internet of Things, Cryptography and Blockchain.

Pragna M S is a Computer Science student at Dr. Ambedkar Institute of Technology, driven by a passion for technology and innovation. Eager to contribute and excel in dynamic world

Sanju Mahawar's educational background is steeped in depth and richness. He boasts an impressive track record of research publications in esteemed journals and has earned accolades such as a best paper award at an international conference. His primary area of expertise centers around Information Technology and e commerce.

Pallabi Mukherjee is an Associate Professor and Head of Research Committee and Head Evaluer at the Institute of Business Management and Research (IBMR) NAAC A ++ and UGC Autonomous College, IPS Academy, Indore, India. She is a Ph.D. in Economics from School of Economics (SOE), Devi Ahilya University (DAVV), Indore. She has done her Masters in Economics from SOE, DAVV and Bachelor of Science in Economics from Calcutta University. She has her diploma in Executive MBA Program from MTF Institute of Management & Technology, Lisbon, Portugal. She has more ten years of teaching experience with more than 30 research papers to her credit published in national and international journals. Her publications are in UGC, ABDC B and C category journals.She is proud author of the book titled ' The Power of Law of Attraction, Techniques To Manifest Your Dream Life' and 'Sustainable Economic Development Assessment – a Measure of Wealth to Well being' and has also written book chapters published in Springer and conference proceedings in Taylor and Francis. She has presented her research papers at esteemed national conferences at IIM Shillong, IIT Gwahati, IIT Roorkee, IIM Indore etc and prominent foreign conferences, including Tennessee State University (TSU), Nashville, United States (Apr 2018), Marshall Center at the University of South Florida, Tampa, United States (Feb 2018) etc.

Kali Charan Modak is a distinguished academician and researcher known for his expertise in the field of Management, particularly in Foreign Trade and Healthcare Product Marketing Strategy. With a Master's degree in Foreign Trade (MBA-FT) and currently pursuing his Doctorate in Management from DAVV Indore, Dr. Modak has dedicated his career to advancing knowledge and understanding in his chosen areas of specialization. Dr. Modak's academic journey began with a strong foundation in commerce and management. Prior to joining IBMR, IPS Academy, he served as a visiting faculty at the School of Commerce, DAVV Indore, where he honed his teaching skills and imparted knowledge to students. His areas of expertise include Marketing Management, Research Methodology, International Business, International Finance, Derivatives, Business Statistics, Economics, International Marketing & Documentation, and Exim Policy. Driven by a passion for research, Dr. Modak has made significant contributions to academia through his extensive publication record. With thirty-two research papers published and presented in various national and international conferences and reputed journals, he has garnered recognition for his scholarly work. Notably, he showcased his research prowess by presenting a paper at the prestigious 1st International Conference on Business Analytics and Intelligence organized by IIM Bangalore. In addition to his research endeavors, Dr. Modak has played a pivotal role in guiding numerous major research projects for MBA students, imparting valuable insights and mentorship. His commitment to continuous learning is evident through his participation in workshops and training programs across different fields of Management and Research. Beyond academia, Dr. Modak is a respected columnist for the renowned daily newspaper, Dainik Dabang Duniya, where he shares his perspectives on current affairs and management-related topics. His clear and insightful writing style has earned him a loyal readership and further solidified his reputation as a thought leader in the field. Dr. Modak's academic achievements also include clearing the UGC NET in management in 2010, a testament to his deep understanding and proficiency in his chosen discipline. His relentless pursuit of excellence, coupled with his dedication to advancing knowledge and empowering students, continues to inspire and influence the academic community. Dr. Kali Charan Modak stands as a beacon of scholarly excellence, shaping the future of management education and research in India and beyond.

Snthil Kumar, Associate Professor, Faculty of Engineering and Technology, Jain Deemed to be University, having rich experience in teaching and research with over 17 years in DBMS, Datamining, Data science, Machine Learning. Also coordinated with Oracle workforce development team, Infosys Campus Connect program, Wipro Mission 10X and AICTE funded training programs for various certifications. The Research interest on Artificial Intelligence and Machine Learning, I have published the research work in various National and International journals including SCI, Web of Science, Scopus Indexed Journal and IEEE Explore.

Rajaprabakaran Rajendran is B.Pharmacy & MSc. (IT&M) graduate and research scholar at CMS Business School, Jain Deemed to-be University, Bengaluru, India. He is an incisive medical communication professional with over 23 years of experience in healthcare professional marketing through multi-channel platforms, brand/medical communication, Continuing Medical Education, client servicing, and KOL management; managing brand/medical communication programmes for healthcare professionals (HCPs) in Asia Pacific, Europe and the Middle East and North Africa region. He has an extensive experience in the designing medical communication strategies and delivering high quality medical communication programmes through multi-channel platforms in collaboration with national and international medical associations, universities and hospitals, and key opinion leaders for the leading pharmaceutical/consumer healthcare companies to facilitate effective engagement with their target audiences (HCPs) across medical specialities.

Gerardo Reyes Ruiz. He is an Actuary by training from the Faculty of Sciences-UNAM; he studied a Specialty in Econometrics in the Postgraduate Studies Division of the Faculty of Economics-UNAM; He obtained a Master's and Doctorate (with a scholarship from CONACYT and the Carolina Foundation) in Business Studies (actuarial profile) from the Faculty of Economics and Business of the University of Barcelona, Spain. In the Doctorate he graduated with the highest honors awarded to a thesis of this nature, that is, he obtained the qualification of Excellent Cum Laude. Later he did a postdoctoral stay at the Center for Economic, Administrative, and Social Studies (CIECAS) of the National Polytechnic Institute (IPN). His work experience has been in public education institutions (UNAM, UAEM, IPN, Centro de Estudios Superiores Navales-CESNAV) where he has taught classes in Bachelor's, Specialty, Master's, and Doctorate degrees. In some of these institutions, he developed several research projects, including Basic Science, forming and creating Research Networks (both nationally and internationally). All this accumulated experience allowed him to enter the National System of Researchers (SNI), Social Area, of Mexico (he has the appointment of Level I National Researcher). He is currently attached to the Center for Superior Naval Studies (CESNAV), in Mexico.

Jaya Rubi stands as a luminary in the field of Biomedical Engineering, currently pursuing her PhD at VISTAS. Alongside her academic pursuits, she serves as an Assistant Professor in the Department of Biomedical Engineering at VELS Institute of Science, Technology, and Advanced Studies, Chennai, India. With a wealth of experience spanning over five years in industry and academia, she has emerged as a guiding force in the discipline. Jaya's research is at the vanguard of Robot-assisted surgeries, dedicated to creating a cost-effective approach for widespread implementation in the service sector. Her ingenuity extends to patented creations, including a groundbreaking Smart Shield for women, reflecting her resolute commitment to engineering solutions that enhance lives. Jaya's extensive repertoire of published works encompasses a range of topics from robotic surgical assistance to web-based blood donation systems and sensory aids for the visually impaired. She boasts a substantial portfolio of journal publications, conference contributions, and authored book chapters. As an esteemed editor and reviewer for peer-reviewed impact factor journals, she plays an active role in shaping scholarly discourse. Jaya Rubi's affiliations as a Life Member of esteemed professional societies IFERP and IAENG underscore her dedication to advancing the field. Her tireless efforts in merging technology with healthcare stand as a testament to her unwavering commitment to making advanced medical solutions accessible to all.

Syesha Singh is working as an Assistant Professor (Senior) in Department of Psychology, Manipal University Jaipur. She has an experience of over 13 years in teaching, research and Life Skills Training. Her research interests include Clinical Psychology, Counselling and Psychotherapy, Applied Psychology & Organizational Behaviour. She is Certified Counsellor and an Art Analyst.

Ranjit Singha is a Doctorate Research Fellow at Christ (Deemed to be University) and a distinguished American Psychological Association (APA) member. His expertise lies in research and development across various domains, including Mindfulness, Addiction Psychology, Women Empowerment, UN Sustainable Development Goals, and Data Science. He has earned certifications from renowned institutions, including IBM and The University of Oxford Mindfulness Centre, UK, in Mindfulness. Additionally, he holds certifications as a Microsoft Innovative Educator, Licensed Yoga Professional, Certified Mindfulness Teacher, and CBCT Teachers Training from Emory University, USA. Mr Ranjit's educational qualifications include PGDBA (GM), MBA (IB), MSc in Counseling Psychology, and completion of a Senior Diploma in Tabla

(Musical Instrumentation). His dedication to continuous learning is evident through his involvement in the SEE Learning® (Social, Emotional, and Ethical) Learning program. As a committed researcher and educator, Mr Ranjit focuses on mindfulness and compassion-based interventions. He has an impressive publication record, having authored twenty-three research papers, ten chapters, four books, and five edited books. His research interests encompass various aspects of mindfulness, such as assessment, benefits of mindfulness-based programs, change mechanisms, professional training, mindfulness ethics, cognitive and neuropsychology, and studies related to high-risk behaviours. Apart from his research endeavours, Mr Ranjit has extensive teaching experience, instructing courses in diverse subjects like Forensic Psychology, Positive Psychology, Organizational Planning, Strategic Management, Psycho Metric Tests, Counseling Skills, Disaster Management, Basic Computer Science, Business Planning, Business Law, and Auditing. He has mentored numerous Postgraduate and undergraduate research projects, demonstrating his commitment to nurturing young minds in psychology. Ad Hoc Reviewer at International Journal of Cyber Behavior, Psychology and Learning (IJCBPL), Reviewer and author at IGI Global, and Editor and Reviewer at TNT Publication. Furthermore, Mr Ranjit actively provides personal counselling services, showcasing his genuine concern for his students' well-being and academic success. His unwavering dedication to research and education has solidified his position as a valuable contributor to psychology.

Surjit Singha is an academician with a broad spectrum of interests, including UN Sustainable Development Goals, Organizational Climate, Workforce Diversity, Organizational Culture, HRM, Marketing, Finance, IB, Global Business, Business, AI, Women Studies, and Cultural Studies. Currently a faculty member at Kristu Jayanti College, Dr. Surjit also serves as an Editor, reviewer, and author for prominent global publications and journals, including being on the Editorial review board of Information Resources Management Journal and a contributor to IGI Global. With over 13 years of experience in Administration, Teaching, and Research, Dr. Surjit is dedicated to imparting knowledge and guiding students in their research pursuits. As a research mentor, Dr. Surjit has nurtured young minds and fostered academic growth. Dr. Surjit has an impressive track record of over 75 publications, including articles, book chapters, and textbooks, holds two US Copyrights, and has successfully completed and published two fully funded minor research projects from Kristu Jayanti College.

Yavana Rani Subramanian, Professor of MBA in the Decision Science area at CMS Business School, Jain Deemed-to-be University, Bangalore. Since receiving her MBA and Ph.D. in Management, she has devoted her career to Research and Teaching. She also has a Master's degree in Structural Engineering. She is the University rank holder in MBA. She has 16 years of teaching experience. Dr. Rani has received Young Scientist Fellowship Award from Tamilnadu State Council for Science and Technology (TNSCST). She has completed her fellowship from Indian Institute of Science (IISc), Bangalore. She is the life time member in Indian Society for Technical Education (ISTE). Dr. Yavana Rani has done two research projects sponsored by Indian Council for Social Science and Research (ICSSR). She has published more than 10 research articles in Scopus indexed and Springer journals. She has presented papers in National and International conferences in India and abroad. She is the editor for many reputed journals. She has delivered key note address in countries like Egypt, Malaysia. Prof. Rani holds many administrative roles such as Dean Student Affairs, Director Coordination for various activities. She has been project Director for Entrepreneurship Cell (EDC) sponsored by Department of Science and Technology (DST). She also coordinated many programmes. Professor has got funding for conducting conferences, International visit from various funding agencies like DST and ICSSR.

Shivani Venkatesan is a Biomedical undergraduate at Vels Institute of Science and Technology, passionately pursuing a B.E. in Biomedical Engineering. Her interests lie at the intersection of technology and healthcare, where she aspires to innovate and improve patient well-being. With a strong academic foundation and a commitment to research, she is poised to make a meaningful impact in the biomedical field. Her journey is fueled by an unwavering curiosity and a dedication to pushing the boundaries of medical science.

Index

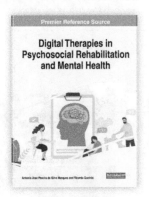
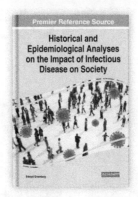
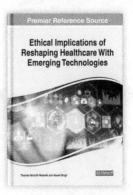
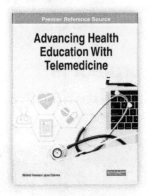
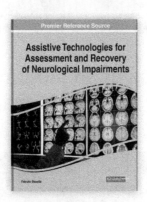
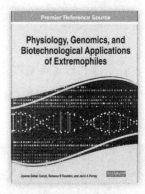
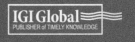

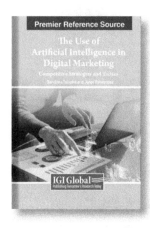
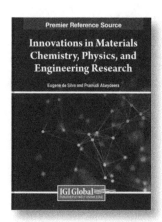
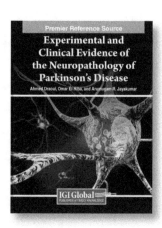
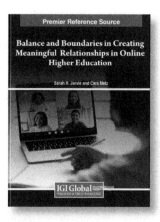

Submit an Open Access Book Proposal

Have Your Work Fully & Freely Available Worldwide After Publication

Seeking the Following Book Classification Types:

Authored & Edited Monographs • Casebooks • Encyclopedias • Handbooks of Research

Gold, Platinum, & Retrospective OA Opportunities to Choose From

Easily Track Your Work in Our Advanced Manuscript Submission System With **Rapid Turnaround Times**

Double-Blind Peer Review by Notable Editorial Boards (*Committee on Publication Ethics* (COPE) Certified

Publications Adhere to All **Current OA Mandates & Compliances**

Affordable APCs *(Often 50% Lower Than the Industry Average)* Including Robust Editorial Service Provisions

Direct Connections with **Prominent Research Funders** & OA Regulatory Groups

Institution Level OA Agreements Available (Recommend or Contact Your Librarian for Details)

Join a **Diverse Community of 150,000+ Researchers Worldwide** Publishing With IGI Global

Content Spread Widely to Leading Repositories (AGOSR, ResearchGate, CORE, & More)

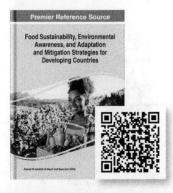
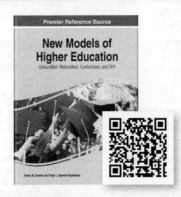
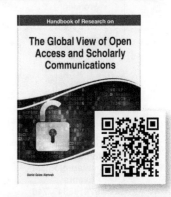

Retrospective Open Access Publishing

You Can Unlock Your Recently Published Work, Including Full Book & Individual Chapter Content to Enjoy All the Benefits of Open Access Publishing

Learn More

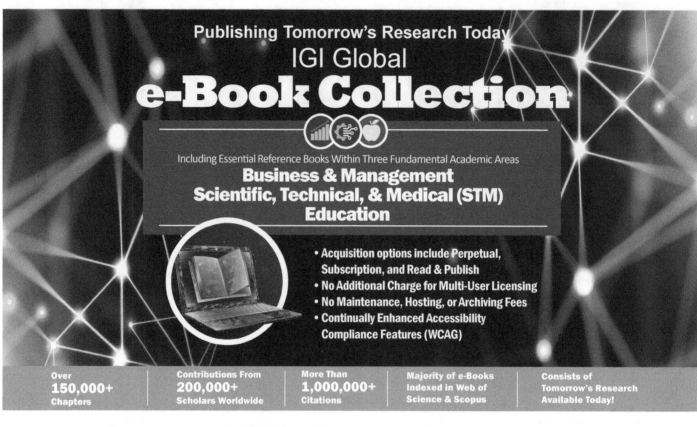
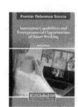
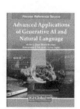
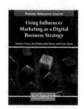
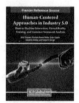
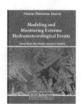
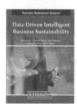
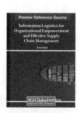